HERE'S AMERICA'S FAVORITE DIET GUIDE

CALORIES AND CARBOHYDRATES

THE BOOK THAT MAKES IT FUN TO LOSE THOSE EXTRA POUNDS

Whether you aim to lose five pounds or fifty, the only safe, healthy way is to eat an adequate, well-balanced diet, choosing your calories from many different kinds of foods in order to ensure that you're getting sufficient vitamins, minerals, and other nutrients. CALORIES AND CARBOHY-DRATES contains the most accurate and dependable caloric and carbohydrate counts for practically everything you will eat and drink—thousands and thousands of brand names and basic foods, including alcoholic beverages and take-out foods such as your favorites from McDONALD'S or BURGER KING.

So diet—and enjoy it!

BARBARA KRAUS

CALORIES AND CARBOHYDRATES

SIXTH REVISED EDITION

A PLUME BOOK

NEW AMERICAN LIBRARY

NEW YORK AND SCARBOROUGH, ONTARIO

NAL BOOKS ARE AVAILABLE AT QUANTITY DISCOUNTS
WHEN USED TO PROMOTE PRODUCTS OR SERVICES. FOR
INFORMATION PLEASE WRITE TO PREMIUM MARKETING DIVISION,
NEW AMERICAN LIBRARY, 1633 BROADWAY,
NEW YORK, NEW YORK 10019.

PLUME TRADEMARK REG. U.S. PAT. OFF. AND FOREIGN COUNTRIES
REG. TRADEMARK—MARCA REGISTRADA
HECHO EN HARRISONBURG, VA., U.S.A.

SIGNET, SIGNET CLASSIC, MENTOR, PLUME, MERIDIAN
and NAL BOOKS are published *in the United States*
by New American Library,
1633 Broadway, New York, New York 10019,
in Canada by The New American Library of Canada Limited,
81 Mack Avenue, Scarborough, Ontario M1L 1M8

Sixth Revised Edition

[Eleventh Plume Printing], May, 1985

12   13   14   15   16   17   18   19

PRINTED IN THE UNITED STATES OF AMERICA

Contents

Introduction

This dictionary of foods lists several thousand brand-name products and basic foods with their caloric and carbohydrate content. The calorie yield of your diet versus the amount of energy you expend is the key to whether you maintain your ideal weight, gain too many pounds or lose weight.

Because of the relationship of weight to health, many individuals are "counting calories" at every meal. Interest has also been directed to the carbohydrate content of the diet in relation to weight control. Comprehensive information on these values in basic foods and brand-name products is not readily available in any one source. Nor is the information regularly reported in portions that are usually eaten or bought at the grocery store. To compound the problem, hundreds of new food items appear in our stores every year.

Arrangement of This Book

Foods are listed alphabetically by brand name or by the name of the food. The singular form is used for the entries, that is, blackberry instead of blackberries. Most items are listed individually though a few are grouped (see p. xii); for example, all candies are listed together so that if you are looking for *Mars* bar, you look first under Candy, then under *M* in alphabetical order. But, if you are looking for a breakfast food such as Oatmeal, you will find it under *O* in the main alphabet. Many cross references are included to assist in finding items called by different names.

Under the main headings, it was often not possible nor even desirable to follow an alphabetical arrangement. For basic foods such as apricots, for example, the first entries are for the fresh product weighed with seeds as it is purchased in the store, then the fruit in small portions as they may be eaten or measured. These entries are followed by the processed products, canned (although it may actually be a bottle or jar), dehydrated, dried and frozen. This basic plan, with adaptations where necessary, was followed for fruits, vegetables and meats.

In almost all entries where data were available the U.S. Department of Agriculture figures are shown first. The Department values represent averages from several manufacturers and are shown for comparison with the values from individual companies or for use where particular brands are not available.

All brand-name products have been italicized and company names appear in parentheses.

Portions Used

The portion column is a most important one to read and note. Common household measures are used insofar as possible. For some items, the amounts given are those commonly purchased in the store, such as 1 pound of meat. These quantities can be divided into the number of servings used in the home and the nutritive values available to each person served can then be readily determined. Of course, any ingredients added to preparing such products must also be taken into account.

The smaller portions given are for foods as served or measured in moderate amounts, such as ½ cup of juice reconstituted, or 4 ounces of meat. Be sure to adjust the calories and carbohydrates to the actual portions you use. For example, if you serve 1 cup of juice instead of ½ cup, multiply the calories and carbohydrates shown for the smaller amount by 2.

Don't fool yourself about the size of portions you use. If you are serious about controlling the calories and carbohydrates in your diet, weigh your foods until you can accurately gauge the weight visually. Remember, the calories and carbohydrates go up with any increase in the weight of foods. Remember, too, that 4 ounces by weight may be very different from 4 fluid ounces or ½ cup. Ounces in the table are always ounces by weight unless specified as fluid ounces, or fractions of a cup or other volumetric measure. Foods that are fluffy in texture, such as flaked coconut and bean sprouts, vary greatly in weight per cup depending on how tightly they are packed into the cup. Such foods as canned green beans also vary when weighed with or without liquid; for example, canned green beans with liquid weigh 4.2 ounces for ½ cup, but drained beans weigh 2.5 ounces for the same ½ cup. Check the weights of your serving portions regularly. Bear in mind that you can cut calories and carbohydrates by cutting the serving size.

It was impossible to convert all the portions to a uniform basis. Some sources were only able to report data in terms of weights with no information on cup or other volumetric measures. I have shown small portions in quantities that might reasonably be expected to be served or measured in the home or institution. Package sizes are useful to show the composition of products as they are purchased and may be divided into the number of serving portions prepared from the entire product, taking into account any added ingredients.

You will find in the portion column the phrases "weighed with bone," or "weighed with skin and seeds" or other inedible parts. These descriptions apply to the products as you purchase them in the markets but the caloric values and the carbohydrate content as shown are for the amount of edible food after you discard the bone, skin, seed or other inedible part. The weight given in the "measure or quantity" column is to the nearest gram or fraction of an ounce.

Data on the composition of foods are constantly changing for many reasons. Better sampling and analytical methods, improvements in marketing procedures and changes in formulas of mixed products, all may alter values for carbohydrates and other nutrients as well as caloric values. Weights of packaged foods are frequently changed. It is essential to read label information to be informed about these matters and to make intelligent use of food tables.

I will be constantly revising and updating this book along with my individual calorie and carbohydrate annual guides (*The Barbara Kraus 1985 Calorie, Carbohydrate, and Sodium Guides to Brand Names and Basic Foods*) to help keep you as up-to-date as possible.

Calories

What is a calorie? It is not a nutrient nor is it a good guide to the nutritive value of food. It is more like a yardstick to measure the energy that a food will yield in the body. You need energy for your body functions as well as for exercise. If your diet contains more calories than your body uses for these purposes, the extra "energy" will be stored as fat.

If your plan is to cut down on calories, the easiest way to do so is to consult the calorie column of this counter and keep an accurate count of your total intake of food and beverages for a period of seven days. If you have not gained or lost weight during that week divide that number by seven and you'll have your maintenance diet expressed in calories. To lose weight, you must reduce your daily or weekly intake of calories below this maintenance level. (To gain, increase the intake.)

One pound of fat is equal to 3,500 calories. Add this number of calories to those you need to balance your energy requirements and you will gain one pound; subtract it, and you will lose a pound.

Carbohydrates

The carbohydrate column shows the amount of this nutrient in grams for the quantities of foods indicated in the portion column. Some dietitians are giving special attention to this nutrient at present in connection with weight control. Carbohydrates include sugars, starches, acids and other nutrients. The values in this book are total carbohydrates, by difference, the basis on which calories from carbohydrates are calculated in the U.S. diet.

Other Nutrients

Do not forget that other nutrients are extremely important in diet planning—protein, fat, minerals and vitamins. Calories yielded by alcohol must also be taken into consideration. From a nutrition viewpoint, perhaps the best advice that can be given to the dieter is to eat a varied diet with all classes of foods represented. Meat, fish, chicken, fats and oils, milk, vegetables, fruits and grain products are all important sources of essential nutrients and some foods from each of these classes of foods should be included in the diet every day. With the great abundance and variety of foods on the grocer's shelves, there is no reason why the dieter should not enjoy a tasty, nutritious and attractive diet. Just eat in moderation and there is no need to eliminate any one food altogether, except in special conditions under a doctor's directions. Choose wisely and eat well.

Sources of Data

Values in this dictionary are based on publications issued by the U.S. Department of Agriculture and on data submitted by manufacturers and processors. The U.S. Department of Agriculture issues basic tables on food composition for use in the United States. The commercial products from U.S.D.A. publications represent average values obtained on products of more than one company. The figures designated "home recipe" are based on recipes on file with the Department of Agriculture. Data on commercial products listed by brand name in this publication are based on values supplied by manufacturers and processors for their own individual products. Very few supermarket brand names, such as Pathmark or private labels were included in this book inasmuch as they are not usually analyzed under these trade names. Every care has been taken to interpret the data and the descriptions supplied by the companies as fully and accurately as possible. Many values have been recalculated to different portions from those submitted in order to bring about greater uniformity among similar items.

Calories in these different sources are not always on a strictly uniform basis. In the Department of Agriculture, calories are calculated using specific factors, which make allowances for losses in digestion and metabolism. The technical explanation of these factors is given in Handbook 74 of the United States Department of Agriculture. Most manufacturers use average factors of 4, 9 and 4 for calories yielded by each gram of protein, fat and carbohydrate respectively; a factor of 7 is used as an average value to calculate the calories from one gram of alcohol. These differences in procedure will give somewhat different results for products of similar composition. Some manufacturers have adopted the values from U.S. Department of Agriculture publications as representative of their own products. In these cases, it will be apparent in the table that the data from the companies match exactly those from U.S.D.A. publications.

Analyses of foods to provide information on nutritive values are extremely expensive to conduct. Many small companies have not been able to afford to have their products analyzed and thus were unable to provide data for this book or were able to provide only the calories or only the carbohydrates. Other companies have simply never gotten around to having the analysis done. New requirements for labeling nutritive values of products may provide information on additional items in the future. Therefore, wherever data for carbohydrates were unavailable, blank spaces were left which may be filled in by the reader at a later time.

Bear in mind that small differences in calorie values on similar products of the same weight are not important in diet planning. They may be due to different methods of calculating the calories or to small differences in the nutritive values of the samples analyzed because no two foods ever have exactly the same composition. Some differences may also be due to the way the food was measured as noted in the case of green beans earlier.

Carbohydrates in this book are usually total carbohydrates by difference. A few manufacturers reported only "available carbohydrates." These values were omitted.

Foods Listed by Groups

Certain foods are reported together rather than as individual items in the main alphabet. For example: Baby Food; Bread; Cake; Cake Icing; Cake Icing Mix; Cake Mix; Candy; Cheese; Cookie; Cookie Mix; Cracker; Gravy; Pie; Pie Filling; Salad Dressing; Sauce; Sausage; Soft Drinks and Syrup.

BARBARA KRAUS

Abbreviations and Symbols

(USDA) = United States Department of Agriculture
(HEW/FAO) = Health, Education and Welfare/Food and Agriculture Organization
* = prepared as package directs[1]
< = less than
& = and
″ = inch
canned = bottles or jars as well as cans
dia. = diameter
fl. = fluid

liq. = liquid
lb. = pound
med. = medium
oz. = ounce
pkg. = package
pt. = pint
qt. = quart
sq. = square
T. = tablespoon
Tr. = trace
tsp. = teaspoon
wt. = weight

italics or name in parentheses = registered trademark, ®
the letters DNA indicate that no data are available.

Equivalents

By Weight
1 pound = 16 ounces
1 ounce = 28.35 grams
3.52 ounces = 100 grams

By Volume
1 quart = 4 cups
1 cup = 8 fluid ounces
1 cup = ½ pint
1 cup = 16 tablespoons
2 tablespoons = 1 fluid ounce
1 tablespoon = 3 teaspoons

[1]If the package directions call for whole or skim milk, the data given here are for whole milk, unless otherwise stated.

Food and Description	Measure or Quantity	Calories	Carbo-hydrates (grams)

A

ABALONE (USDA):
Raw, meat only	4 oz.	111	3.9
Canned	4 oz.	91	2.6

AC'CENT ¼ tsp.   3   0.

ACEROLA, fresh fruit ¼ lb. (weighed with seeds)   52   12.6

ALBACORE, raw, meat only (USDA) 4 oz.   201   0.

ALE (See **BEER**)

ALLSPICE (French's) 1 tsp.   6   1.3

ALMOND:
Fresh (USDA):
In shell	10 nuts	60	2.0
Shelled, raw, natural, with skins	1 oz.	170	5.5

Roasted:
Dry (Planters)	1 oz.	170	6.0
Oil (Fisher)	1 oz.	178	5.5

ALMOND EXTRACT (Virginia Dare) pure 1 tsp.   10   0.

ALPHA-BITS, cereal (Post) 1 cup (1 oz.)   113   24.6

AMARANTH, raw, trimmed (USDA) 4 oz.   41   7.4

(USDA): United States Department of Agriculture
(HEW/FAO):   Health, Education and Welfare/Food and Agriculture
                Organization
* Prepared as Package Directs

Food and Description	Measure or Quantity	Calories	Carbo-hydrates (grams)
AMARETTO DI SARONNO, 28% alcohol	1 fl. oz.	82	9.0
ANCHOVY, PICKLED, canned (USDA) flat or rolled, not heavily salted, drained	2-oz. can	79	.1
ANISE EXTRACT (Virginia Dare) 76% alcohol	1 tsp.	22	0.
ANISETTE:			
(DeKuyper)	1 fl. oz.	95	11.4
(Mr. Boston)	1 fl. oz.	88	10.8
APPLE:			
Fresh (USDA):			
Eaten with skin	2½" dia. (4.1 oz.)	61	15.3
Eaten without skin	2½" dia. (4.1 oz.)	53	13.9
Canned (Comstock):			
Rings, drained	1 ring (1.1 oz.)	30	7.0
Sliced	⅙ of 21-oz. can	45	10.0
Dried:			
(Del Monte)	2-oz. serving	140	37.0
(Sun-Maid/Sunsweet) chunks	2-oz. serving	150	42.0
Frozen, sweetened, slices	10-oz. pkg.	264	68.9
APPLE BROWN BETTY, home recipe (USDA)	1 cup	325	63.9
APPLE BUTTER (Smucker's) cider	1 T.	38	9.0
APPLE-CHERRY JUICE COCKTAIL, canned, *Musselman's*	8 fl. oz.	110	28.0
APPLE CIDER:			
Canned (Mott's) sweet	½ cup	59	14.6
*Mix:			
Country Time	8 fl. oz.	98	24.5
(Hi-C)	6 fl. oz.	72	18.0

Food and Description	Measure or Quantity	Calories	Carbo-hydrates (grams)
APPLE-CRANBERRY JUICE, canned (Lincoln)	6 fl. oz.	100	25.0
APPLE DRINK: Canned:			
Capri Sun, natural	6¾ fl. oz.	90	22.7
(Hi-C)	6 fl. oz.	92	23.0
*Mix (Hi-C)	6 fl. oz.	72	18.0
APPLE DUMPLINGS, frozen (Pepperidge Farm)	1 dumpling (3.1 oz.)	260	33.0
APPLE, ESCALLOPED, frozen (Stouffer's)	4-oz. serving	140	28.0
APPLE-GRAPE JUICE, canned:			
Musselman's	6 fl. oz.	82	21.0
(Red Cheek)	6 fl. oz.	69	22.6
APPLE JACKS, cereal (Kellogg's)	1 cup (1 oz.)	110	26.0
APPLE JAM (Smucker's)	1 T.	53	13.5
APPLE JELLY:			
Sweetened (Smucker's)	1 T. (.7 oz.)	57	14.0
Dietetic:			
(Dia-Mel; Featherweight; Louis Sherry)	1 T. (.6 oz.)	6	0.
(Diet Delight)	1 T. (.6 oz.)	12	3.0
APPLE JUICE:			
Canned:			
(Lincoln)	6 fl. oz.	100	24.0
(Mott's)	6 fl. oz.	80	19.0
Musselman's	6 fl. oz.	80	21.0
(Ocean Spray)	6 fl. oz.	90	23.0

(USDA): United States Department of Agriculture
(HEW/FAO):   Health, Education and Welfare/Food and Agriculture
                    Organization
* Prepared as Package Directs

Food and Description	Measure or Quantity	Calories	Carbohydrates (grams)
(Red Cheek)	6 fl. oz.	83	21.2
(Seneca Foods)	6 fl. oz.	90	22.0
Chilled (Minute Maid)	6 fl. oz.	100	24.0
*Frozen:			
(Minute Maid)	6 fl. oz.	100	24.0
(Seneca Foods):			
Regular or no sugar added	6 fl. oz.	90	22.0
Natural	6 fl. oz.	84	22.0
APPLE PIE (See **PIE,** Apple)			
APPLE SAUCE, canned:			
Regular:			
(Del Monte)	½ cup (4 oz.)	90	24.0
(Mott's):			
Natural style	½ cup (4 oz.)	115	27.5
With ground cranberries	½ cup (4 oz.)	110	27.0
Musselman's	½ cup (4.5 oz.)	96	23.5
Dietetic:			
(Del Monte, Lite; Diet Delight)	½ cup	50	13.0
(Mott's) natural style	4-oz. serving	50	11.0
(S&W) *Nutradiet,* white or blue label	½ cup	55	14.0
APPLE STRUDEL, frozen (Pepperidge Farm)	3-oz. serving	240	35.0
APRICOT:			
Fresh (USDA):			
Whole	1 lb. (weighed with pits)	217	54.6
Whole	3 apricots (about 12 per lb.)	55	13.7
Halves	1 cup (5½ oz.)	79	19.8
Canned, regular pack, solids & liq.:			
(USDA):			
Juice pack	4 oz.	61	15.4
Extra heavy syrup	4 oz.	115	29.5
(Del Monte):			
Whole	½ cup (4¼ oz.)	100	26.0
Halves, peeled	½ cup	200	27.0

Food and Description	Measure or Quantity	Calories	Carbo-hydrates (grams)
(Stokely-Van Camp)	½ cup (4.6 oz.)	110	27.0
Canned, dietetic, solids & liq.:			
(Del Monte) Lite	½ cup (4¼ oz.)	60	16.0
(Diet Delight):			
Juice pack	½ cup (4.4 oz.)	60	15.0
Water pack	½ cup (4.3 oz.)	35	9.0
(Featherweight):			
Juice pack	½ cup	50	12.0
Water pack	½ cup	35	9.0
(Libby's) Lite	½ cup (4.4 oz.)	60	15.0
(S&W) *Nutradiet:*			
Halves, white or blue label	½ cup	35	9.0
Whole, juice pack	½ cup	28	7.0
Dried (Del Monte; Sun-Maid; Sunsweet) uncooked	2-oz. serving	140	35.0
APRICOT, CANDIED (USDA)	1 oz.	96	24.5
APRICOT LIQUEUR			
(DeKuyper) 60 proof	1 fl. oz.	82	8.3
APRICOT NECTAR, canned:			
(Del Monte)	6 fl. oz.	100	26.0
(Libby's)	6 fl. oz.	110	27.0
APRICOT-PINEAPPLE NECTAR, canned, dietetic (S&W) *Nutradiet*, blue label	6 oz.	35	12.0
APRICOT & PINEAPPLE PRESERVE OR JAM:			
Sweetened (Smucker's)	1 T. (.7 oz.)	53	13.5
Dietetic:			
(Diet Delight; Louis Sherry)	1 T. (.6 oz.)	6	3.0
(Featherweight)	1 T.	6	1.0
(SW&) *Nutradiet,* red label	1 T.	12	3.0
(Tillie Lewis) *Tasti Diet*	1 T.	12	3.0

(USDA): United States Department of Agriculture
(HEW/FAO):   Health, Education and Welfare/Food and Agriculture
                        Organization
* Prepared as Package Directs

Food and Description	Measure or Quantity	Calories	Carbo-hydrates (grams)
ARBY'S:			
Bac'n Cheddar Deluxe	1 sandwich	560	35.0
Beef & Cheddar Sandwich	1 sandwich	450	46.0
Chicken breast sandwich	7¼-oz. sandwich	584	55.0
French Dip	5½-oz. sandwich	386	47.0
French fries	1½-oz. serving	216	26.0
Ham 'N Cheese	1 sandwich	380	46.0
Potato cakes	2 pieces	190	24.0
Roast Beef:			
Regular	5 oz. sandwich	350	32.0
Deluxe	8¼-oz. sandwich	486	43.0
Junior	3-oz. sandwich	220	21.0
Super	9¼-oz. sandwich	620	61.0
Sauce:			
Arby's	1 oz.	30	7.0
Horsey	1 oz.	100	5.0
Shake:			
Chocolate	14-oz. serving	370	61.0
Jamocha	14-oz. serving	400	73.0
Vanilla	14-oz. serving	330	49.0
ARTICHOKE:			
Fresh (USDA):			
Raw, whole	1 lb. (weighed untrimmed)	85	19.2
Boiled, without salt, drained	15-oz. artichoke	187	42.1
Canned (Cara Mia) marinated, drained	6-oz. jar	175	12.6
Frozen (Bird Eye) hearts, deluxe	⅓ pkg. (3 oz.)	39	6.6
ASPARAGUS:			
Fresh (USDA):			
Raw, spears	1 lb. (weighed untrimmed)	66	12.7
Boiled, without salt, drained	1 spear (½″ dia. at base)	3	.5
Canned, regular pack, solids & liq.:			
(Del Monte) spears, green or white	½ cup (4 oz.)	20	3.0
(Green Giant):			
Cuts	½ of 8-oz. can	20	2.0
Spears, green	½ cup (4 oz.)	23	3.2

Food and Description	Measure or Quantity	Calories	Carbo-hydrates (grams)
(Le Sueur) green spears	½ of 8-oz. can	30	4.0
Mussleman's	½ cup (4.5 oz.)	20	3.0
Canned, dietetic pack (USDA) drained solids, cut	1 cup (8.3 oz.)	47	7.3
Canned, dietetic pack, solids & liq.:			
(Diet Delight)	½ cup	16	2.0
(S&W) *Nutradiet,* green label	½ cup	17	3.0
Frozen:			
(USDA) cuts & tips, boiled, drained	1 cup (6.3 oz.)	40	6.3
(Birds Eye):			
Cuts	⅓ pkg. (3.3 oz.)	29	3.8
Spears, regular or jumbo deluxe	⅓ pkg. (3.3 oz.)	30	3.9
(Green Giant) cuts, in butter sauce	½ cup	70	6.0
(McKenzie)	⅓ pkg. (3.3 oz.)	25	4.0
(Seabrook Farms)	3.3-oz. serving	30	3.8
(Stouffer's) souffle	⅓ pkg. (4 oz.)	115	8.0

AUNT JEMIMA SYRUP (See **SYRUP**)

AVOCADO, all varieties (USDA):			
Whole	1 fruit (10.7 oz.)	378	14.3
Cubed	1 cup (5.3 oz.)	251	9.5
***AWAKE** (Birds Eye)	6 fl. oz. (6.5 oz.)	84	20.5
AYDS:			
Butterscotch	1 piece (.2 oz.)	27	5.7
Chocolate, chocolate mint, vanilla	1 piece (.2 oz.)	26	5.5

(USDA): United States Department of Agriculture
(HEW/FAO):   Health, Education and Welfare/Food and Agriculture Organization
* Prepared as Package Directs

Food and Description	Measure or Quantity	Calories	Carbo-hydrates (grams)

B

BABY FOOD:

Advance (Similac)	1 fl. oz.	15	1.5
Apple & apricot (Beech-Nut):			
Junior	7¾-oz. jar	93	24.4
Strained	4¾-oz. jar	57	14.0
Apple-banana juice (Gerber) strained	4.2 fl. oz.	57	13.7
Apple-betty (Beech-Nut):			
Junior	7¾-oz. jar	173	41.4
Strained	4¾-oz. jar	106	25.4
Apple-blueberry (Gerber):			
Junior	7½-oz. jar	111	26.2
Strained	4½-oz. jar	74	17.5
Apple-cherry juice:			
Strained:			
(Beech-Nut)	4⅕ fl. oz.	50	14.0
(Gerber)	4.2 fl. oz.	57	13.7
Toddler (Gerber)	4 fl. oz.	52	12.7
Apple-cranberry juice (Beech-Nut) strained	4½ fl. oz.	55	13.6
Apple dessert, Dutch (Gerber):			
Junior	7¾-oz. jar	160	35.0
Strained	4¾-oz. jar	97	21.1
Apple-grape juice:			
Strained:			
(Beech-Nut)	4⅕ fl. oz.	56	13.9
(Gerber)	4.2 fl. oz.	57	14.0
Toddler (Gerber)	4 fl. oz.	56	13.6
Apple juice:			
Strained:			
(Beech-Nut)	4⅕ fl. oz.	54	13.6
(Gerber)	4.2 fl. oz.	59	14.0
Toddler (Gerber)	4 fl. oz.	54	13.3
Apple-peach juice, strained:			
(Beech-Nut)	4⅕ fl. oz.	59	14.6
(Gerber)	4.2 fl. oz.	55	13.4

Food and Description	Measure or Quantity	Calories	Carbo- hydrates (grams)
Apple-plum juice (Gerber) strained	4.2 fl. oz.	60	14.4
Apple-prune juice (Gerber) strained	4.2 fl. oz.	61	14.7
Applesauce:			
Junior:			
(Beech-Nut)	7¾-oz. jar	97	24.1
(Gerber)	7½-oz. jar	95	22.4
Strained:			
(Beech-Nut)	4¾-oz. jar	60	14.8
(Gerber)	4½-oz. jar	59	13.8
Applesauce & apricots (Gerber):			
Junior	7½-oz. jar	98	22.8
Strained	4½-oz. jar	66	15.5
Applesauce & bananas (Beech-Nut) strained	4¾-oz. jar	63	15.4
Applesauce & cherries (Beech-Nut):			
Junior	7¾-oz. jar	115	28.4
Strained	4¾-oz. jar	61	15.1
Applesauce with pineapple (Gerber) strained	4½-oz. jar	63	14.8
Applesauce & raspberries (Beech-Nut):			
Junior	7¾-oz. jar	102	24.6
Strained	4¾-oz. jar	61	15.1
Apple & yogurt (Gerber) strained	4½-oz. jar	95	21.2
Apricot with tapioca:			
Junior:			
(Beech-Nut)	7½-oz. jar	113	27.9
(Gerber)	7¾-oz. jar	162	38.5
Strained (Gerber)	4¾-oz. jar	97	23.2
Apricot with tapioca & apple juice (Beech-Nut) strained	4¾-oz. jar	72	17.6
Banana-apple dessert (Gerber):			
Junior	7¾-oz. jar	166	38.5

(USDA): United States Department of Agriculture
(HEW/FAO): Health, Education and Welfare/Food and Agriculture Organization
* Prepared as Package Directs

Food and Description	Measure or Quantity	Calories	Carbo-hydrates (grams)
Strained	4¾-oz. jar	94	22.7
Banana dessert (Beech-Nut) junior	7½-oz. jar	165	40.1
Banana with pineapple & tapioca (Gerber):			
Junior	7½-oz. jar	112	26.0
Strained	4½-oz. jar	64	14.7
Banana & pineapple with tapioca & apple juice (Beech-Nut):			
Junior	7¾-oz. jar	109	26.6
Strained	4¾-oz. jar	67	16.3
Banana with tapioca:			
Junior:			
(Beech-Nut)	7¾-oz. jar	72	27.5
(Gerber)	7½-oz. jar	128	30.0
Strained:			
(Beech-Nut)	4¾-oz. jar	72	16.9
(Gerber)	7½-oz. jar	69	15.9
Banana & yogurt (Gerber) strained	4 1.2-oz. jar	80	16.7
Bean, green:			
Junior (Beech-Nut)	7¼-oz. jar	62	13.0
Strained:			
(Beech-Nut)	4½-oz. jar	38	8.1
(Gerber)	4½-oz. jar	31	5.9
Bean, green, creamed (Gerber) junior	7½-oz. jar	87	17.7
Bean, green, potatoes & ham casserole (Gerber) toddler	6¼-oz. jar	132	14.6
Beef (Gerber):			
Junior	3½-oz. jar	98	.4
Strained	3½-oz. jar	93	.3
Beef & beef broth (Beech-Nut):			
Junior	7½-oz. jar	235	.4
Strained	4½-oz. jar	152	.3
Beef with beef heart (Gerber) strained	3½-oz. jar	90	.5
Beef dinner, high meat, with vegetables (Gerber):			
Junior	4½-oz. jar	125	8.4
Strained	4½-oz. jar	111	7.4

Food and Description	Measure or Quantity	Calories	Carbo-hydrates (grams)
Beef & egg noodle (Beech-Nut):			
Junior	7½-oz. jar	122	17.0
Strained	4 1.2-oz. jar	72	9.9
Beef & egg noodles with vegetable (Gerber):			
Junior	7½-oz. jar	137	18.9
Strained	4½-oz. jar	85	11.9
Beef lasagna (Gerber) toddler	6¼-oz. jar	109	15.6
Beef liver (Gerber) strained	3½-oz. jar	98	2.9
Beef & rice with tomato sauce (Gerber) toddler	6¼-oz. jar	131	17.0
Beef stew (Gerber) toddler	6-oz. jar	110	12.4
Beef with vegetables & cereal, high meat (Beech-Nut):			
Junior	4½-oz. jar	132	8.0
Strained	4½-oz. jar	132	8.1
Beef (Gerber) strained	4½-oz. jar	47	10.0
Biscuit (Gerber)	11-gram piece	42	8.5
Carrot:			
Junior:			
(Beech-Nut)	7½-oz. jar	67	13.8
(Gerber)	7½-oz. jar	54	10.7
Strained:			
(Beech-Nut)	4½-oz. jar	40	8.3
(Gerber)	4½-oz. jar	31	6.3
Cereal, dry:			
Barley:			
(Beech-Nut)	½-oz. serving	54	9.9
(Gerber)	4 T. (½ oz.)	53	10.4
High protein:			
(Beech-Nut)	½-oz. serving	55	7.1
(Gerber)	4 T. (½ oz.)	53	5.9
High protein with apple & orange (Gerber)	4 T. (½ oz.)	55	7.7
Mixed:			
(Beech-Nut)	½-oz. serving	55	9.9
(Gerber)	4 T. (½ oz.)	54	9.7
Mixed with banana (Gerber)	4 T. (½ oz.)	55	10.6

(USDA): United States Department of Agriculture
(HEW/FAO): Health, Education and Welfare/Food and Agriculture Organization
* Prepared as Package Directs

Food and Description	Measure or Quantity	Calories	Carbo-hydrates (grams)
Oatmeal:			
(Beech-Nut)	½-oz. serving	56	9.7
(Gerber)	4 T. (½ oz.)	56	9.2
Oatmeal & banana (Gerber)	4 T. (½ oz.)	56	9.8
Rice:			
(Beech-Nut)	½-oz. serving	49	9.9
(Gerber)	4 T. (½ oz.)	55	10.7
Cereal, dry:			
Rice with banana (Gerber)	4 T. (½ oz.)	56	10.7
Cereal or mixed cereal:			
With applesauce & banana:			
Junior (Gerber)	7½-oz. jar	131	26.4
Strained:			
(Beech-Nut)	4½-oz. jar	80	17.3
(Gerber)	4½-oz. jar	83	16.7
& egg yolk (Gerber):			
Junior	7½-oz. jar	109	15.1
Strained	4½-oz. jar	70	9.6
With egg yolks & bacon (Beech-Nut):			
Junior	7½-oz. jar	163	14.9
Strained	4½-oz. jar	113	8.9
Oatmeal with applesauce & banana (Gerber):			
Junior	7½-oz. jar	119	23.0
Strained	4½-oz. jar	73	18.8
Rice with applesauce & banana, strained:			
(Beech-Nut)	4¾-oz. jar	96	21.4
(Gerber)	4¾-oz. jar	96	21.3
Rice with mixed fruit (Gerber) junior	7¾-oz. jar	161	36.1
Cherry vanilla pudding (Gerber):			
Junior	7½-oz. jar	147	32.0
Strained	4½-oz. jar	87	18.9
Chicken (Gerber):			
Junior	3½-oz. jar	137	.2
Strained	3½-oz. jar	139	.3
Chicken & chicken broth (Beech-Nut):			
Junior	7½-oz. jar	228	.4
Strained	4½-oz. jar	128	.3

Food and Description	Measure or Quantity	Calories	Carbo-hydrates (grams)
Chicken & noodles:			
Junior:			
(Beech-Nut)	7½-oz. jar	86	16.6
(Gerber)	7½-oz. jar	117	16.8
Strained:			
(Beech-Nut)	4½-oz. jar	59	10.5
(Gerber)	4½-oz. jar	77	11.1
Chicken & rice (Beech-Nut) strained	4½-oz. jar	72	12.0
Chicken with vegetables, high meat (Gerber):			
Junior	4½-oz. jar	132	7.5
Strained	4½-oz. jar	126	7.8
Chicken with vegetables & cereal (Beech-Nut):			
Junior	7½-oz. jar	150	14.9
Strained	4½-oz. jar	90	8.9
Chicken soup, cream of (Gerber) strained	4½-oz. jar	77	10.4
Chicken stew (Gerber) toddler	6-oz. jar	145	12.3
Chicken sticks (Gerber) junior	2½-oz. jar	120	1.0
Cookie (Gerber):			
Animal-shaped	6½-gram piece	28	4.3
Arrowroot	5½-gram piece	25	3.7
Corn, creamed:			
Junior:			
(Beech-Nut)	7½-oz. jar	142	30.9
(Gerber)	7½-oz. jar	128	26.2
Strained:			
(Beech-Nut)	4½-oz. jar	85	18.5
(Gerber)	4½-oz. jar	82	16.8
Cottage cheese with pineapple juice (Beech-Nut):			
Junior	7¾-oz. jar	178	32.1
Strained	4¾-oz. jar	111	22.3
Custard:			
Apple (Beech-Nut):			
Junior	7½-oz. jar	132	27.7
Strained	4½-oz. jar	79	16.6

(USDA): United States Department of Agriculture
(HEW/FAO):   Health, Education and Welfare/Food and Agriculture
                       Organization
* Prepared as Package Directs

Food and Description	Measure or Quantity	Calories	Carbo-hydrates (grams)
Chocolate (Gerber) strained	4½-oz. jar	106	19.3
Vanilla:			
Junior:			
(Beech-Nut)	7½-oz. jar	166	29.0
(Gerber)	7¾-oz. jar	186	33.7
Strained:			
(Beech-Nut)	4½-oz. jar	92	15.7
(Gerber)	4½-oz. jar	106	19.6
Egg yolk (Gerber):			
Junior	3⅓-oz. jar	184	.2
Strained	3⅓-oz. jar	186	.9
Fruit dessert:			
Junior:			
(Beech-Nut):			
Regular	7¾-oz. jar	162	40.3
Tropical	7¾-oz. jar	137	34.1
(Gerber)	7¾-oz. jar	160	38.3
Strained:			
(Beech-Nut)	4½-oz. jar	97	24.0
(Gerber)	4¾-oz. jar	92	22.0
Fruit juice, mixed:			
Strained:			
(Beech-Nut)	4⅕ fl. oz.	59	14.5
(Gerber)	4.2 fl. oz.	58	13.6
Toddler (Gerber)	4 fl. oz.	54	13.2
Fruit, mixed with yogurt:			
Junior (Beech-Nut)	7½-oz. jar	120	27.3
Strained:			
(Beech-Nut)	4¾-oz. jar	76	17.3
(Gerber)	4½-oz. jar	100	21.6
Guava (Gerber) strained	4½-oz. jar	84	19.9
Guava & papaya (Gerber) strained	4½-oz. jar	85	20.3
Ham (Gerber):			
Junior	3½-oz. jar	114	.4
Strained	3½-oz. jar	105	.5
Ham & ham broth (Beech-Nut) strained	4½-oz. jar	143	.3
Ham with vegetables, high meat (Gerber):			
Junior	4½-oz. jar	105	9.5
Strained	4½-oz. jar	99	8.3

Food and Description	Measure or Quantity	Calories	Carbo-hydrates (grams)
Ham with vegetables & cereal (Beech-Nut):			
Junior	4½-oz. jar	126	7.9
Strained	4½-oz. jar	126	7.9
Hawaiian Delight (Gerber):			
Junior	7¾-oz. jar	187	40.7
Strained	4½-oz. jar	111	24.3
Isomil (similac) ready-to-feed	1 fl. oz.	20	1.9
Lamb (Gerber):			
Junior	3½-oz. jar	99	.5
Strained	3½-oz. jar	99	.6
Lamb & lamb broth (Beech-Nut):			
Junior	7½-oz. jar	265	.4
Strained	4½-oz. jar	157	.2
Macaroni & cheese (Gerber):			
Junior	7½-oz. jar	135	18.8
Strained	4½-oz. jar	80	10.9
Macaroni & tomato with beef:			
Junior:			
(Beech-Nut)	7½-oz. jar	117	16.4
(Gerber)	7½-oz. jar	119	21.3
Strained:			
(Beech-Nut)	4½-oz. jar	81	10.7
(Gerber)	4½-oz. jar	71	11.5
Mango (Gerber) strained	4¾-oz. jar	97	23.3
MBF (Gerber):			
Concentrate	1 fl. oz. (2 T.)	39	3.7
Concentrate	15-fl.-oz. can	598	56.6
*Diluted, 1 to 1	1 fl. oz. (2 T.)	20	1.9
Meat sticks (Gerber) junior	2½-oz. jar	104	.9
Orange-apple juice, strained:			
(Beech-Nut)	4½ fl. oz.	55	13.5
(Gerber)	4.2 fl. oz.	58	13.5
Orange-apricot juice (Beech-Nut) strained	4.2 fl. oz.	60	13.2
Orange-banana juice (Beech-Nut) strained	4⅕ fl. oz.	58	13.9

(USDA): United States Department of Agriculture
(HEW/FAO): Health, Education and Welfare/Food and Agriculture Organization
* Prepared as Package Directs

Food and Description	*Measure or Quantity*	*Calories*	*Carbo-hydrates (grams)*
Orange juice, strained:			
(Beech-Nut)	4⅕ fl. oz.	56	13.2
(Gerber)	4.2 fl. oz.	57	12.5
Orange-pineapple dessert (Beech-Nut) strained	4¾-oz. jar	107	26.4
Orange-pineapple juice, strained:			
(Beech-Nut)	4⅕-fl. oz.	57	13.6
(Gerber)	4.2 fl. oz.	64	14.8
Orange pudding (Gerber) strained	4¾-oz. jar	101	24.0
Papaya & applesauce (Gerber) strained	4½-oz. jar	82	19.9
Pea:			
Junior:			
(Beech-Nut)	7¼-oz. jar	114	19.1
(Gerber)	7½-oz. jar	127	21.5
Strained:			
(Beech-Nut)	4½-oz. jar	67	11.2
(Gerber)	4½-oz. jar	56	8.6
Pea & carrot (Beech-Nut) strained	4½-oz. jar	61	11.1
Peach:			
Junior:			
(Beech-Nut)	7¾-oz. jar	97	22.9
(Gerber)	7½-oz. jar	94	20.7
Strained:			
(Beech-Nut)	4¾-oz. jar	59	14.0
(Gerber)	4½-oz. jar	64	14.4
Peach & apple with yogurt (Beech-Nut):			
Junior	7½-oz. jar	113	25.1
Strained	4½-oz. jar	68	15.1
Peach cobbler (Gerber):			
Junior	7¾-oz. jar	155	36.8
Strained	4¾-oz. jar	94	22.1
Peach melba (Beech-Nut):			
Junior	7¾-oz. jar	161	39.4
Strained	4¾-oz. jar	99	24.2
Pear:			
Junior:			
(Beech-Nut)	7½-oz. jar	106	26.2
(Gerber)	7½-oz. jar	110	25.4

Food and Description	Measure or Quantity	Calories	Carbo-hydrates (grams)
Strained:			
(Beech-Nut)	4½-oz. jar	64	15.7
(Gerber)	7½-oz. jar	66	15.2
Pear & pineapple:			
Junior:			
(Beech-Nut)	7½-oz. jar	121	29.6
(Gerber)	7½-oz. jar	109	25.4
Strained:			
(Beech-Nut)	4½-oz. serving	73	17.8
(Gerber)	4½-oz. jar	68	15.7
Pineapple dessert (Beech-Nut) strained	4¾-oz. jar	107	26.4
Pineapple with yogurt (Beech-Nut):			
Junior	7½-oz. jar	133	30.0
Strained	4¾-oz. jar	84	19.0
Plum with tapioca (Gerber):			
Junior	7¾-oz. jar	157	37.4
Strained	4¾-oz. jar	91	21.9
Plum with tapioca & apple juice (Beech-Nut):			
Junior	7¾-oz. jar	120	29.3
Strained	4¾-oz. jar	73	17.9
Pork (Gerber) strained	3½-oz. jar	106	.3
Pretzel (Gerber)	6-gram piece	23	4.7
Prune-orange juice (Beech-Nut) strained	4⅕ fl. oz.	66	15.7
Prune with tapioca:			
Junior:			
(Beech-Nut)	7¾-oz. jar	174	40.5
(Gerber)	7¾-oz. jar	172	40.1
Strained:			
(Beech-Nut)	4¾-oz. jar	107	24.8
(Gerber)	4¾-oz. jar	98	22.7
Similac:			
Ready-to-feed or concentrated liquid, with or without added iron	1 fl. oz.	20	2.0
*Powder, regular or with iron	1 fl. oz.	20	2.0

(USDA): United States Department of Agriculture
(HEW/FAO):   Health, Education and Welfare/Food and Agriculture
                         Organization
* Prepared as Package Directs

Food and Description	Measure or Quantity	Calories	Carbo-hydrates (grams)
Spaghetti & meatballs (Gerber) toddler	6½-oz. jar	127	18.6
Spaghetti, tomato & beef (Beech-Nut) junior	7½-oz. jar	131	19.4
Spaghetti with tomato sauce & beef (Gerber) junior	7½-oz. jar	136	22.2
Spinach, creamed (Gerber) strained	4½-oz. jar	56	6.9
Split pea & ham, junior:			
(Beech-Nut)	7½-oz. jar	149	23.4
(Gerber)	7½-oz. jar	151	23.0
Squash:			
Junior:			
(Beech-Nut)	7½-oz. jar	57	11.7
(Gerber)	7½-oz. jar	56	11.1
Strained:			
(Beech-Nut)	4½-oz. jar	34	7.0
(Gerber)	4½-oz. jar	33	6.6
Sweet potato:			
Junior:			
(Beech-Nut)	7¾-oz. jar	118	27.5
(Gerber)	7¾-oz. jar	132	29.5
Strained:			
(Beech-Nut)	4½-oz. jar	68	15.9
(Gerber)	4¾-oz. jar	82	18.2
Turkey (Gerber):			
Junior	3½-oz. jar	130	Tr.
Strained	3½-oz. jar	127	.3
Turkey & rice (Beech-Nut):			
Junior	7½-oz. jar	83	16.6
Strained	4½-oz. jar	59	12.0
Turkey & rice with vegetables (Gerber):			
Junior	4½-oz. jar	132	8.1
Strained	4½-oz. jar	127	7.4
Turkey with vegetables & cereal (Beech-Nut) high meat:			
Junior	4½-oz. jar	112	8.9
Strained	4½-oz. jar	112	8.9
Turkey sticks (Gerber) junior	2½-oz. jar	122	1.1
Turkey & turkey broth (Beech-Nut) strained	4½-oz. jar	140	.2

Food and Description	Measure or Quantity	Calories	Carbo-hydrates (grams)
Veal (Gerber):			
Junior	3½-oz. jar	98	.1
Strained	3½-oz. jar	90	.2
Veal & vegetables (Gerber):			
Junior	4½-oz. jar	92	9.2
Strained	4½-oz. jar	85	7.8
Veal with vegetable & cereal, high meat (Beech-Nut) junior or strained	4½-oz. jar	108	8.1
Veal & veal broth (Beech-Nut) strained	4½-oz. jar	143	.2
Vegetable & bacon:			
Junior:			
(Beech-Nut)	7½-oz. jar	141	18.9
(Gerber)	7½-oz. jar	166	19.2
Strained:			
(Beech-Nut)	4½-oz. jar	83	9.9
(Gerber)	4½-oz. jar	96	10.6
Vegetable & beef:			
Junior:			
(Beech-Nut)	7½-oz. jar	123	18.1
(Gerber)	7½-oz. jar	139	20.7
Strained:			
(Beech-Nut)	4½-oz. jar	79	10.9
(Gerber)	4½-oz. jar	84	10.6
Vegetable & chicken:			
Junior:			
(Beech-Nut)	7½-oz. jar	89	15.9
(Gerber)	* 7½-oz. jar	109	16.8
Strained:			
(Beech-Nut)	4½-oz. jar	58	9.9
(Gerber)	4½-oz. jar	61	8.6
Vegetable & ham, strained:			
(Beech-Nut)	4½-oz. jar	75	10.9
(Gerber)	4½-oz. jar	73	10.7
Vegetable & lamb with rice & barley (Beech-Nut):			
Junior	7½-oz. jar	120	17.0
Strained	4½-oz. jar	74	10.0

(USDA): United States Department of Agriculture
(HEW/FAO):   Health, Education and Welfare/Food and Agriculture
            Organization
* Prepared as Package Directs

Food and Description	Measure or Quantity	Calories	Carbo-hydrates (grams)
Vegetable & liver (Gerber):			
Junior	7½-oz. jar	90	16.4
Strained	4½-oz. jar	60	9.7
Vegetable & liver with rice & barley (Beech-Nut):			
Junior	7½-oz. jar	91	16.8
Strained	4½-oz. jar	58	9.8
Vegetable & ham (Gerber) junior	7½-oz. jar	126	17.9
Vegetable, mixed:			
Junior:			
(Beech-Nut)	7½-oz. jar	79	17.0
(Gerber)	7½-oz. jar	83	17.0
Strained:			
(Beech-Nut):			
Regular	4½-oz. jar	55	12.0
Garden	4½-oz. jar	66	12.5
(Gerber):			
Regular	4½-oz. jar	52	10.4
Garden	4½-oz. jar	43	6.8
Vegetable & turkey:			
Junior (Gerber)	7½-oz. jar	112	18.3
Strained:			
(Beech-Nut)	4½-oz. jar	77	12.1
(Gerber)	4½-oz. jar	65	9.3
Vegetable & turkey casserole (Gerber) toddler	6¼-oz. jar	147	14.2
BACON, broiled:			
(USDA):			
Medium slice	1 slice (7½ grams)	43	.2
Thick slice	1 slice (12 grams)	72	.4
Thin slice	1 slice (5 grams)	30	.2
(Hormel):			
Black Label	1 slice	30	0.
Range Brand	1 slice	55	0.
(Oscar Mayer):			
Regular slice	6-gram slice	35	.1
Thick slice	1 slice (11 grams)	64	.2
Wafer thin	1 slice (4 grams)	23	.1

Food and Description	Measure or Quantity	Calories	Carbo-hydrates (grams)
BACON BITS:			
Bac*Os (Betty Crocker)	1 tsp.	13	.6
(Durkee) imitation	1 tsp.	8	.5
(French's) imitation	1 tsp.	6	Tr.
(Hormel)	1 tsp.	10	0.
(Libby's) crumbles	1 tsp.	8	.7
(McCormick) imitation	1 tsp.	9	.7
(Oscar Mayer) real	1 tsp.	6	.1
BACON, CANADIAN, unheated:			
(USDA)	1 oz.	61	Tr.
(Eckrich)	1-oz. slice	35	1.0
(Hormel) sliced	1 oz.	45	0.
(Oscar Mayer) 93% fat free:			
Thin	.7-oz. slice	30	0.
Thick	1-oz. slice	40	0.
BACON, SIMULATED, cooked:			
(Oscar Mayer) *Lean 'N Tasty:*			
Beef	1 slice (.3 oz.)	39	.2
Pork	1 slice (.3 oz.)	45	.2
(Swift's) *Sizzlean*	1 strip (.4 oz.)	50	0.
BAGEL (USDA):			
Egg	3-inch dia. bagel, 1.9 oz.	162	28.3
Water	3-inch dia. bagel, 1.9 oz.	163	30.5
BAKING POWDER: (USDA):			
Phosphate	1 tsp. (3.8 grams)	5	1.1
SAS	1 tsp. (3 grams)	4	.9
Tartrate	1 tsp. (2.8 grams)	2	.5

(USDA): United States Department of Agriculture
(HEW/FAO): Health, Education and Welfare/Food and Agriculture
              Organization
* Prepared as Package Directs

Food and Description	Measure or Quantity	Calories	Carbo-hydrates (grams)
(Calumet)	1 tsp. (3.6 grams)	2	1.0
(Featherweight) low sodium, cereal free	1 tsp.	8	2.0
BALSAMPEAR, fresh (Hew/FAO):			
Whole	1 lb. (weighed with cavity contents)	69	16.3
Flesh only	4 oz.	22	5.1
BAMBOO SHOOTS:			
Raw, trimmed (USDA)	4 oz.	31	5.9
Canned, drained (La Choy)	¼ cup (1.5 oz.)	6	1.0
BANANA (USDA):			
Common yellow:			
Fresh:			
Whole	1 lb. (weighed with skin)	262	68.5
Small size	5.9-oz. banana (7¾″ × 1¹¹⁄₃₂″)	81	21.1
Medium size	6.3-oz. banana (8¾″ × 1¹³⁄₃₂″)	101	26.4
Large size	7-oz. banana 9¾″ × 1⁷⁄₁₆″)	116	30.2
Mashed	1 cup (about 2 med.)	191	50.0
Sliced	1 cup (about 1¼ med.)	128	33.3
Dehydrated flakes	½ cup (1.8 oz.)	170	44.3
Red, fresh, whole	1 lb. (weighed with skin)	278	72.2
BANANA EXTRACT (Durkee) imitation	1 tsp.	15	DNA
BANANA NECTAR, canned (Libby's)	6 fl. oz.	60	14.0

BANANA PIE (See **PIE**, Banana)

Food and Description	Measure or Quantity	Calories	Carbo-hydrates (grams)
BARBECUE SEASONING (French's)	1 tsp. (.1 oz.)	6	1.0
BARBERA WINE (Louise M. Martini) 12½% alcohol	3 fl. oz.	66	.2
BARDOLINO WINE (Antinori) 12% alcohol	3 fl. oz.	84	6.3
BARLEY, pearled, dry:			
Light (USDA)	¼ cup (1.8 oz.)	174	39.4
Pot or Scotch:			
(USDA)	2 oz.	197	43.8
(Quaker) Scotch	¼ cup (1.7 oz.)	172	36.3
BASIL:			
Fresh (HEW/FAO) sweet, leaves	½ oz.	6	1.0
Dried (French's)	1 tsp.	3	.7
BASS (USDA):			
Black Sea:			
Raw, whole	1 lb. (weighed whole)	165	0.
Baked, stuffed, home recipe	4 oz.	294	12.9
Smallmouth & largemouth, raw:			
Whole	1 lb. (weighed whole)	146	0.
Meat only	4 oz.	118	0.
Striped:			
Raw, whole	1 lb. (weighed whole)	205	0.
Raw, meat only	4 oz.	119	0.
Oven-fried	4 oz.	222	7.6
White, raw, meat only	4 oz.	111	0.
BAY LEAF (French's)	1 tsp.	5	1.0

(USDA): United States Department of Agriculture
(HEW/FAO):   Health, Education and Welfare/Food and Agriculture
            Organization
* Prepared as Package Directs

Food and Description	Measure or Quantity	Calories	Carbo-hydrates (grams)
B & B LIQUEUR, 86 proof	1 fl. oz.	94	5.7
B.B.Q. SAUCE & BEEF, frozen (Banquet) *Cookin' Bag,* sliced	4-oz. pkg.	133	13.0
BEAN, BAKED:			
(USDA):			
With pork & molasses sauce	1 cup (9 oz.)	382	53.8
With pork & tomato sauce	1 cup (9 oz.)	311	48.5
With tomato sauce	1 cup (9 oz.)	306	58.7
Canned:			
(B&M):			
Pea bean with pork in brown sugar sauce	8 oz.	345	50.0
Red kidney or yellow eye bean in brown sugar sauce	8 oz.	325	50.0
(Campbell):			
Home style	8-oz. can	270	48.0
With pork & tomato sauce	8-oz. can	270	49.0
Old fashioned, in molasses & brown sugar sauce	8-oz. can	250	44.0
(Friend's)			
Pea	9-oz. serving	363	61.4
Red kidney	9-oz. serving	343	56.3
Yellow eye	9-oz. serving	353	58.8
(Grandma Brown's) home baked	8-oz. serving	289	54.1
(Howard Johnson's)	1 cup	340	21.1
(Van Camp):			
& pork	8-oz. serving	226	41.3
Vegetarian	8-oz. serving	216	41.9
BEAN, BARBECUE (Campbell)	7⅞-oz. can	250	43.0
BEAN, BLACK OR BROWN, dry (USDA)	1 cup	678	122.4
BEAN, & FRANKFURTER, canned:			
(USDA)	1 cup (9 oz.)	367	32.1
(Campbell) in tomato and molasses sauce	7⅞-oz. can	350	42.0

Food and Description	Measure or Quantity	Calories	Carbo-hydrates (grams)
(Hormel) *Short Orders*, 'n wieners	7½-oz. can	280	39.0
BEAN & FRANKFURTER DINNER, frozen:			
(Banquet)	10¼-oz. dinner	500	64.0
(Morton)	10¾-oz. dinner	530	79.0
(Swanson) *TV Brand*	11¼-oz. dinner	490	62.0
BEAN, GARBANZO, canned, dietetic (S&W) *Nutradiet,* low sodium, green label	½ cup	105	19.0
BEAN, GREEN:			
Fresh (USDA):			
Whole	1 lb. (weighed untrimmed)	128	28.3
French style	½ cup (1.4 oz.)	13	2.8
Boiled (USDA):			
Whole, drained	½ cup (2.2 oz.)	16	3.3
Boiled, 1½" to 2" pieces, drained	½ cup (2.4 oz.)	17	3.7
Canned, regular pack:			
(USDA):			
Whole, solids & liq.	½ cup (4.2 oz.)	22	5.0
Whole, drained solids	4 oz.	27	5.9
Cut, drained solids	½ cup (2.5 oz.)	17	3.6
Drained liquid only	4 oz.	11	2.7
(Comstock) solids & liq.	½ cup (4 oz.)	23	4.0
(Del Monte) solids & liq.	4 oz.	20	4.0
(Green Giant) french or whole, solids & liq.	½ cup	21	4.2
(Libby's) french, solids & liq.	½ cup (4 oz.)	21	4.0
(Sunshine) solids & liq.	½ cup (4.2 oz.)	20	3.8
Canned, dietetic or low calorie:			
(USDA):			
Solids & liq.	4 oz.	18	4.1
Drained solids	4 oz.	25	5.4

(USDA): United States Department of Agriculture
(HEW/FAO):   Health, Education and Welfare/Food and Agriculture
                    Organization
* Prepared as Package Directs

Food and Description	Measure or Quantity	Calories	Carbo-hydrates (grams)
(Del Monte) No Salt Added, solids & liq.	½ cup (4 oz.)	19	4.0
(Diet Delight) solids & liq.	½ cup (4.2 oz.)	20	3.0
(Featherweight) solids & liq.	½ cup (4 oz.)	25	5.0
(S&W) *Nutradiet* green label, solids & liq.	½ cup	20	4.0
Frozen:			
(Birds Eye):			
Cut or French	⅓ of pkg (3 oz.)	30	5.9
French, with almonds	⅓ of pkg. (3 oz.)	58	8.4
Whole, deluxe	⅓ of pkg.	26	5.1
(Green Giant):			
Cut or french, with butter sauce	½ cup	40	6.0
Cut, *Harvest Fresh*	½ cup	25	4.0
With mushroom in cream sauce	½ cup	80	10.0
Polybag	½ cup	20	4.0
(Seabrook Farms)	⅓ of pkg. (3 oz.)	29	5.8
(Southland) cut or french	⅕ of 16-oz. pkg.	25	5.0
BEAN, GREEN & MUSHROOM CASSEROLE, frozen (Stouffer's)	½ of 9½-oz. pkg.	150	12.0
BEAN, GREEN, WITH POTATOES, canned (Sunshine) solids & liq.	½ cup (4.3 oz.)	34	7.0
BEAN, ITALIAN:			
Canned (Del Monte) cut, solids & liq.	4 oz.	25	6.0
Frozen (Birds Eye)	⅓ of pkg. (3 oz.)	38	7.3
BEAN, KIDNEY OR RED			
(USDA):			
Dry	½ cup (3.3 oz.)	319	57.6
Cooked	½ cup (3.3 oz.)	109	19.8
Canned, regular pack, solids & liq.			
(Furman) red, fancy, light	½ cup (4½ oz.)	121	21.2
(Van Camp):			
Dark	8 oz.	192	35.0

Food and Description	Measure or Quantity	Calories	Carbo- hydrates (grams)
Light	8 oz.	194	35.9
New Orleans Style	8 oz.	188	33.8
Red	8 oz.	213	37.9
Canned, dietetic (S&W) Nutradiet, low sodium, green label	½ cup	90	16.0
BEAN, LIMA:			
Raw (USDA):			
Young, whole	1 lb. (weighed in pod)	223	40.1
Mature, dry	½ cup (3.4 oz.)	331	61.4
Young, without shell	1 lb. (weighed shelled)	558	100.2
Boiled (USDA) drained	½ cup	94	
Canned, regular pack,: (USDA):			
Solids & liq.	4 oz.	81	15.2
Drained solids	4 oz.	109	20.8
(Del Monte) solids & liq.	4 oz.	70	14.0
(Libby's) solids & liq.	½ cup (4.3 oz.)	91	16.0
(Sultana) butter bean, solids & liq.	¼ of 15-oz. can	82	
Canned, dietetic (Featherweight) solids & liq.	½ cup	80	16.0
Frozen:			
(Birds Eye):			
Baby	⅓ of 10-oz. pkg.	130	24.3
Baby butter	⅓ of 10-oz. pkg.	139	26.0
Fordhook	⅓ of 10-oz. pkg.	103	18.7
Tiny, deluxe	⅓ of 10-oz. pkg.	111	20.3
(Green Giant):			
In butter sauce	½ cup	120	20.0
Harvest Fresh, or polybag	½ cup	100	19.0
(McKenzie):			
Baby	3.3 oz.	130	24.0
Fordhook	3.3 oz.	100	19.0
Speckled butter	3.3 oz.	120	23.0
Tiny	3.3 oz.	110	21.0

(USDA): United States Department of Agriculture
(HEW/FAO):   Health, Education and Welfare/Food and Agriculture
                        Organization
* Prepared as Package Directs

Food and Description	Measure or Quantity	Calories	Carbohydrates (grams)
(Southland) speckled butter	1.5 of 16-oz. pkg.	110	20.0
BEAN, MUNG (USDA) dry	½ cup (3.7 oz.)	357	63.3
BEAN, PINTO:			
Dry (USDA)	4 oz.	396	72.2
Canned (Del Monte) spicy	½ cup (4.3 oz.)	120	19.0
Frozen (McKenzie)	3.2-oz. serving	160	29.0
BEAN, REFRIED, canned:			
(Del Monte) regular or spicy	½ cup (4.3 oz.)	130	20.0
Old El Paso:			
Plain	4 oz.	106	17.0
With green chili peppers	4 oz.	100	18.2
With sausage	4 oz.	224	14.8
(Ortega) lightly spicy or true bean	½ cup	170	25.0
BEAN SALAD, canned (Green Giant) three bean, solids & liq.	¼ of 17-oz. can	80	18.0
BEAN SOUP (see SOUP, Bean)			
BEAN SPROUT:			
Fresh (USDA):			
Mung, raw	½ lb.	80	15.0
Mung, boiled, drained	¼ lb.	32	5.9
Soy, raw	½ lb.	104	12.0
Soy, boiled, drained	¼ lb.	43	4.2
Canned (La Choy) drained solids	⅔ cup	8	1.0
BEAN, YELLOW OR WAX:			
Raw, whole (USDA)	1 lb. (weighed untrimmed)	108	24.0
Boiled (USDA) 1″ pieces, drained	½ cup (2.9 oz.)	18	3.7
Canned, regular pack, solids & liq.:			
(Comstock)	½ cup (4 oz.)	22	4.5
(Del Monte) cut or french	½ cup (4 oz.)	20	4.0

Food and Description	Measure or Quantity	Calories	Carbo-hydrates (grams)
(Libby's) cut	4 oz.	23	4.4
(Stokely Van Camp) cut	½ cup	23	4.0
Canned, dietetic, (Featherweight) cut stringless, solids & liq.	½ cup (4 oz.)	25	5.0
Frozen (McKenzie) cut	3 oz.	25	5.0

BEEF. Values for beef cuts are given below for "leans and fat" and for "lean only." Beef purchased by the consumer at the retail store usually is trimmed to about one-half inch layer of fat. This is the meat described as "lean and fat." If all the fat that can be cut off with a knife is removed, the remainder is the "lean only." These cuts still contain flecks of fat known as "marbling" distributed through the meat. Cooked meats are medium done. Choice grade cuts (USDA):

Brisket:			
Raw	1 lb. (weighed with bone)	1284	0.
Braised:			
Lean & fat	4 oz.	467	0.
Lean only	4 oz.	252	0.
Chuck:			
Raw	1 lb. (weighed with bone)	984	0.
Braised or pot-roasted:			
Lean & fat	4 oz.	371	0.
Lean only	4 oz.	243	0.
Dried (see **BEEF, CHIPPED**)			
Fat, separable, cooked	1 oz.	207	0.

Filet mignon. There is no data available on its composition.

(USDA): United States Department of Agriculture
(HEW/FAO):   Health, Education and Welfare/Food and Agriculture Organization
* Prepared as Package Directs

Food and Description	Measure or Quantity	Calories	Carbo-hydrates (grams)
For dietary estimates, the data for sirloin steak, lean only, afford the closest approximation.			
Flank:			
Raw	1 lb.	653	0.
Braised	4 oz.	222	0.
Foreshank:			
Raw	1 lb. (weighed with bone)	531	0.
Simmered:			
Lean & fat	4 oz.	310	0.
Lean only	4 oz.	209	0.
Ground:			
Lean:			
Raw	1 lb.	812	0.
Raw	1 cup (8 oz.)	405	0.
Broiled	4 oz.	248	0.
Regular:			
Raw	1 lb.	1216	0.
Raw	1 cup (8 oz.)	606	0.
Broiled	4 oz.	324	0.
Heal of round:			
Raw	1 lb.	966	0.
Roasted:			
Lean & fat	4 oz.	296	0.
Lean only	4 oz.	204	0.
Hindshank:			
Raw	1 lb. (weighed with bone)	604	0.
Simmered:			
Lean & fat	4 oz.	409	0.
Lean only	4 oz.	209	0.
Neck:			
Raw	1 lb. (weighed with bone)	820	0.
Pot-roasted:			
Lean & fat	4 oz.	332	0.
Lean only	4 oz.	222	0.
Plate:			
Raw	1 lb. (weighed with bone)	1615	0.

Food and Description	Measure or Quantity	Calories	Carbo-hydrates (grams)
Simmered:			
Lean & fat	4 oz.	538	0.
Lean only	4 oz.	252	0.
Rib roast:			
Raw	1 lb. (weighed with bone)	1673	0.
Roasted:			
Lean & fat	4 oz.	499	0.
Lean only	4 oz.	273	0.
Round:			
Raw	1 lb. (weighed with bone)	863	0.
Broiled:			
Lean & fat	4 oz.	296	0.
Lean only	4 oz.	214	0.
Rump:			
Raw	1 lb. (weighed with bone)	1167	0.
Roasted:			
Lean & fat	4 oz.	393	0.
Lean only	4 oz.	236	0.
Steak, club:			
Raw	1 lb. (weighed without bone)	1724	0.
Broiled:			
Lean & fat	4 oz.	515	0.
Lean only	4 oz.	277	0.
One 8-oz. steak (weighed without bone before cooking) will give you:			
Lean & fat	5.9 oz.	754	0.
Lean only	3.4 oz.	234	0.
Steak, porterhouse:			
Raw	1 lb. (weighed with bone)	1603	0.
Broiled:			
Lean & fat	4 oz.	527	0.
Lean only	4 oz.	254	0.

(USDA): United States Department of Agriculture
(HEW/FAO):   Health, Education and Welfare/Food and Agriculture
Organization
* Prepared as Package Directs

Food and Description	Measure or Quantity	Calories	Carbo-hydrates (grams)
One 16-oz. steak (weighed with bone before cooking) will give you:			
Lean & fat	10.2 oz.	1339	0.
Lean only	5.9 oz.	372	0.
Steak, ribeye, broiled:			
One 10-oz. steak (weighed before cooking without bone) will give you:			
Lean & fat	7.3 oz.	911	0.
Lean only	3.8 oz.	258	0.
Steak, sirloin, double-bone:			
Raw	1 lb. (weighed with bone)	1240	0.
Broiled:			
Lean & fat	4 oz.	463	0.
Lean only	4 oz.	245	0.
One 16-oz. steak (weighed before cooking with bone) will give you:			
Lean & fat	8.9 oz.	1028	0.
Lean only	5.9 oz.	359	0.
One 12-oz. steak (weighed before cooking with bone) will give you:			
Lean & fat	6.6 oz.	767	0.
Lean only	4.4 oz.	268	0.
Steak, sirloin, hipbone:			
Raw	1 lb. (weighed with bone)	1585	0.
Broiled:			
Lean & fat	4 oz.	552	0.
Lean only	4 oz.	272	0.
Steak, sirloin, wedge & round-bone:			
Raw	1 lb. (weighed with bone)	1316	0.
Broiled:			
Lean & fat	4 oz.	439	0.
Lean only	4 oz.	235	0.
Steak, T-bone:			
Raw	1 lb. (weighed with bone)	1596	0.

Food and Description	Measure or Quantity	Calories	Carbo-hydrates (grams)
Broiled:			
Lean & fat	4 oz.	536	0.
Lean only	4 oz.	253	0.
One 16-oz. steak (weighed before cooking with bone) will give you:			
Broiled:			
Lean & fat	4 oz.	463	0.
Lean only	4 oz.	245	0.
BEEF BOUILLON:			
(Herb-Ox):			
Cube	1 cube	6	.7
Packet	1 packet	8	.9
(Maggi)	1 cube	6	0.
MBT	1 packet	14	2.0
Low sodium (Featherweight)	1 tsp.	18	2.0
BEEF, CHIPPED:			
Cooked, home recipe (USDA) creamed	½ cup (4.3 oz.)	188	8.7
Frozen, creamed:			
(Banquet) *Cookin' Bag*	4-oz. pkg.	125	8.0
(Morton)	5-oz. pkg.	160	9.0
(Stouffer's)	5½-oz. serving	235	10.0
(Swanson)	10½-oz. entree	330	16.0
BEEF DINNER or ENTREE,			
frozen:			
(Banquet):			
American Favorites:			
Chopped	11-oz. dinner	434	23.0
With gravy	10-oz. dinner	345	19.0
Extra Helping:			
Regular	16-oz. dinner	864	72.0
Chopped	18-oz. dinner	1028	70.0
(Green Giant)			
Baked, boneless ribs in BBQ sauce with corn on the cob	1 meal	390	40.0

(USDA): United States Department of Agriculture
(HEW/FAO):   Health, Education and Welfare/Food and Agriculture
                        Organization
* Prepared as Package Directs

Food and Description	Measure or Quantity	Calories	Carbo-hydrates (grams)
Baked, stir fry, teriyaki	10-oz. entree	320	36.0
Twin pouch, burgundy, with rice & carrots	9-oz. entree	280	33.0
(Morton):			
Regular:			
Dinner	10-oz. dinner	260	20.0
Entree, patty	5-oz. pkg.	200	8.0
Country Table, sliced	14-oz. dinner	510	57.0
Steak House:			
Chopped sirloin	9½-oz. dinner	760	43.0
Rib eye	9-oz. dinner	820	38.0
Sirloin strip	9½-oz. dinner	760	43.0
Tenderloin	9½-oz. dinner	890	43.0
(Stouffer's) *Lean Cuisine,* oriental	8⅝-oz. pkg.	280	32.0
(Swanson):			
Hungry Man:			
Chopped	18-oz. dinner	690	50.0
Sliced	17-oz. dinner	500	55.0
Sliced	12¼-oz. dinner	300	20.0
3-course	15-oz. dinner	450	50.0
TV Brand:			
Regular	11½-oz. dinner	310	30.0
Chopped sirloin	10-oz. dinner	380	33.0
(Weight Watchers):			
Beefsteak, 2-compartment meal	9¼-oz. pkg.	320	14.0
Oriental	10-oz. meal	260	32.1
Sirloin in mushroom sauce, 3-compartment meal	13-oz. pkg.	410	16.0
BEEF, DRIED, packaged:			
(Hormel)	1 oz.	45	0.
(Swift)	1 oz.	47	0.
BEEF GOULASH (Hormel) *Short Orders*	7½-oz. can	230	17.0
BEEF, GROUND, SEASONING MIX:			
*(Durkee):			
Regular	1 cup	653	9.0
With onion	1 cup	659	6.5
(French's) with onion	1⅛-oz. pkg.	100	24.0

Food and Description	Measure or Quantity	Calories	Carbo-hydrates (grams)
BEEF HASH, ROAST:			
Canned, *Mary Kitchen* (Hormel):			
Regular	7½-oz. serving	350	18.0
Short Orders	7½-oz. can	360	18.0
Frozen (Stouffer's)	½ of 11½-oz. pkg.	265	11.0
BEEF PEPPER ORIENTAL, frozen (La Choy):			
Dinner	12-oz. dinner	250	45.0
Entree	12-oz. entree	160	18.0
BEEF PIE, frozen:			
(Banquet):			
Regular	8-oz. pie	557	47.0
Supreme	8-oz. pie	380	38.0
(Morton)	8-oz. pie	320	31.0
(Stouffer's)	10-oz. pie	550	38.0
(Swanson):			
Regular	8-oz. pie	400	40.0
Hungry Man:			
Regular	16-oz. pie	720	65.0
Steak burger	16-oz. pie	760	61.0
BEEF, POTTED (USDA)	1 oz.	70	0.
BEEF PUFFS, frozen (Durkee)	1 piece (.5 oz.)	47	3.0
BEEF ROLL (Hormel) Lumberjack	1 oz.	101	0.
BEEF, SHORT RIBS, frozen (Stouffer's) boneless, with vegetable gravy	½ of 11½-oz. pkg.	350	2.0
BEEF SOUP (See SOUP, Beef)			

(USDA): United States Department of Agriculture
(HEW/FAO):   Health, Education and Welfare/Food and Agriculture
                      Organization
* Prepared as Package Directs

Food and Description	Measure or Quantity	Calories	Carbohydrates (grams)
BEEF SPREAD, ROAST,			
canned:			
(Hormel)	1 oz.	62	0.
(Underwood)	½ of 4¾-oz. can	140	Tr.
BEEF STEAK, BREADED			
(Hormel) frozen	4-oz. serving	370	13.0
BEEF STEW:			
Home recipe, made with lean beef chuck	1 cup (8.6 oz.)	218	15.2
Canned, regular pack:			
Dinty Moore (Hormel):			
Regular	⅓ of 24-oz. can	220	15.0
Short Orders	7½-oz. can	180	14.0
(Libby's)	7½-oz. serving	160	18.0
(Swanson's)	7⅝-oz. serving	150	16.0
Canned, dietetic:			
(Dia-Mel)	8-oz. serving	200	19.0
(Featherweight)	7½-oz. serving	220	24.0
Frozen:			
(Banquet) *Buffet Supper*	2-lb. pkg.	1016	84.0
(Green Giant) Boil 'N Bag	9-oz. entree	180	20.0
(Morton) Family Meal	2-lb. pkg.	760	56.0
(Stouffer's)	10-oz. serving	310	16.0
BEEF STEW SEASONING MIX:			
*(Durkee)	1 cup	379	16.7
(French's)	1⅛-oz. pkg.	150	30.0
BEEF STOCK BASE (French's)	1 tsp (.13 oz.)	8	2.0
BEEF STROGANOFF, frozen:			
(Green Giant) with noodles	9-oz. entree	380	35.0
(Stouffer's) with parsley noodles	9¾-oz. pkg.	390	31.0
***BEEF STROGANOFF SEASONING MIX** (Durkee)	1 cup	820	71.2
BEER & ALE:			
Regular:			
Black Horse Ale	12 fl. oz.	162	13.8

Food and Description	Measure or Quantity	Calories	Carbo-hydrates (grams)
Budweiser: Busch Bavarian	12 fl. oz.	148	12.4
Michelob	12 fl. oz.	162	14.3
Pearl Premium	12 fl. oz.	148	12.5
Stroh Bohemian	12 fl. oz.	148	13.6
Light or low carbohydrate:			
Budweiser Light:			
Natural Light	12 fl. oz.	108	6.7
Michelob Light	12 fl. oz.	134	11.5
Stroh Light	12 fl. oz.	115	7.1
BEER, NEAR:			
Goetz Pale	12 fl. oz.	78	3.9
Kingsbury (Heileman)	12 fl. oz.	59	11.4
(Metbrew)	12 fl. oz.	73	13.7
BEET:			
Raw (USDA):			
Whole	1 lb. (weighed with skins, without tops)	137	31.4
Diced	½ cup (2.4 oz.)	29	6.6
Boiled (USDA) drained:			
Whole	2 beets (2″ dia., 3.5 oz.)	32	7.2
Diced	½ cup (3 oz.)	27	6.1
Sliced	½ cup (3.6 oz.)	33	7.3
Canned, regular pack, solids & liq.:			
(Del Monte)			
Pickled	4 oz.	80	19.0
Sliced, tiny or whole	4 oz.	35	8.0
(Greenwood)			
Harvard	½ cup	70	16.0
Pickled	½ cup	110	27.5
Pickled, with onion	½ cup	115	27.5
(Stokely-Van Camp) pickled	½ cup	95	22.5
Canned, dietetic, solids & liq.:			
(Blue Boy) whole	½ cup (4 oz.)	39	9.2

(USDA): United States Department of Agriculture
(HEW/FAO):   Health, Education and Welfare/Food and Agriculture Organization
* Prepared as Package Directs

Food and Description	Measure or Quantity	Calories	Carbohydrates (grams)
(Comstock)	½ cup	30	6.5
(Del Monte) No Salt Added	½ cup (4 oz.)	35	8.0
(Featherweight) sliced	½ cup	45	10.0
(S&W) *Nutradiet*, sliced, green label	½ cup	35	9.0
BEET GREENS (USDA):			
Raw, whole	1 lb. (weighed untrimmed)	61	11.7
Boiled, halves & stems, drained	½ cup (2.6 oz.)	13	2.4
BENEDICTINE LIQUEUR			
(Julius Wile) 86 proof	1 fl. oz.	112	10.3
BIG H, burger sauce			
(Hellmann's)	1 T. (.5 oz.)	71	1.6
BIG MAC (See **McDONALD'S**)			
BIG WHEEL (Hostess)	1 piece (1⅓ oz.)	172	21.5
BISCUIT DOUGH (Pillsbury):			
Baking Powder, *1869 Brand*	1 biscuit	100	13.5
Big Country	1 biscuit	95	15.5
Big Country, Good 'N Buttery	1 biscuit	100	14.0
Buttermilk:			
Regular	1 biscuit	50	10.0
Ballard, Oven Ready	1 biscuit	50	10.0
Extra Lights	1 biscuit	60	10.5
Extra rich, *Hungry Jack*	1 biscuit	65	9.0
Fluffy, *Hungry Jack*	1 biscuit	100	12.0
Butter Tastin', *1869 Brand*	1 biscuit	100	13.5
Dinner	1 biscuit	55	7.5
Flaky, *Hungry Jack*	1 biscuit	90	11.5
Oven Ready, Ballard	1 biscuit	50	10.0
BITTERS (Angostura)	1 tsp.	14	2.1
BLACKBERRY:			
Fresh (USDA) includes boysenberry, dewberry, youngsberry:			
Will hulls	1 lb. (weighed untrimmed)	250	55.6

Food and Description	Measure or Quantity	Calories	Carbohydrates (grams)
Hulled	½ cup (2.6 oz.)	41	9.4
Canned, regular pack (USDA) solids & liq.:			
Juice pack	4-oz. serving	61	13.7
Light syrup	4-oz. serving	82	19.6
Heavy syrup	½ cup (4.6 oz.)	118	28.9
Extra heavy syrup	4-oz. serving	125	30.7
Frozen (USDA):			
Sweetened, unthawed	4-oz. serving	109	27.7
Unsweetened, unthawed	4-oz. serving	55	12.9
BLACKBERRY JELLY:			
Sweetened (Smucker's)	1 T. (.7 oz.)	53	13.5
Dietetic:			
(Diet Delight)	1 T. (.6 oz.)	12	3.0
(Featherweight) imitation	1 T.	16	4.0
BLACKBERRY LIQUEUR			
(Bols)	1 fl. oz.	95	8.9
BLACKBERRY PRESERVE OR JAM:			
Sweetened (Smucker's)	1 T. (.7 oz.)	53	13.5
Dietetic:			
(Dia-Mel; Louis Sherry)	1 T. (.6 oz.)	6	0.
(Featherweight)	1 T.	16	4.0
(S&W) *Nutradiet*, red label	1 T.	12	3.0
BLACKBERRY WINE (Mogen David)	3 fl. oz.	135	18.7
BLACK-EYED PEAS:			
Canned, with pork, solids & liq. (Sunshine)	½ cup	90	16.1
Frozen:			
(Birds Eye)	⅓ of pkg. (3.3 oz.)	133	23.5

(USDA): United States Department of Agriculture
(HEW/FAO):   Health, Education and Welfare/Food and Agriculture Organization
* Prepared as Package Directs

Food and Description	Measure or Quantity	Calories	Carbo-hydrates (grams)
(McKenzie; Seabrook Farms)	⅓ of pkg. (3.3 oz.)	130	23.0
(Southland)	⅕ of 16-oz. pkg.	120	21.0
BLINTZE, frozen (King Kold)			
cheese	2½-oz. piece	132	21.4
BLOODY MARY MIX:			
Dry (Bar-Tender's)	1 serving	26	5.7
Liquid (Sacramento)	5½-fl.-oz. can	39	9.1
BLUEBERRY:			
Fresh (USDA):			
Whole	1 lb. (weighed untrimmed)	259	63.8
Trimmed	½ cup (2.6 oz.)	45	11.2
Canned (USDA) solids & liq.:			
Syrup pack, extra heavy	½ cup (4.4 oz.)	126	32.5
Water pack	½ cup (4/3 oz.)	47	11.9
Frozen (USDA):			
Sweetened, solids & liq.	½ cup (4 oz.)	120	30.2
Unsweetened, solids & liq.	½ cup (2.9 oz.)	45	11.2
BLUEBERRY PIE (See **PIE,** Blueberry)			
BLUEBERRY PRESERVE OR JAM:			
Sweetened (Smucker's)	1 T.	53	13.5
Dietetic (Dia-Mel; Louis Sherry)	1 T.	6	0.
BLUEFISH (USDA):			
Raw:			
Whole	1 lb. (weighed whole)	271	0.
Meat only	4 oz.	133	0.
Baked or broiled	4.4-oz. piece (3½" × 3" × ½")	199	0.
Fried	5.3-oz. piece (3½" × 3" × ½")	308	7.0

Food and Description	Measure or Quantity	Calories	Carbo-hydrates (grams)
BODY BUDDIES, cereal (General Mills):			
Brown sugar & honey	1 cup (1 oz.)	110	24.0
Natural fruit flavor	¾ cup (1 oz.)	110	24.0
BOLOGNA:			
(Eckrich):			
Beef:			
Regular	1 oz.	90	2.0
Smorgas Pak	¾-oz. slice	70	1.0
Thick slice	1½-oz. slice	140	2.0
Thin slice	1 slice	55	1.0
Garlic	1-oz. slice	90	2.0
German brand, sliced or chub	1-oz. slice	80	1.0
Lunch chub	1-oz. serving	100	2.0
Meat:			
Regular	1-oz. slice	90	2.0
Thick slice	1.7-oz. slice	160	3.0
Thin slice	1 slice	55	1.0
Ring or sandwich	1-oz. slice	90	2.0
(Hormel):			
Beef:			
Regular	1 slice	85	.5
Coarse grind	1 oz.	80	.5
Meat	1 slice	90	0.
(Oscar Mayer):			
Beef	.8-oz. slice	73	.6
Beef	1-oz. slice	90	.8
Beef	1.3-oz. slice	120	1.1
Meat	1-oz. slice	91	.5
Meat	2-oz. slice	183	1.0
(Swift)	1-oz. slice	95	1.5
BOLOGNA & CHEESE:			
(Eckrich)	.7-oz. slice	90	2.0
(Oscar Mayer)	.8-oz. slice	73	.6

(USDA): United States Department of Agriculture
(HEW/FAO):   Health, Education and Welfare/Food and Agriculture
                        Organization
* Prepared as Package Directs

Food and Description	Measure or Quantity	Calories	Carbo-hydrates (grams)
BONITO:			
Raw (USDA) meat only	4 oz.	191	0.
Canned (Star-Kist):			
Chunk	6½-oz. can	605	0.
Solid	7-oz. can	650	0.
BOO*BERRY, cereal			
(General Mills)	1 cup (1 oz.)	110	24.0
BORSCHT, canned:			
Regular:			
(Gold's)	8-oz. serving	72	17.5
(Mother's) old fashioned	8-oz. serving	90	21.3
Dietetic or low calorie:			
(Gold's)	8-oz. serving	24	17.5
(Mother's):			
Artificially sweetened	8-oz. serving	29	6.1
Unsalted	8-oz. serving	107	25.1
(Rokeach)	8-oz. serving	27	6.7
BOSCO (See **SYRUP**)			
BOYSENBERRY:			
Fresh (See **BLACKBERRY**)			
Frozen (USDA) sweetened	10-oz. pkg.	273	69.3
BOYSENBERRY JELLY:			
Sweetened (Smucker's)	1 T. (.7 oz.)	53	13.5
Dietetic (S&W) *Nutradiet*, red			
label	1 T.	12	3.0
BRAINS, all animals			
(USDA) raw	4 oz.	142	.9
BRAN:			
Crude (USDA)	1 oz.	60	17.5
Miller's (Elam's)	1 T. (.2 oz.)	17	2.8
BRAN BREAKFAST CEREAL:			
(Kellogg's):			
All Bran or *Bran Buds*	⅓ cup (1 oz.)	70	22.0
Cracklin' Oat Bran	½ cup (1 oz.)	120	20.0
40% bran flakes	¾ cup (1 oz.)	90	23.0

Food and Description	Measure or Quantity	Calories	Carbo-hydrates (grams)
Fruitful Bran	¾ cup (1 oz.)	110	27.0
Raisin	¾ cup	110	30.0
(Nabisco)	½ cup (1 oz.)	70	21.0
(Post):			
40% bran flakes	⅔ cup (1 oz.)	107	22.5
With raisins	½ cup (1 oz.)	101	21.5
With raisins, *Honey Nut*			
Crunch	½ cup (1 oz.)	102	22.7
(Quaker) *Corn Bran*	⅔ cup (1 oz.)	109	23.3
(Ralston-Purina):			
Bran Chex	⅔ cup (1 oz.)	90	23.0
40% bran	¾ cup (1 oz.)	100	23.0
Honey bran	⅞ cup (1 oz.)	100	24.0
Raisin	¾ cup (1.3 oz.)	120	30.0

BRANDY, FLAVORED (Mr.
Boston) 35% alcohol:
Apricot	1 fl. oz.	94	8.9
Blackberry	1 fl. oz.	92	8.6
Cherry	1 fl. oz.	87	7.4
Coffee	1 fl. oz.	72	10.6
Ginger	1 fl. oz.	72	3.5
Peach	1 fl. oz.	94	8.9

BRAUNSCHWEIGER:
(Eckrich) chub	1 oz.	70	1.0
(Hormel)	1 oz.	80	0.
(Oscar Mayer) chub	1 oz.	98	1.0
(Swift) 8-oz. chub	1 oz.	109	1.4

BRAZIL NUT:
Raw (USDA):
Whole, in shell	1 cup (4.3 oz.)	383	6.4
Shelled	½ cup (2.5 oz.)	458	7.6
Shelled	4 nuts (.6 oz.)	114	1.9
Roasted (Fisher) salted	1 oz. (¼ cup).	193	3.1

(USDA): United States Department of Agriculture
(HEW/FAO): Health, Education and Welfare/Food and Agriculture
Organization
* Prepared as Package Directs

Food and Description	Measure or Quantity	Calories	Carbo-hydrates (grams)
BREAD:			
Apple (Pepperidge Farm) with cinnamon	.9-oz. slice	70	13.0
Boston Brown (USDA)	3″ × ¾″ slice (1.7 oz.)	101	21.9
Bran:			
(Arnold) *Bran'nola*	1.2-oz. slice	90	15.5
(Pepperidge Farm) with raisins	.9-oz. slice	65	12.5
Cinnamon (Pepperidge Farm)	.9-oz. slice	80	12.5
Cinnamon apple & walnut (Pepperidge Farm)	.9-oz. slice	70	14.0
Corn & molasses (Pepperidge Farm)	.9-oz. slice	75	15.0
Cracked wheat:			
(Pepperidge Farm) thin sliced	.9-oz. slice	75	13.0
(Wonder)	1-oz. slice	75	13.6
Crispbread, *Wasa:*			
Mora	3.2-oz. slice	333	70.5
Rye:			
Golden	.3-oz. slice	37	7.8
Lite	.3-oz. slice	30	6.2
Sesame	.5-oz. slice	50	10.6
Sport	.4-oz. slice	42	9.1
Date nut roll (Dromedary)	1-oz. slice	80	13.0
Date walnut (Pepperidge Farm)	.9-oz. slice	75	11.5
Flatbread, *Ideal:*			
Bran	.2-oz. slice	19	4.1
Extra thin	.1-oz. slice	12	2.5
Whole grain	.2-oz. slice	19	4.0
French:			
(Arnold) *Francisco*	¹⁄₁₆ of loaf (1 oz.)	80	14.5
(Pepperidge Farm):			
Brown & serve	2-oz. slice	180	34.0
Fully baked	2-oz. slice	150	28.0
Twin	2-oz. slice	140	25.0
(Wonder)	1-oz. slice	71	13.6
Hillbilly	1-oz. slice	72	13.6
Hollywood:			
Dark	1-oz. slice	72	12.5
Light	1-oz. slice	71	13.1
Honey bran (Pepperidge Farm)	1 slice (1.2 oz.)	95	13.0

Food and Description	Measure or Quantity	Calories	Carbo-hydrates (grams)
Honey wheat berry:			
(Arnold)	1.2-oz. slice	90	16.0
(Pepperidge Farm)	.9-oz. slice	70	13.5
Italian:			
(USDA)	1-oz. slice	78	18.5
(Pepperidge Farm) brown & serve	2-oz. slice	150	27.0
Low sodium (Wonder)	1-oz. slice	71	13.6
Multi-grain (Pepperidge Farm)	.5-oz. slice	35	7.0
Oat (Arnold) *Bran'nola*	1.3-oz. slice	110	19.0
Oatmeal (Pepperidge Farm)	.9-oz. slice	70	12.5
Onion (Pepperidge Farm) party	.2-oz. slice	15	2.8
Orange & Raisin			
(Pepperidge Farm)	.9-oz. slice	70	12.5
Protein (Thomas')	.7-oz. slice	46	7.4
Pumpernickel:			
(Arnold)	1-oz. slice	75	14.0
(Levy's)	1.1-oz. slice	85	15.5
(Pepperidge Farm):			
Regular	1.1-oz. slice	85	15.5
Party	.2-oz. slice	17	3.0
Raisin:			
(Arnold) tea	.9-oz. slice	70	13.0
(Pepperidge Farm)	1 slice	75	14.0
(Sun-Maid)	1-oz. slice	80	14.5
(Thomas') cinnamon	.8-oz. slice	60	11.7
Roman Meal	1-oz. slice	77	13.6
Rye:			
(Arnold):			
Jewish	1.1-oz. slice	75	14.0
Melba Thin	.7-oz. slice	50	9.5
(Levy's) real	1-oz. slice	80	14.5
(Pepperidge Farm)			
Family	1.1-oz. slice	85	15.5
Family	1.2-oz. slice	85	16.5
Jewish	1.1-oz. slice	90	16.5
Party	.2-oz. slice	17	3.2
Sandwich	1.2-oz. slice	95	16.5
Very thin slice	.6-oz. slice	45	8.5

(USDA): United States Department of Agriculture
(HEW/FAO):   Health, Education and Welfare/Food and Agriculture
                        Organization
* Prepared as Package Directs

Food and Description	Measure or Quantity	Calories	Carbo-hydrates (grams)
(Wonder)	1-oz. slice	69	12.8
Sahara (Thomas'):			
Wheat	1-oz. piece	85	13.7
White	1-oz. piece	85	16.0
Salt Rising (USDA)	.9-oz. slice	67	13.0
Z-Grain, *Home Pride*	1-oz. slice	72	12.8
Sourdough, *Di Carlo*	1-oz. slice	70	13.6
Sprouted wheat:			
(Arnold)	.9-oz. slice	65	12.0
(Pepperidge Farm)	.9-oz. slice	70	11.5
Vienna (Pepperidge Farm)	.9-oz. slice	75	13.5
Wheat (see also Cracked Wheat or Whole Wheat):			
(Arnold) *Bran'nola,* hearty	1.3-oz. slice	105	17.5
Fresh Horizons	1-oz. slice	54	9.6
Fresh & Natural	1-oz. slice	77	13.6
Home Pride	1-oz. slice	73	13.1
(Pepperidge Farm):			
Family	.9-oz. slice	70	13.0
Sandwich	.8-oz. slice	55	10.0
(Wonder) family	1-oz. slice	75	13.6
Wheatberry, *Home Pride:*			
Honey	1-oz. slice	74	13.3
Regular	1-oz. slice	70	12.5
Wheat Germ (Pepperidge Farm)	.9-oz. slice	70	12.5
White:			
(Arnold):			
Brick Oven	.8-oz. slice	65	11.0
Brick Oven	1.1-oz. slice	85	24.5
Country	1.2-oz. slice	95	17.0
Heartstone	1.1-oz. slice	85	15.0
Measure Up	.5-oz. slice	40	7.0
Fresh Horizons	1-oz. slice	54	10.0
Home Pride	1-oz. slice	72	13.1
(Pepperidge Farm):			
Regular	1.2-oz. slice	85	15.5
Large loaf, thin slice	.9-oz. slice	75	13.5
Sandwich	.8-oz. slice	65	11.5
Sliced, thin	.9-oz. slice	75	13.0
Toasting	1.2-oz. slice	85	16.0
Very thin slice	.6-oz. slice	45	8.5

Food and Description	Measure or Quantity	Calories	Carbo-hydrates (grams)
(Wonder):			
Regular	1-oz. slice	70	13.4
Buttermilk	1-oz. slice	73	13.4
White & cracked wheat			
(Pepperidge Farm)	1.2-oz. slice	95	17.5
Whole wheat:			
(Arnold):			
Brick Oven	.8-oz. slice	60	9.5
Measure Up	.5-oz. slice	40	6.5
Stone ground	.8-oz. slice	55	9.5
Home Pride	1-oz. slice	70	12.2
(Pepperidge Farm):			
Thin slice	.9-oz. slice	70	12.0
Very thin slice	.6-oz. slice	45	7.5
(Thomas') 100%	.8-oz. slice	56	10.1
(Wonder) 100%	1-oz. slice	69	11.9
BREAD, CANNED, brown,			
plain or raisin (B&M)	½" slice (1.6 oz.)	80	18.2
BREAD CRUMBS:			
(Contadina) seasoned	½ cup (2.1 oz.)	211	40.6
(4C):			
Plain	4 oz.	405	85.2
Seasoned	4 oz.	384	77.3
(Pepperidge Farm) regular			
or seasoned	1 oz.	110	22.0
***BREAD DOUGH:**			
Frozen:			
(Pepperidge Farm):			
Country rye or white	⅒ of loaf (1 oz.)	80	13.5
Stone ground wheat	⅒ of loaf (1 oz.)	75	13.0
(Rich's):			
French	1/20 of loaf	59	11.0
Italian	1/20 of loaf	60	11.0
Raisin	1/20 of loaf	66	12.3
Wheat	.5-oz. slice	60	10.5
White	.8-oz. slice	56	9.4

(USDA): United States Department of Agriculture
(HEW/FAO):   Health, Education and Welfare/Food and Agriculture
                    Organization
* Prepared as Package Directs

Food and Description	Measure or Quantity	Calories	Carbo-hydrates (grams)
Refrigerated (Pillsbury) *Poppin' Fresh*:			
Rye or wheat	¹⁄₁₆ of loaf	110	21.0
White	¹⁄₁₆ of loaf	110	20.0
*BREAD MIX (Pillsbury):			
Applesauce spice or banana	¹⁄₁₂ of loaf	150	27.0
Apricot nut	¹⁄₁₂ of loaf	150	27.0
Blueberry nut	¹⁄₁₂ of loaf	150	26.0
Carrot nut	¹⁄₁₂ of loaf	150	27.0
Cherry nut	¹⁄₁₂ of loaf	170	30.0
Cranberry	¹⁄₁₂ of loaf	160	30.0
Date	¹⁄₁₂ of loaf	160	31.0
Nut	¹⁄₁₂ of loaf	160	31.0
BREAD PUDDING, with raisins, home recipe (USDA)	1 cup (9.3 oz.)	496	75.3
*BREAD STICK DOUGH (Pillsbury) *Pipin' Hot,* soft	1 piece	100	18.0
*BREAKFAST DRINK (Pillsbury)	1 pouch	290	38.0
BREAKFAST SQUARES (General Mills) all flavors	1 bar (1.5 oz.)	190	22.5
BROCCOLI:			
Raw (USDA):			
Whole	1 lb. (weighed untrimmed)	69	16.3
Large leaves removed	1 lb.	113	20.9
Boiled (USDA):			
½" pieces, drained	½ cup (2.8 oz.)	20	3.5
Whole, drained	1 med. stalk (6.3 oz.)	47	8.1
Frozen:			
(Birds Eye):			
With almonds & selected seasonings	¹⁄₃ of pkg. (3.3 oz.)	62	5.7

Food and Description	Measure or Quantity	Calories	Carbo-hydrates (grams)
In cheese sauce	⅓ of pkg. (3.3 oz.)	87	8.4
Chopped, cuts or florets	⅓ of pkg. (3.3 oz.)	31	4.5
Spears:			
Regular	⅓ of pkg. (3.3 oz.)	33	4.9
In butter sauce	⅓ of pkg. (3.3 oz.)	58	5.3
Deluxe	⅓ of pkg. (3.3 oz.)	37	4.9
& water chestnuts with selected seasonings	⅓ of pkg. (3.3 oz.)	35	5.8
(Green Giant):			
In cheese sauce	½ cup	70	8.0
Cuts, *Harvest Fresh*	½ cup	30	4.0
Cuts, polybag	½ cup	18	
Spears:			
In butter sauce	3⅓ oz.	40	5.0
Harvest Fresh	½ cup	30	4.0
Mini, Harvest Fresh	⅛ of pkg.	16	3.0
In white cheddar cheese sauce	½ cup	70	8.0
(McKenzie) chopped, cuts or spears	3.3 oz.	25	5.0
(Seabrook Farms) chopped or spears	⅓ of pkg.	30	4.1
(Stouffer's) in cheese sauce	½ of 9-oz. pkg.	130	8.0
BRUSSELS SPROUT:			
Raw (USDA) trimmed	1 lb.	204	37.6
Boiled (USDA) drained	3-4 sprouts	28	4.9
Frozen:			
(USDA) boiled, drained	4 oz.	37	7.4
(Birds Eye):			
Regular	⅓ of 10-oz. pkg.	46	7.4
In butter sauce	⅓ of 10-oz. pkg.	59	7.2

(USDA): United States Department of Agriculture
(HEW/FAO):   Health, Education and Welfare/Food and Agriculture
                      Organization
* Prepared as Package Directs

Food and Description	Measure or Quantity	Calories	Carbo-hydrates (grams)
Baby, with cheese sauce	⅓ of 10-oz. pkg.	84	8.7
Baby, deluxe	⅓ of 10-oz. pkg.	49	7.3
(Geen Giant):			
In butter sauce	½ cup	60	9.0
Halves in cheese sauce	½ cup	80	13.0
Polybag	½ cup	30	5.0
(McKenzie)	3.3-oz. serving	35	7.0

BUCKWHEAT:
Flour (See **FLOUR**)
Groats (Pocono):

Brown, whole	1 oz.	104	19.4
White, whole	1 oz.	102	20.1

BUC*WHEATS cereal

(General Mills)	1 oz. (¾ cup)	110	24.0

BULGUR (form hard red winter wheat) (USDA):

Dry	1 lb.	1605	343.4
Canned:			
Unseasoned	4-oz. serving	191	39.7
Seasoned	4-oz. serving	206	37.2

***BULLWINKLE PUDDING STIX**, Good Humor*

	2½-fl. oz. bar	120	20.0

BURGER KING:

Apple pie	3-oz. pie	240	32.0
Cheeseburger	1 burger	350	30.0
Cheeseburger, double meat	1 burger	530	32.0
Coca Cola	1 medium-sized drink	121	31.0
French fries	1 regular order	210	25.0
Hamburger	1 burger	290	29.0
Onion rings	1 regular order	270	29.0
Pepsi, diet	1 medium-sized drink	7	1.6
Shake:			
Chocolate	1 shake	340	57.0
Vanilla	1 shake	340	53.0
Whopper:			
Regular	1 burger	630	50.0

Food and Description	Measure or Quantity	Calories	Carbo-hydrates (grams)
Regular, with cheese	1 burger	740	52.0
Double beef	1 burger	850	52.0
Double beef, with cheese	1 burger	950	54.0
Junior	1 burger	370	31.0
Junior with cheese	1 burger	420	32.0
BURGUNDY WINE:			
(Louis M. Martini)			
12½% alcohol	3 fl. oz.	60	.2
(Paul Masson) 12% alcohol	3 fl. oz.	70	2.2
(Taylor) 12½% alcohol	3 fl. oz.	75	3.3
BURGUNDY WINE, SPARKLING:			
(B&G) 12% alcohol	3 fl. oz.	69	2.2
(Great Western) 12% alcohol	3 fl. oz.	82	5.1
(Taylor) 12% of alcohol	3 fl. oz.	78	4.2
BURRITO:			
*Canned (Del Monte)	1 burrito	310	39.0
Frozen:			
(Hormel):			
Beef	1 burrito	205	31.0
Cheese	1 buritto	210	32.0
Chicken & rice	1 burrito	200	32.0
Hot chili	1 burrito	240	33.0
(Van de Kamp's):			
Regular, crispy fried & guacamole sauce	6-oz. serving	350	40.0
Beef & bean	6-oz. serving	280	44.0
BURRITO FILLING MIX, canned (Del Monte)	½ cup (403 oz.)	110	20.0
BUTTER, salted or unsalted:			
Regular:			
(USDA)	¼ lb.	812	.5
(USDA)	1 T. (.5 oz.)	102	.1

(USDA): United States Department of Agriculture
(HEW/FAO): Health, Education and Welfare/Food and Agriculture
                      Organization
* Prepared as Package Directs

Food and Description	Measure or Quantity	Calories	Carbo-hydrates (grams)
(USDA)	1 pat (5 grams)	36	Tr.
(Breakstone)	1 T.	100	Tr.
(Meadow Gold)	1 tsp.	35	0.
Whipped (Breakstone)	1 T.	67	Tr.
BUTTERFISH, raw (USDA):			
Gulf:			
Whole	1 lb. (weighed whole)	220	0.
Meat only	4 oz.	108	0.
Northern:			
Whole	1 lb. (weighed whole)	391	0.
Meat only	4 oz.	192	0.
BUTTERSCOTCH MORSELS			
(Nestlé)	1 oz.	150	

Food and Description	Measure or Quantity	Calories	Carbo-hydrates (grams)

C

CABBAGE:
  White (USDA):
    Raw:

Whole	1 lb. (weighed untrimmed)	86	19.3
Finely shredded or chopped	1 cup (3.2 oz.)	22	4.9
Coarsely shredded or sliced	1 cup (2.5 oz.)	17	3.8
Wedge	3½" × 4½"	24	5.4

    Boiled:

Shredded, in small amount of water, short time drained	½ cup (2.6 oz.)	15	3.1
Wedges, in large amount of water, long time, drained	½ cup (3.2 oz.)	17	3.7
Dehydrated	1 oz.	87	20.9

  Red:

Raw (USDA) whole	1 lb. (weighed untrimmed)	111	24.7
Canned, solids & liq:			
(Comstock) sweet & sour	½ cup	60	13.0
(Greenwood)	½ cup	60	13.0
Savory (USDA) raw, whole	1 lb. (weighed untrimmed)	86	16.5

CABBAGE, STUFFED, frozen

(Green Giant)	½ of pkg.	220	19.0

CABERNET SAUVIGNON:

(Louis M. Martini) 12½% alcohol	3 fl. oz.	63	.2
(Paul Masson) 11.9% alcohol	3 fl. oz.	70	.2

(USDA): United States Department of Agriculture
(HEW/FAO):   Health, Education and Welfare/Food and Agriculture
                Organization
* Prepared as Package Directs

Food and Description	Measure or Quantity	Calories	Carbo-hydrates (grams)
CAFE COMFORT, 55 proof	1 fl. oz.	79	8.8
CAKE:			
Non Frozen:			
Plain:			
Home recipe, with butter & boiled white icing	⅑ of 9″ square	401	70.5
Home recipe, with butter & chocolate icing	⅑ of 9″ square	453	73.1
Angel food, home recipe	1/12 of 8″ cake	108	24.1
Caramel, home recipe:			
Without icing	⅑ of 9″ square	331	46.2
With caramel icing	⅑ of 9″ square	322	50.2
Chocolate, home recipe, with chocolate icing, 2-layer	1/12 of 9″ cake	365	55.2
Crumb (see also **ROLL** or **BUN**) (Hostess)	1¼-oz. piece	131	21.7
Devil's food, home recipe:			
Without icing	3″ × 2″ × 1½″ piece	201	28.6
Without chocolate icing, 2-layer	1/16 of 9″ cake	277	41.8
Fruit, home recipe:			
Dark	1/30 of 8″ loaf	57	9.0
Light, made with butter	1/30 of 8″ loaf	58	8.6
Honey (Holland Honey Cake) low sodium:			
Fruit and raisin	½″ slice (.9 oz.)	80	19.0
Orange and premium unsalted	½″ slice (.9 oz.)	70	17.0
Pound, home recipe:			
Equal weights flour, sugar butter and eggs	3½″ × 3½″ slice (1.1 oz.)	142	14.1
Traditional, made with butter	3½″ × 3½″ slice (1.1 oz.)	123	16.4
Sponge, home recipe	1/12 of 10″ cake	196	35.7
White, home recipe:			
Made with butter, without icing, 2-layer	⅑ of 9″ wide, 3″ high cake	353	50.8
Made with butter, with coconut icing, 2-layer	1/12 of 9″ wide, 3″ high cake	386	63.1

Food and Description	Measure or Quantity	Calories	Carbo-hydrates (grams)
Yellow, home recipe, made with butter, without icing, 2-layer	⅑ of cake	351	56.3
Frozen:			
Apple walnut:			
(Pepperidge Farm) with cream cheese icing	⅛ of 11¾-oz. cake	150	18.0
(Sara Lee)	⅛ of 12½-oz. cake	165	21.6
Banana (Sara Lee)	⅛ of 13¾-oz. cake	175	26.9
Banana nut (Sara Lee)	⅛ of 20-oz. cake	232	26.5
Black Forest (Sara Lee)	⅛ of 21-oz. cake	203	27.9
Boston Cream			
(Pepperidge Farm)	¼ of 11¾-oz. cake	290	39.0
Carrot:			
(Pepperidge Farm) with cream cheese icing	⅛ of 11¾-oz. cake	140	17.0
(Sara Lee)	⅛ of 12¼-oz. cake	152	18.9
(Weight Watchers)	2⅝-oz. serving	153	26.1
Cheesecake:			
(Morton) Great Little Desserts:			
Cherry	6-oz. cake	460	47.0
Cream cheese	6-oz. cake	480	42.0
Pineapple	6-oz. cake	460	48.0
Strawberry	6-oz. cake	460	50.0
(Rich's) Viennese	1/14 of 42-oz. cake	230	24.1
(Sara Lee):			
Blueberry, For 2	½ of 11.3-oz. cake	425	66.6
Cream cheese:			
Regular	⅓ of 10-oz. cake	281	29.9
Large	⅙ of 17-oz. cake	231	25.9

(USDA): United States Department of Agriculture
(HEW/FAO): Health, Education and Welfare/Food and Agriculture Organization
* Prepared as Package Directs

Food and Description	Measure or Quantity	Calories	Carbo-hydrates (grams)
Cherry	⅙ of 19-oz. cake	225	35.2
Cherry, *For 2*	½ of 11.3-oz. cake	423	69.3
French	⅛ of 23.5-oz. cake	274	24.9
Strawberry	⅙ of 19-oz. cake	223	33.6
Strawberry, *For 2*	½ of 11.3-oz. cake	420	67.9
(Weight Watchers):			
Regular	4-oz. serving	172	27.1
Black cherry	4-oz. serving	148	23.1
Strawberry	4-oz. serving	153	22.2
Chocolate:			
(Pepperidge Farm):			
Layer:			
Fudge	⅒ of 17-oz. cake	190	23.0
German	⅒ of 17-oz. cake	180	23.0
Rich 'N Moist:			
With chocolate frosting	⅛ of 14¼-oz. cake	190	23.0
With vanilla frosting	⅛ of 14¼-oz. cake	180	23.0
Supreme	¼ of 11½-oz. cake	310	37.0
(Sara Lee):			
Regular	⅛ of 13¼-oz. cake	199	28.1
Bavarian	⅛ of 22½-oz. cake	285	22.6
German	⅛ of 12¼-oz. cake	173	19.3
Layer:			
N'cream	⅛ of 18-oz. cake	215	23.8
Double	⅛ of 18-oz. cake	217	24.1
Coconut (Pepperidge Farm) layer	⅒ of 17-oz. cake	180	25.0
Coffee (Sara Lee):			
Almond	⅛ of 11¾-oz. cake	165	20.2
Almond ring	⅛ of 9½-oz. cake	135	16.8
Apple	⅛ of 15-oz. cake	175	24.1
Apple, *For 2*	½ of 9-oz. cake	419	58.1
Blueberry ring	⅛ of 9¾-oz. cake	134	17.6

Food and Description	Measure or Quantity	Calories	Carbo-hydrates (grams)
Butter, *For 2*	½ of 6½-oz. cake	356	41.9
Maple crunch ring	⅛ of 9¾-oz. cake	138	17.3
Pecan	⅛ of 11¼-oz. cake	163	19.1
Raspberry ring	⅛ of 9¾-oz. cake	133	18.5
Streusel, butter	⅛ of 11½-oz. cake	164	20.3
Streusel, cinnamon	⅛ of 10.9-oz. cake	154	19.0
Crumb (See **ROLL** or **BUN,** Crumb)			
Devil's food (Pepperidge Farm) layer	⅒ of 17-oz. cake	180	24.0
Golden (Pepperidge Farm) layer	⅒ of 17-oz. cake	180	24.0
Lemon coconut (Pepperidge Farm)	¼ of 12¼-oz. cake	280	38.0
Orange (Sara Lee)	⅛ of 13¾-oz. cake	179	25.3
Pineapple cream (Pepperidge Farm)	1/12 of 24-oz. cake	180	27.0
Pound:			
(Pepperidge Farm) butter	⅒ of 10¾-oz. cake	130	16.0
(Sara Lee):			
Regular	⅒ of 10¾-oz. cake	125	14.2
Banana nut	⅒ of 11-oz. cake	117	15.1
Chocolate	⅒ of 10¾-oz. cake	122	14.4
Chocolate swirl	⅒ of 11.8-oz. cake	116	16.0

(USDA): United States Department of Agriculture
(HEW/FAO):   Health, Education and Welfare/Food and Agriculture
Organization
* Prepared as Package Directs

Food and Description	Measure or Quantity	Calories	Carbo-hydrates (grams)
Family size	1/15 of 16½-oz. cake	127	14.8
Homestyle	1/10 of 9½-oz. cake	114	13.1
Raisin	1/10 of 12.9-oz. cake	126	19.6
Spice (Weight Watchers)	2⅝-oz. serving	157	27.2
Strawberry cream (Pepperidge Farm) Supreme	1/12 of 12-oz. cake	190	27.0
Strawberries'n cream, layer (Sara Lee)	1/8 of 20½-oz. cake	218	29.4
Strawberry shortcake (Sara Lee)	1/8 of 21-oz. cake	193	25.9
Torte (Sara Lee):			
Apples'n cream	1/8 of 21-oz. cake	203	26.2
Fudge & nut	1/8 of 15¾-oz. cake	200	21.0
Vanilla (Pepperidge Farm) layer	1/10 of 17-oz. cake	180	25.0
Walnut:			
(Pepperidge Farm)	1/4 of 10-oz. cake	300	33.0
(Sara Lee) layer	1/8 of 18-oz. cake	210	22.8
Yellow (Pepperidge Farm) *Rich 'N Moist*, with chocolate frosting	1/8 of 12½-oz. cake	170	23.0
CAKE OR COOKIE ICING			
(Pillsbury) all flavors	1 T.	70	12.0
CAKE ICING:			
Butter pecan (Betty Crocker) *Creamy Deluxe*	1/12 of can	170	27.0
Caramel, home recipe (USDA)	4 oz.	408	86.8
Caramel pecan (Pillsbury) *Frosting Supreme*	1/12 of can	160	21.0
Cherry (Betty Crocker) *Creamy Deluxe*	1/12 of can	170	28.0
Chocolate:			
(USDA) home recipe	½ cup (4.9 oz.)	519	93.0

Food and Description	Measure or Quantity	Calories	Carbo-hydrates (grams)
(Betty Crocker) *Creamy Deluxe:*			
Regular or milk	1/12 of can	170	25.0
Chip	1/12 of can	170	27.0
Fudge, dark dutch	1/12 of can	160	24.0
Nut	1/12 of can	170	24.0
Sour cream	1/12 of can	160	25.0
(Duncan Hines):			
Regular	1/12 of can	163	25.0
Fudge, dark dutch	1/12 of can	160	24.3
Milk	1/12 of can	162	24.7
(Pillsbury) *Frosting Supreme,* fudge, milk or mint	1/12 of can	150	24.0
Coconut almond (Pillsbury) *Frosting Supreme*	1/12 of can	150	17.0
Coconut pecan (Pillsbury) *Frosting Supreme*	1/12 of can	160	17.0
Cream cheese:			
(Betty Crocker) *Creamy Deluxe*	1/12 of can	170	27.0
(Pillsbury) *Frosting Supreme*	1/12 of can	160	27.0
Double dutch (Pillsbury) *Frosting Supreme*	1/12 of can	150	22.0
Lemon:			
(Betty Crocker) *Sunkist, Creamy Deluxe*	1/12 of can	170	28.0
(Pillsbury) *Frosting Supreme*	1/12 of can	160	26.0
Orange (Betty Crocker) *Creamy Deluxe*	1/12 of can	170	28.0
Strawberry (Pillsbury) *Frosting Supreme*	1/12 of can	160	26.0
Vanilla:			
(Betty Crocker) *Creamy Deluxe*	1/12 of can	170	28.0
(Duncan Hines)	1/12 of can	163	25.5
(Pillsbury) *Frosting Supreme,* regular or sour cream	1/12 of can	160	

(USDA): United States Department of Agriculture
(HEW/FAO):   Health, Education and Welfare/Food and Agriculture
                        Organization
* Prepared as Package Directs

Food and Description	Measure or Quantity	Calories	Carbo-hydrates (grams)
White:			
Home recipe, boiled (USDA)	4 oz.	358	91.1
Home recipe, uncooked (USDA)	4 oz.	426	92.5
(Betty Crocker) *Creamy Deluxe*, sour cream	1/12 of can	160	27.0
*CAKE ICING MIX:			
Regular:			
Banana (Betty Crocker) *Chiquita*, creamy	1/12 of pkg.	170	30.0
Butter Brickle (Betty Crocker) creamy	1/12 of pkg.	170	30.0
Butter pecan (Betty Crocker) creamy	1/12 of pkg.	170	30.0
Caramel (Pillsbury) *Rich'n Easy*	1/12 of pkg.	140	24.0
Cherry (Betty Crocker) creamy	1/12 of pkg.	170	30.0
Chocolate:			
(Betty Crocker) creamy:			
Almond fudge	1/12 of pkg.	180	27.0
Fudge, regular or dark	1/12 of pkg.	170	30.0
Milk or sour cream	1/12 of pkg.	170	30.0
(Pillsbury) *Rich'n Easy* fudge or milk	1/12 of pkg.	150	26.0
Coconut almond:			
(Betty Crocker) creamy	1/12 of pkg.	140	18.0
(Pillsbury)	1/12 of pkg.	160	16.0
Coconut pecan:			
(Betty Crocker) creamy	1/12 of pkg.	140	18.0
(Pillsbury)	1/12 of pkg.	150	20.0
Cream cheese & nut (Betty Crocker) creamy	1/12 of pkg.	150	24.0
Doubledutch (Pillsbury) *Rich 'n Easy*	1/12 of pkg.	150	26.0
Lemon:			
(Betty Crocker) *Sunkist*, creamy	1/12 of pkg.	170	30.0
(Pillsbury) *Rich 'n Easy*	1/12 of pkg.	140	25.0
Strawberry (Pillsbury) *Rich 'n Easy*	1/12 of pkg.	140	25.0

Food and Description	Measure or Quantity	Calories	Carbo-hydrates (grams)
Vanilla (Pillsbury) *Rich 'n Easy*	1/12 of pkg.	150	25.0
White:			
(Betty Crocker):			
Creamy	1/12 of pkg.	180	31.0
Fluffy	1/12 of pkg.	60	16.0
Sour cream, creamy	1/12 of pkg.	170	31.0
(Pillsbury) fluffy	1/12 of pkg.	60	15.0
CAKE MIX:			
Regular:			
Angel Food:			
(Betty Crocker):			
Chocolate, lemon custard or one-step	1/12 of pkg.	140	32.0
Confetti or strawberry	1/12 of pkg.	150	34.0
Traditional	1/12 of pkg.	130	30.0
(Duncan Hines)	1/12 of pkg.	124	28.9
*(Pillsbury) raspberry or white	1/12 of cake	140	32.0
*Apple (Pillsbury) *Streusel Swirl*	1/16 of cake	260	38.0
*Apple cinnamon (Betty Crocker)	1/12 of cake	260	36.0
Applesauce raisin (Betty Crocker) *Snackin' Cake*	1/9 of pkg.	180	33.0
*Applesauce spice (Pillsbury)	1/12 of cake	250	36.0
*Banana:			
(Betty Crocker) *Supermoist*	1/12 of cake	260	36.0
(Pillsbury):			
Pillsbury Plus	1/12 of cake	250	36.0
Streusel Swirl	1/12 of cake	260	38.0
*Banana walnut (Betty Crocker) *Snackin' Cake*	1/9 of cake	190	31.0
*Boston cream (Pillsbury) *Bundt*	1/16 of cake	270	43.0

(USDA): United States Department of Agriculture
(HEW/FAO):   Health, Education and Welfare/Food and Agriculture
                       Organization
* Prepared as Package Directs

Food and Description	Measure or Quantity	Calories	Carbo-hydrates (grams)
*Butter (Pillsbury):			
Pillsbury Plus	¹/₁₂ of cake	240	36.0
Streusel Swirl, rich	¹/₁₆ of cake	260	38.0
Butter Brickle (Betty			
Crocker) *Supermoist*	¹/₁₂ of cake	260	37.0
Butter pecan (Betty			
Crocker):			
Snackin' Cake	¹/₉ of pkg.	190	31.0
Supermoist	¹/₁₂ of cake	250	35.0
*Carrot (Betty Crocker):			
Stir N' Frost	¹/₆ of cake	230	42.0
Supermoist	¹/₁₂ of cake	260	34.0
Carrot nut (Betty Crocker)			
Snackin' Cake	¹/₉ of pkg.	180	30.0
*Carrot'n spice (Pillsbury)			
Pillsbury Plus	¹/₁₂ of cake	260	36.0
*Cheesecake (Jello-O)	⅛ of cake	283	36.5
*Cherry chip (Betty Crocker)			
Supermoist	¹/₁₂ of cake	180	36.0
Chocolate:			
(Betty Crocker):			
*Pudding	¹/₆ of cake	230	45.0
Snackin' Cake:			
Almond	¹/₉ of pkg.	200	31.0
Fudge Chip	¹/₉ of pkg.	190	32.0
German coconut pecan	¹/₉ of pkg.	180	32.0
Stir 'N Frost:			
Chocolate chip, with			
chocolate frosting	¹/₆ of pkg.	220	40.0
Fudge, with vanilla			
frosting	¹/₆ of pkg.	220	41.0
Stir 'N Streusel, German	¹/₆ of pkg.	240	42.0
Supermoist:			
Chocolate chip	¹/₁₂ of cake	250	33.0
Fudge	¹/₁₂ of cake	250	35.0
German	¹/₁₂ of cake	260	36.0
Milk	¹/₁₂ of cake	250	35.0
Sour cream	¹/₁₂ of cake	260	36.0
*(Pillsbury):			
Bundt:			
Fudge nut crown	¹/₁₆ of cake	220	31.0
Fudge, tunnel of	¹/₁₆ of cake	270	37.0
Macaroon	¹/₁₆ of cake	250	37.0

Food and Description	Measure or Quantity	Calories	Carbo-hydrates (grams)
Pillsbury Plus:			
Fudge, dark	1/12 of cake	260	35.0
Fudge, marble	1/12 of cake	270	36.0
German	1/12 of cake	250	36.0
Mint	1/12 of cake	260	35.0
Streusel Swirl, German	1/16 of cake	260	36.0
Stir 'N Streusel	1/6 of pkg.	240	42.0
*Cinnamon (Pillsbury)			
Streusel Swirl	1/16 of cake	260	38.0
Coconut pecan (Betty			
Crocker) *Snackin' Cake*	1/9 of pkg.	190	30.0
Coffee cake:			
*(Aunt Jemima)	1/8 of cake	170	29.0
*(Pillsbury):			
Apple cinnamon	1/8 of cake	240	40.0
Butter pecan	1/8 of cake	310	39.0
Cinnamon streusel	1/8 of cake	250	41.0
Sour cream	1/8 of cake	270	35.0
Date nut (Betty Crocker)			
Snackin' Cake	1/9 of pkg.	190	32.0
Devil's food:			
*(Betty Crocker)			
Supermoist	1/12 of cake	260	34.0
(Duncan Hines) deluxe	1/12 of pkg.	190	35.6
*(Pillsbury) *Pillsbury Plus*	1/12 of cake	250	35.0
Fudge (see Chocolate)			
Golden chocolate chip (Betty			
Crocker) *Snackin' Cake*	1/9 of pkg.	190	34.0
Lemon:			
(Betty Crocker):			
*Chiffon	1/12 of cake	190	35.0
*Pudding	1/6 of cake	230	45.0
Stir 'N Frost, with lemon			
frosting	1/12 of pkg.	230	39.0
Supermoist	1/12 of cake	260	36.0
*(Pillsbury):			
Bundt, tunnel of	1/16 of cake	270	45.0

(USDA): United States Department of Agriculture
(HEW/FAO):   Health, Education and Welfare/Food and Agriculture
           Organization
* Prepared as Package Directs

Food and Description	Measure or Quantity	Calories	Carbo-hydrates (grams)
Pillsbury Plus	1/12 of cake	260	36.0
Streusel Swirl	1/16 of cake	260	39.0
*Lemon blueberry (Pillsbury)			
Bundt	1/16 of cake	200	28.0
Marble:			
*(Betty Crocker)			
Supermoist	1/12 of cake	260	36.0
*(Pillsbury):			
Bundt, supreme ring	1/16 of cake	250	38.0
Streusel Swirl, fudge	1/16 of cake	260	38.0
*Oats'n brown sugar			
(Pillsbury) Pillsbury Plus	1/12 of cake	260	35.0
*Orange (Betty Crocker)			
Supermoist	1/12 of cake	260	36.0
*Pecan brown sugar			
(Pillsbury) Streusel Swirl	1/16 of cake	260	37.0
Pound:			
*(Betty Crocker) golden	1/12 of cake	200	27.0
*(Dromedary)	3/4″ slice		
	(1/12 of pkg.)	210	29.0
*(Pillsbury) Bundt	1/16 of cake	230	33.0
Spice (Betty Crocker):			
Snackin' Cake, raisin	1/9 of pkg.	180	32.0
Stir 'N Frost, with vanilla			
frosting	1/6 of pkg.	270	47.0
Supermoist	1/12 of cake	260	36.0
Strawberry:			
*(Betty Crocker)			
Supermoist	1/12 of cake	260	36.0
*(Pillsbury) Pillsbury Plus	1/12 of cake	260	37.0
*Upside down			
(Betty Crocker) pineapple	1/9 of cake	270	43.0
White:			
*(Betty Crocker):			
Stir 'N Frost, with milk			
chocolate frosting	1/6 of cake	220	38.0
Supermoist	1/12 of cake	230	35.0
Supermoist, sour cream	1/12 of cake	180	36.0
(Duncan Hines) deluxe	1/12 of pkg.	188	36.1
*(Pillsbury) Pillsbury Plus	1/12 of cake	240	35.0
Yellow:			
(Betty Crocker):			
Stir 'N Frost	1/6 of pkg.	220	38.0

Food and Description	Measure or Quantity	Calories	Carbo-hydrates (grams)
Supermoist	¹⁄₁₂ of cake	260	36.0
Supermoist, butter recipe	¹⁄₁₂ of cake	260	37.0
(Duncan Hines) deluxe	¹⁄₁₂ of pkg.	188	37.0
*(Pillsbury) *Pillsbury Plus*	¹⁄₁₂ of cake	260	36.0
*Dietetic (Dia-Mel; Estee)	¹⁄₁₀ of cake	100	17.0
CAMPARI, 45 proof	1 fl. oz.	66	7.1

CANDY. The following values of candies from the U.S. Department of Agriculture are representative of the types sold commercially. These values may be useful when individual brands or sizes are not known:

Almond:			
Chocolate-coated	1 cup (6.3 oz.)	1024	71.3
Chocolate-coated	1 oz.	161	11.2
Sugar-coated or Jordan	1 oz.	129	19.9
Butterscotch	1 oz.	113	26.9
Candy corn	1 oz.	103	25.4
Caramel:			
Plain	1 oz.	113	21.7
Plain with nuts	1 oz.	121	20.0
Chocolate	1 oz.	113	21.7
Chocolate with nuts	1 oz.	121	20.0
Chocolate-flavored roll	1 oz.	112	23.4
Chocolate:			
Bittersweet	1 oz.	135	13.3
Milk:			
Plain	1 oz.	147	16.1
With almonds	1 oz.	151	14.5
With peanuts	1 oz.	154	12.6
Semisweet	1 oz.	144	16.2
Sweet	1 oz.	150	16.4
Chocolate discs, sugar coated	1 oz.	132	20.6
Coconut center, chocolate-coated	1 oz.	124	20.4
Fondant, plain	1 oz.	103	25.4

(USDA): United States Department of Agriculture
(HEW/FAO): Health, Education and Welfare/Food and Agriculture Organization
* Prepared as Package Directs

Food and Description	Measure or Quantity	Calories	Carbo-hydrates (grams)
Fondant, chocolate-covered	1 oz.	116	23.0
Fudge:			
Chocolate fudge	1 oz.	113	21.3
Chocolate fudge, chocolate-coated	1 oz.	122	20.7
Chocolate fudge with nuts	1 oz.	121	19.6
Chocolate fudge with nuts, chocolate-coated	1 oz.	128	19.1
Vanilla fudge	1 oz.	113	21.2
Vanilla fudge with nuts	1 oz.	120	19.5
With peanuts & caramel, chocolate-coated	1 oz.	130	16.6
Gum drops	1 oz.	98	24.8
Hard	1 oz.	109	27.6
Honeycombed hard candy, with peanut butter, chocolate-covered	1 oz.	131	20.0
Jelly beans	1 oz.	104	26.4
Marshmallows	1 oz.	90	22.8
Mints, uncoated	1 oz.	103	25.4
Nougat & caramel, chocolate-covered,	1 oz.	118	20.6
Peanut bar	1 oz.	146	13.4
Peanut brittle	1 oz.	119	23.0
Peanuts, chocolate-covered	1 oz.	159	11.1
Raisins, chocolate-covered	1 oz.	120	20.0
Vanilla creams, chocolate-covered	1 oz.	123	19.9
CANDY, REGULAR:			
Almond, chocolate covered (Hershey's) *Golden Almond*	1 oz.	163	12.4
Almond, Jordan (Banner)	1¼-oz. box	154	27.9
Apricot Delight (Sahadi)	1 oz.	100	25.0
Baby Ruth	1.8-oz. piece	260	31.0
Butterfinger	1.6-oz. bar	220	28.0
Butterscotch Skimmers (Nabisco)	1 piece (6 grams)	25	5.7
Caramel:			
Caramel Flipper (Wayne)	1 oz.	128	19.0
Caramel Nip (Pearson)	1 piece	29	5.6
Charleston Chew	1½-oz. bar	179	32.6

Food and Description	Measure or Quantity	Calories	Carbo-hydrates (grams)
Cherry, chocolate-covered (Nabisco; *Welch's*)	1 piece (.6 oz.)	67	13.0
Chocolate bar:			
Crunch (Nestle)	1⅙-oz. bar	159	19.1
Milk:			
(Hershey's)	.35-oz. bar	55	5.7
(Hershey's)	1.2-oz. bar	187	19.4
(Hershey's)	4-oz. bar	623	64.7
(Nestlé)	.35-oz. bar	53	6.0
(Nestlé)	1¹⁄₁₆-oz. bar	159	18.1
Special Dark (Hershey's)	1.05-oz. bar	160	18.4
Special Dark (Hershey's)	4-oz. bar	611	70.2
Chocolate bar with almonds:			
(Hershey's) milk	.35-oz. bar	55	5.4
(Hershey's) milk	1.15-oz. bar	180	17.6
(Nestlé)	1-oz.	150	17.0
Chocolate Parfait (Pearson)	1 piece (6.5 grams)	31	5.2
Chuckles	1 oz.	92	23.0
Clark Bar	1.4-oz. bar	188	28.4
Coffee Nip (Pearson)	1 piece (6.5 grams)	29	5.6
Coffioca (Pearson)	1 piece (6.5 grams)	31	5.2
Crispy Bar (Clark)	1¼-oz. bar	187	24.2
Crows (Mason)	1 piece (.1 oz.)	11	2.7
Dots (Mason)	1 piece (.1 oz.)	11	2.7
Dutch Treat Bar (Clark)	1¹⁄₁₆-oz. bar	160	20.3
Good & Plenty	1 oz.	100	24.8
Halvah (Sahadi) original and marble	1 oz.	150	13.0
Hollywood	1½-oz. bar	185	28.9
Jelly bean (Curtiss)	1 piece (3.5 grams)	12	3.0
Jelly rings, *Chuckles*	1 piece (.4 oz.)	37	9.0
JuJubes, *Chuckles*	1 piece (4 grams)	13	3.3

(USDA): United States Department of Agriculture
(HEW/FAO): Health, Education and Welfare/Food and Agriculture Organization
* Prepared as Package Directs

Food and Description	Measure or Quantity	Calories	Carbo-hydrates (grams)
Ju Jus:			
Assorted	1 piece (2 grams)	7	2.0
Coins or raspberries	1 piece (4.3 grams)	15	4.0
Kisses (Hershey's)	1 piece (.2 oz.)	27	2.8
Kisses (Hershey's)	8-oz. piece	1250	129.3
Kit Kat	.6-oz. bar	80	9.4
Kit Kat	1.25-oz. bar	179	21.0
Krackle Bar	.35-oz. bar	52	5.9
Krackle Bar	1.2-oz. bar	178	20.3
Licorice:			
Licorice Nips (Pearson)	1 piece (6.5 grams)	29	5.6
(Switzer) bars, bites or stix:			
Black	1 oz.	94	22.1
Cherry or strawberry	1 oz.	98	23.2
Chocolate	1 oz.	97	22.7
Lollipops (Life Savers)	.9-oz. pop	99	24.0
Mallo Cup (Boyer)	.6-oz. piece	54	11.2
Mars Bar (M&M/Mars)	1.7-oz. bar	233	29.4
Marshmallow (Campfire)	1 oz.	111	24.9
Mary Jane (Miller):			
Small size	¼-oz. piece	19	3.5
Large size	1½-oz. bar	110	20.3
Milk Duds (Clark)	¾-oz. bar	89	17.8
Milky Way (M&M/Mars)	2.1-oz. bar	267	42.2
Mint or peppermint:			
Jamaica or Liberty Mints (Nabisco)	1 piece (6 grams)	24	5.8
Mint Parfait (Pearson)	1 piece (6.5 grams)	31	5.2
Junior mint pattie (Nabisco)	1 piece (.1 oz.)	10	2.0
Peppermint pattie (Nabisco)	1 piece (.5 oz.)	64	12.5
M & M's:			
Peanut	1.67-oz. pkg.	242	32.3
Plain	1.69-oz. pkg.	236	32.6
Mr. Goodbar (Hershey's)	.35-oz. bar	54	4.9
Mr. Goodbar (Hershey's)	1½-oz. bar	233	20.8
$100,000 Bar (Nestlé)	1¼-oz. bar	175	23.8
Orange slices, *Chuckles*	1 piece	29	7.2

Food and Description	Measure or Quantity	Calories	Carbo-hydrates (grams)
Peanut, chocolate-covered:			
(Curtiss)	1 piece	5	1.0
(Nabisco)	1 piece		
	(4.1 grams)	24	1.6
Peanut brittle (Planters):			
Jumbo Peanut Block bar	1 oz.	119	23.0
Jumbo Peanut Block Bar	1 piece		
	(12.2 grams)	61	12.0
Peanut butter cup:			
(Boyer)	1.5-oz. pkg.	148	17.4
(Reese's)	.6-oz. cup	92	8.7
Peanut crunch (Sahadi)	¾-oz. bar	110	10.0
Raisin, chocolate-covered			
(Nabisco)	1 piece	4	.6
Reggie Bar	2-oz. bar	290	29.0
Rolo (Hershey's)	1 piece		
	(6 grams)	30	4.1
Royals, mint chocolate			
(M&M/Mars)	1.52-oz. pkg.	212	29.5
Sesame Crunch (Sahadi)	¾-oz. bar	110	7.0
Snickers (M&M/Mars)	2-oz. bar	275	33.5
Spearmint leaves (Curtiss)	1 piece (.7 oz.)	32	8.0
Starburst (M&M/Mars)	1-oz. serving	118	24.2
Sugar Babies (Nabisco):	1 piece		
	(1.5 grams)	6	1.3
Sugar Daddy (Nabisco):			
Caramel sucker	1 piece (1.1 oz.)	121	26.4
Nugget	1 piece		
	(7 grams)	27	6.0
Sugar Mama (Nabisco)	1 piece (.8 oz.)	101	18.6
Summit bar (M&M/Mars)	¾-oz. bar	115	12.0
Taffy, Turkish (Bonomo)	1 oz.	108	24.4
3 Musketeers	.8-oz. bar	99	17.3
3 Musketeers	2.06-oz. bar	256	44.6
Tootsie Roll:			
Chocolate	.23-oz. midgee	26	5.3
Chocolate	1/16-oz. bar	72	14.3
Chocolate	1-oz. bar	115	22.9

(USDA): United States Department of Agriculture
(HEW/FAO):   Health, Education and Welfare/Food and Agriculture
          Organization
* Prepared as Package Directs

Food and Description	Measure or Quantity	Calories	Carbo-hydrates (grams)
Flavored	.6-oz. square	19	3.8
Pop, all flavors	.49-oz. pop	55	12.5
Pop drop, all flavors	4.7-gram piece	19	4.2
Whatchamacallit (Hershey's)	1.15-oz. bar	176	18.7
World Series Bar	1 oz.	128	21.3
Zagnut Bar (Clark)	.7-oz. bar	92	14.6
CANDY, DIETETIC:			
Carob bar, *Joan's Natural:*			
Coconut	3-oz. bar	516	28.4
Fruit & nut	3-oz. bar	559	31.2
Honey bran	3-oz. bar	487	34.0
Peanut	3-oz. bar	521	27.4
Chocolate or chocolate flavored bar:			
(Estee):			
Coconut, fruit & nut, milk or toasted bran	.2-oz. square	30	2.5
Crunch	.2-oz. square	22	2.0
(Louis Sherry):			
Coffee or orange flavored	.2-oz. square	22	2.0
Bittersweet or milk	.2-oz. square	30	2.5
Estee-ets, with peanuts (Estee)	1 piece (1.4 grams)	7	.8
Gum drops (Estee) any flavor	1 piece (1.8 grams)	3	.7
Hard candy:			
(Estee) assorted fruit	1 piece (.1 oz.)	11	2.7
(Featherweight) assorted	1 piece	12	3.0
(Louis Sherry)	1 piece (.1 oz.)	12	3.0
Lollipop (Estee; Louis Sherry)	1 piece (.2 oz.)	18	5.0
Mint:			
(Estee)	1 piece (1.1 grams)	4	1.0
(Sunkist):			
Mini mint	1 piece (.2 grams)	<1	.2
Roll Mint	1 piece (.9 grams)	4	.9
Peanut butter cup (Estee)	1 cup (.3 oz.)	45	3.3
Raisins, chocolate-covered (Estee)	1 piece (1.2 grams)	5	.7

Food and Description	Measure or Quantity	Calories	Carbo-hydrates (grams)
Rice crisp bar (Featherweight)	1 piece	50	4.5
T.V. Mix (Estee)	1 piece (1.6 grams)	9	.7
CANNELONI, frozen: (Stouffer's):			
Beef & pork with mornay sauce	9⅝-oz. pkg.	240	22.0
Cheese with tomato sauce	9⅛-oz. pkg.	260	18.0
(Weight Watchers) florentine, one-comparment meal	13-oz. meal	450	52.0
CANTALOUPE, fresh (USDA):			
Whole, medium	1 lb. (weighed with skin & cavity contents)	68	17.0
Cubed or diced	½ cup (2.9 oz.)	24	6.1
CAP'N CRUNCH, cereal (Quaker):			
Regular	¾ cup (1 oz.)	121	22.9
Crunchberry	¾ cup (1 oz.)	120	22.9
Peanut butter	¾ cup (1 oz.)	127	20.9
CAPOCOLLO (Hormel)	1 oz.	80	0.
CARAWAY SEED (French's)	1 tsp (1.8 grams)	8	.8
CARNATION INSTANT BREAKFAST: Bar:			
Chocolate chip	1 bar (1.44 oz.)	200	20.0
Chocolate crunch	1 bar (1.34 oz.)	190	20.0
Honey nut	1 bar (1.35 oz.)	190	18.0
Peanut butter with chocolate chips	1 bar (1.4 oz.)	200	20.0
Peanut butter crunch	1 bar (1.35 oz.)	200	20.0

(USDA): United States Department of Agriculture
(HEW/FAO): Health, Education and Welfare/Food and Agriculture Organization
* Prepared as Package Directs

Food and Description	Measure or Quantity	Calories	Carbo-hydrates (grams)
Packets:			
Chocolate or egg nog	1 packet	130	23.0
Chocolate malt	1 packet	130	22.0
Coffee, strawberry or vanilla	1 packet	130	24.0
CARROT:			
Raw (USDA):			
Whole	1 lb. (weighed with full tops)	112	26.0
Partially trimmed	1 lb. (weighed without tops, with skins)	156	36.1
Trimmed	5½″ × 1″ carrot (1.8 oz.)	21	4.8
Trimmed	25 thin strips (1.8 oz.)	21	4.8
Chunks	½ cup (2.4 oz.)	29	6.7
Diced	½ cup (1½ oz.)	30	7.0
Grated or shredded	½ cup (1.9 oz.)	23	5.3
Slices	½ cup (2.2 oz.)	27	6.2
Strips	½ cup (2 oz.)	24	5.6
Boiled, drained (USDA):			
Chunks	½ cup (2.9 oz.)	25	5.8
Diced	½ cup (2½ oz.)	24	5.2
Slices	½ cup (2.7 oz.)	24	5.4
Canned, regular pack, solids & liq.:			
(Del Montes) diced, sliced or whole	½ cup (4 oz.)	30	7.0
(Libby's) diced	½ cup (4.3 oz.)	20	4.1
Canned, dietetic pack, solids & liq.:			
(Featherweight) sliced	½ cup	30	6.0
(S&W) *Nutradiet*, green label	½ cup	30	7.0
Frozen:			
(Birds Eye) whole, baby deluxe	⅓ of pkg. (3.3 oz.)	43	9.1
(Green Giant) cuts, in butter sauce	½ cup	80	16.0
(McKenzie)	3.3-oz. serving	40	9.0
(Seabrook Farms) whole	⅓ pkg. (3.3 oz.)	39	8.1

Food and Description	Measure or Quantity	Calories	Carbo-hydrates (grams)
CASABA MELLON (USDA):			
Whole	1 lb. (weighed whole)	61	14.7
Flesh only, cubed or diced	4 oz.	31	7.4
CASHEW NUT:			
(USDA)	1 oz.	159	8.3
(USDA)	½ cup (2.5 oz.)	393	20.5
(USDA)	5 large or 8 med.	60	3.1
(Fisher):			
Dry roasted	¼ cup (1.2 oz.)	187	9.9
Oil roasted	¼ cup (1.2 oz.)	196	9.9
(Planters):			
Dry roasted, salted or unsalted	1 oz.	160	9.0
Oil roasted	1 oz.	170	8.0
CATFISH, freshwater (USDA) raw fillet	4 oz.	117	0.
CATSUP:			
Regular:			
(Del Monte)	1 T. (.5 oz.)	17	3.9
(Del Monte)	¼ cup (2 oz.)	60	16.0
(Smucker's)	1 T.	21	4.5
Dietetic or low calorie:			
(Del Monte) No Salt Added	1 T.	15	4.0
(Dia-Mel)	1 T. (.5 oz.)	6	1.0
(Featherweight)	1 T. (.6 oz.)	6	1.0
(Tillie Lewis) *Tasti Diet*	1 T. (.5 oz.)	8	2.0
CAULIFLOWER:			
Raw (USDA):			
Whole	1 lb. (weighed untrimmed)	49	9.2
Flowerbuds	½ cup (1.8 oz.)	14	2.6
Slices	½ cup (1.5 oz.)	11	2.2

(USDA): United States Department of Agriculture
(HEW/FAO):   Health, Education and Welfare/Food and Agriculture
                        Organization
* Prepared as Package Directs

Food and Description	Measure or Quantity	Calories	Carbo-hydrates (grams)
Boiled (USDA) flowerbuds, drained	½ cup (2.2 oz.)	14	2.5
Frozen:			
(Birds Eye):			
Regular or florets, deluxe	⅓ of 10-oz. pkg.	28	4.6
With almonds & selected seasonings	⅓ of 10-oz. pkg.	46	5.1
With cheese sauce	⅓ of 10-oz. pkg.	84	8.2
(Green Giant):			
In cheese sauce	½ cup	60	10.0
Cuts, polybag	½ cup	16	3.0
(McKenzie)	3.3-oz. serving	25	5.0
CAVIAR, STURGEON (USDA):			
Pressed	1 oz.	90	1.4
Whole eggs	1 T. (.6 oz.)	42	.5
CELERIAC ROOT, raw (USDA):			
Whole	1 lb. (weighed unpared)	156	39.2
Pared	4 oz.	45	9.6
CELERY, all varieties (USDA):			
Fresh:			
Whole	1 lb. (weighed untrimmed)	58	13.3
1 large outer stalk	8″ × 1½ at root end (1.4 oz.)	7	1.6
Diced, chopped or cut in chunks	½ cup (2.1 oz.)	10	2.3
Slices	½ cup (1.9 oz.)	9	2.1
Boiled, drained solids:			
Diced or cut in chunks	½ cup (2.7 oz.)	10	2.4
Slices	½ cup (3 oz.)	12	2.6
CELERY SALT (French's)	1 tsp.	2	Tr.
CELERY SEED (French's)	1 tsp.	11	1.1
CERTS	1 piece	6	1.5

Food and Description	Measure or Quantity	Calories	Carbo-hydrates (grams)
CERVELAT:			
(USDA):			
Dry	1 oz.	128	.5
soft	1 oz.	87	.5
(Hormel) Viking	1-oz. serving	90	0.
CHABLIS WINE:			
(Almaden) light	3 fl. oz.	42	DNA
(Louis M. Martini) 12½%			
alcohol	3 fl. oz.	59	.2
(Paul Masson):			
Regular, 11.8% alcohol	3 fl. oz.	71	2.7
Light, 7.1% alcohol	3 fl. oz.	45	2.7
CHAMPAGNE:			
(Great Western):			
Regular, 12% alcohol	3 fl. oz.	71	2.5
Brut, 12% alcohol	3 fl. oz.	74	3.4
Pink, 12% alcohol	3 fl. oz.	81	4.9
(Taylor) dry, 12½% alcohol	3 fl. oz.	78	3.9
CHARD, Swiss (USDA):			
Raw, whole	1 lb. (weighed untrimmed)	104	19.2
Raw, trimmed	4 oz.	29	5.2
Boiled, drained solids	½ cup (3.4 oz.)	17	3.2
CHARDONNAY WINE (Louis M. Martini) 12½% alcohol	3 fl. oz.	61	.2
CHARLOTTE RUSSE, homemade recipe (USDA)	4 oz.	324	38.0
CHEERIOS, cereal:			
Regular	1¼ cups (1 oz.)	110	20.0
Honey & nut	¾ cup (1 oz.)	110	23.0

(USDA): United States Department of Agriculture
(HEW/FAO): Health, Education and Welfare/Food and Agriculture Organization
* Prepared as Package Directs

Food and Description	Measure or Quantity	Calories	Carbo-hydrates (grams)
CHEESE:			
American or cheddar:			
(USDA):			
Regular	1 oz.	105	.5
Cube, natural	1″ cube (.6 oz.)	68	.3
(Featherweight) low sodium	1 oz.	110	1.0
Laughing Cow, natural	1 oz.	100	Tr.
(Sargento):			
Midget, regular or sharp,			
sliced or sticks	1 oz.	114	1.0
Shredded, non-dairy	1 oz.	90	1.0
Wispride	1 oz.	115	
Blue:			
(USDA) natural	1 oz.	104	.6
(Frigo)	1 oz.	100	1.0
Laughing Cow	¾-oz. wedge	55	.5
(Sargento) cold pack or			
crumbled	1 oz.	100	1.0
Bonbino, *Laughing Cow*,			
natural	1 oz.	103	Tr.
Brick:			
(USDA) natural	1 oz.	105	.5
(Sargento) sliced	1 oz.	105	1.0
Brie (Sargento) *Danish Danko*	1 oz.	80	.1
Burgercheese (Sargento)			
Danish Danko	1 oz.	106	1.0
Camembert:			
(USDA) domestic	1 oz.	85	.5
(Sargento) *Danish Danko*	1 oz.	88	.1
Colby:			
(Featherweight) low sodium	1 oz.	100	0.
(Pauly) low sodium	1 oz.	115	.6
(Sargento) shredded or sliced	1 oz.	112	1.0
Cottage:			
Unflavored:			
(USDA) creamed	½ cup (4.3 oz.)	130	3.5
(Bison):			
Regular	1 oz.	29	1.0
Dietetic	1 oz.	22	1.0
(Dairylea)	1 oz.	30	1.0
(Friendship) California			
style	1 oz.	30	1.0

Food and Description	Measure or Quantity	Calories	Carbo-hydrates (grams)
Flavored (Friendship):			
Dutch apple	1 oz.	31	2.5
Garden salad	1 oz.	30	1.0
Pineapple	1 oz.	35	3.8
Cream, plain, unwhipped:			
(USDA)	1 oz.	106	.6
(Friendship)	1 oz.	103	.8
(Frigo)	1 oz.	100	1.0
Edam:			
(House of Gold)	1 oz.	100	1.0
Laughing Cow	1 oz.	101	Tr.
(Sargento)	1 oz.	101	1.0
Farmers:			
Dutch Garden Brand	1 oz.	100	1.0
(Friendship) regular or			
no salt added	1 oz.	40	1.0
(Sargento)	1 oz.	72	1.0
Wispride	1 oz.	100	1.0
Feta (Sargento) Danish, cups	1 oz.	76	1.0
Gjetost (Sargento) Norwegian	1 oz.	118	13.0
Gouda:			
Laughing Cow	1 oz.	100	Tr.
(Sargento) baby, caraway or			
smoked	1 oz.	101	1.0
Wispride	1 oz.	100	Tr.
Gruyere, *Swiss Knight*	1 oz.	100	Tr.
Havarti (Sargento):			
Creamy	1 oz.	90	.2
Creamy, 60% mild	1 oz.	177	.2
Hoop (Friendship) natural	1 oz.	21	.5
Hot pepper (Sargento) sliced	1 oz.	112	1.0
Jarlsberg (Sargento) Norwegian	1 oz.	100	1.0
Kettle Moraine (Sargento)	1 oz.	100	1.0
Limburger (Sargento) natural	1 oz.	93	14.0
Monterey Jack:			
(Frigo)	1 oz.	100	1.0

(USDA): United States Department of Agriculture
(HEW/FAO):   Health, Education and Welfare/Food and Agriculture
                        Organization
* Prepared as Package Directs

Food and Description	Measure or Quantity	Calories	Carbo-hydrates (grams)
(Sargento) midget, Longhorn, shredded or sliced	1 oz.	106	1.0
Mozzarella:			
(Fisher) part skim milk	1 oz.	90	1.0
(Frigo) part skim milk	1 oz.	90	1.0
(Sargento):			
Bar, rounds, shredded regular or with spices, sliced for pizza or square	1 oz.	79	1.0
Whole milk	1 oz.	100	1.0
Meunster:			
(Sargento) red rind	1 oz.	104	1.0
Wispride	1 oz.	100	Tr.
Nibblin Curds (Sargento)	1 oz.	114	1.0
Parmesan:			
(USDA):			
Regular	1 oz.	111	.8
Shredded	½ cup (not packed)	169	1.2
(Frigo):			
Grated	1 T.	23	Tr.
Whole	1 oz.	110	1.0
(Sargento):			
Grated, non-dairy	1 T.	27	2.3
Wedge	1 oz.	110	1.0
Pizza (Sargento) shredded or sliced, non-dairy	1 oz.	90	1.0
Pot (Sargento) regular, French onion or garlic	1 oz.	30	1.0
Provolone:			
(Frigo)	1 oz.	90	1.0
Laughing Cow:			
Cube	⅙ oz.	12	.1
Wedge	¾ oz.	55	.5
(Sargento) sliced	1 oz.	100	1.0
Ricotta:			
(Frigo) part skim milk	1 oz.	43	.9
(Sargento):			
Part skim milk	1 oz.	39	1.0
Whole milk	1 oz.	49	1.0
Romano (Sargento) wedge	1 oz.	110	1.0

Food and Description	Measure or Quantity	Calories	Carbo-hydrates (grams)
Roquefort, natural (USDA)	1 oz.	104	.6
Samsoe (Sargento) Danish	1 oz.	101	.2
Scamorze (Frigo)	1 oz.	79	.3
Semisoft, Laughing Cow:			
Babybel:			
Regular	1 oz.	91	Tr.
Mini	¾ oz.	75	Tr.
Bonbel:			
Regular	1 oz.	99	Tr.
Mini	¾ oz.	75	Tr.
Reduced calorie	1 oz.	62	.3
Stirred curd (Frigo)	1 oz.	110	1.0
String (Sargento)	1 oz.	90	1.0
Swiss:			
(USDA) domestic, natural or process	1 oz.	105	.5
(Fisher) natural	1 oz.	100	0.
(Frigo) domestic	1 oz.	100	0.
(Sargento) domestic or Finland, sliced	1 oz.	107	1.0
Taco (Sargento) shredded	1 oz.	105	1.0
Washed curd (Frigo)	1 oz.	110	1.0
CHEESE FONDUE,			
Swiss Knight	1 oz.	60	1.0
CHEESE FOOD:			
American or cheddar:			
(USDA) process	1 oz.	92	2.0
(Fisher) Ched-O-Mate or Sandwich-Mate	1 oz.	90	1.0
(Sargento)	1 oz.	94	2.0
(Weight Watchers) colored or white	1 oz.-slice	50	1.0
Wispride:			
Regular	1 oz.	90	2.0
& blue cheese	1 oz.	100	2.0

(USDA): United States Department of Agriculture
(HEW/FAO):   Health, Education and Welfare/Food and Agriculture
            Organization
* Prepared as Package Directs

Food and Description	Measure or Quantity	Calories	Carbo-hydrates (grams)
Hickory smoked	1 oz.	90	3.0
& port wine	1 oz.	100	Tr.
Cheez-ola (Fisher)	1 oz.	90	1.0
Chef's Delight (Fisher)	1 oz.	70	4.0
Cracker snack (Sargento)	1 oz.	90	2.0
Mun-chee (Pauly)	1 oz.	100	2.0
Pimiento (Pauly)	.8-oz. slice	73	.8
Pizza-Mate (Fisher)	1 oz.	90	1.0
Swiss (Pauly)	.8-oz. slice	74	1.6
CHEESE PUFFS, frozen			
(Durkee)	1 piece	59	3.0
CHEESE SPREAD:			
American or cheddar:			
(USDA)	1 T. (.5 oz.)	40	1.1
(Fisher)	1 oz.	80	2.0
Laughing Cow	1 oz.	72	.7
(Nabisco) *Snack Mate*	1 tsp.	16	.4
Blue, *Laughing Cow*	1 oz.	72	.7
Cheese 'n Bacon (Nabisco)			
Snack Mate	1 tsp.	16	.4
Cheese Whiz (Kraft)	1 oz.	78	1.8
Gruyere, *Laughing Cow,*			
La Vache Que Rit	1 oz.	72	.7
Pimiento:			
(Nabisco) *Snack Mate*	1 tsp.	15	.3
(Price)	1 oz.	80	2.0
Provolone, *Laughing Cow*	1 oz.	72	.7
Velveeta (Kraft)	1 oz.	85	2.5
CHEESE STRAW, frozen			
(Durkee)	1 piece	29	1.0
CHENIN BLANC WINE (Louis M. Martini) 12½% alcohol	3 fl. oz.	60	.2
CHERRY:			
Sour (USDA):			
Fresh:			
Whole	1 lb. (weighed with stems)	213	52.5

Food and Description	Measure or Quantity	Calories	Carbo-hydrates (grams)
Whole	1 lb. (weighed without stems)	242	59.7
Pitted	½ cup (2.7 oz.)	45	11.1
Canned, syrup pack, pitted:			
Light syrup	4 oz. (with liq.)	84	21.2
Heavy syrup	½ cup (with liq.)	116	29.5
Extra heavy syrup	4 oz. (with liq.)	127	32.4
Canned, water pack, pitted, solid & liq.	½ cup (4.3 oz.)	52	13.1
Frozen, pitted:			
Sweetened	½ cup (4.6 oz.)	146	36.1
Unsweetened	4 oz.	62	15.2
Sweet:			
Fresh (USDA):			
Whole	1 lb. (weighed with stems)	286	71.0
Whole, with stems	½ cup (2.3 oz.)	41	10.2
Pitted	½ cup (2.9 oz.)	57	14.3
Canned, syrup pack: (USDA):			
Light syrup, pitted	4 oz. (with liq.)	74	18.7
Heavy syrup, pitted	½ cup (with liq., 4.2 oz.)	96	24.2
Extra heavy syrup, pitted	4 oz. (with liq.)	113	29.0
(Del Monte) solids & liq.:			
Dark	½ cup (4.3 oz.)	90	23.0
Light	½ cup (4.3 oz.)	100	26.0
(Stokely-Van Camp) pitted, solids & liq.	½ cup (4.2 oz.)	50	11.0
Canned, dietetic or water pack, solids & liq.:			
(Diet Delight)	½ cup (4.4 oz.)	70	17.0
(Featherweight):			
Dark	½ cup	60	13.0
Light	½ cup	50	11.0
CHERRY, CANDIED (USDA)	1 oz.	96	24.6

(USDA): United States Department of Agriculture
(HEW/FAO):   Health, Education and Welfare/Food and Agriculture Organization
* Prepared as Package Directs

Food and Description	Measure or Quantity	Calories	Carbo-hydrates (grams)
CHERRY DRINK:			
Canned:			
(Hi-C)	6 fl. oz.	93	23.0
(Lincoln) cherry berry	6 fl. oz.	100	25.0
*Mix (Hi-C)	6 fl. oz.	72	18.0
CHERRY HEERING			
(Hiram Walker)	1 fl. oz.	80	10.0
CHERRY JELLY:			
Sweetened (Smucker's)	1 T. (.5 oz.)	53	13.5
Dietetic (Featherweight)	1 T.	16	4.0
CHERRY LIQUEUR			
(DeKuyper) 50 proof	1 fl. oz.	75	8.5
CHERRY, MARASCHINO			
(USDA)	1 oz. (with liq.)	33	8.3
CHERRY PRESERVES OR JAM:			
Sweetened (Smucker's)	1 T. (.7 oz.)	53	13.5
Dietetic			
(Dia-Mel)	1 T. (.6 oz.)	6	0.
(Louis Sherry)	1 t. (.6 oz.)	6	0.
(S&W) *Nutradiet*, red label	1 t.	12	3.0
CHESTNUT (USDA):			
Fresh:			
In shell	1 lb. (weighed in shell)	713	154.7
Shelled	4 oz.	220	47.7
Dried:			
In shell	1 lb. (weighed in shell)	1402	292.4
Shelled	4 oz.	428	89.1
CHEWING GUM:			
Sweetened:			
Bazooka, bubble	1 slice	18	4.5
Beechies, Chiclets, tiny size	1 piece	6	1.6
Beech Nut; Beeman's, Big Red; Black Jack;			

Food and Description	Measure or Quantity	Calories	Carbo-hydrates (grams)
Clove; Doublemint; Freedent; Fruit Punch; Juicy Fruit, Spearmint (Wrigley's); *Teaberry*	1 stick	10	2.3
Dentyne	1 piece	4	1.2
Hubba Bubba (Wrigley's)	1 piece (8 grams)	23	5.8
Dietetic:			
(Clark; *Care*Free*)	1 piece	7	1.7
(Estee) bubble or regular	1 piece	5	1.4
(Featherweight) bubble or regular	1 piece	4	1.0
Orbit (Wrigley's)	1 piece	8	Tr.
CHEX, cereal (Ralston Purina):			
Bran (See **BRAN BREAKFAST CEREAL**)			
Corn	1 cup (1 oz.)	110	25.0
Rice	1⅛ cups (1 oz.)	110	25.0
Wheat	⅔ cup (1 oz.)	110	23.0
Wheat & raisins	¾ cup (1.3 oz.)	130	31.0
CHIANTI WINE (Italian Swiss Colony) 13% alcohol	3 fl. oz.	64	1.5
CHICKEN (see also **CHICKEN, CANNED**) (USDA):			
Broiler, cooked, meat only	4 oz.	154	0.
Capon, raw, with bone	1 lb. (weighed ready-to-cook)	937	0.
Fryer:			
Raw:			
Ready-to-cook	1 lb. (weighed ready-to-cook)	382	0.
Breast	1 lb. (weighed with bone)	394	0.
Leg or drumstick	1 lb. (weighed with bone)	313	0.

(USDA): United States Department of Agriculture
(HEW/FAO):   Health, Education and Welfare/Food and Agriculture
          Organization
* Prepared as Package Directs

Food and Description	Measure or Quantity	Calories	Carbo-hydrates (grams)
Thigh	1 lb. (weighed with bone)	435	0.
Fried. A 2½-lb. chicken (weighed before cooking with bone) will give you:			
Back	1 back (2.2 oz.)	139	2.7
Breast	½ breast (3⅓ oz.)	154	1.1
Leg or drumstrick	1 leg (2 oz.)	87	.4
Neck	1 neck (2.1 oz.)	121	1.9
Rib	1 rib (.7 oz.)	42	.8
Thigh	1 thigh (2¼ oz.)	118	1.2
Wing	1 wing (1¾ oz.)	78	.8
Fried skin	1 oz.	199	2.6
Hen and cock:			
Raw	1 lb. (weighed ready-to-cook)	987	0.
Stewed:			
Meat only	4 oz.	236	0.
Chopped	½ cup (2.5 oz.)	150	0.
Diced	½ cup (2.4 oz.)	139	0.
Ground	½ cup (2 oz.)	116	0.
Roaster:			
Raw:	1 lb. (weighed ready-to-cook)	791	0.
Roasted:			
Dark meat without skin	4 oz.	209	0.
Light meat without skin	4 oz.	206	0.
CHICKEN A LA KING:			
Home recipe (USDA)	1 cup (8.6 oz.)	468	12.3
Canned (Swanson)	½ of 10½-oz. can	180	9.0
Frozen:			
(Banquet) *Cookin' Bag*	5-oz. pkg.	159	10.0
(Green Giant) twin pouch, with biscuits	9-oz. entree	370	40.0
(Morton)	5-oz. pkg.	150	8.0
(Stouffer's) with rice	9½-oz. pkg.	330	38.0
(Weight Watchers)	9-oz. pkg.	230	7.0
CHICKEN BOUILLON:			
(Herb-Ox):			
Cube	1 cube	6	.6
Packet	1 packet	12	1.9

Food and Description	Measure or Quantity	Calories	Carbo-hydrates (grams)
(Maggi) cube	1 cube	7	1.0
Low sodium (Featherweight)	1 tsp.	18	2.0
CHICKEN, BONED, CANNED:			
Regular:			
(USDA)	1 cup (7.2 oz.)	406	0.
(Hormel) chunk:			
Breast	6¾-oz. serving	350	0.
White & dark	6¾-oz. serving	340	0.
(Swanson) chunk:			
Regular	2½ oz.	110	0.
Mixin' chicken	2½ oz.	130	0.
White	2½ oz.	110	0.
Low sodium (Featherweight)	2½ oz.	154	0.
CHICKEN, CREAMED, frozen			
(Stouffer's)	6½ oz. pkg.	300	5.9
CHICKEN DINNER OR ENTREE:			
Canned (Swanson) & dumplings	7½ oz.	220	19.0
Frozen:			
(Banquet):			
American Favorites	11-oz. dinner	359	46.0
Extra Helping:			
& dressing	19-oz. dinner	808	89.0
& dumpling	19-oz. dinner	883	91.0
Fried	17-oz. dinner	744	92.0
(Green Giant):			
Baked:			
In BBQ sauce with corn on the cob	1 meal	350	45.0
In herb butter with stuffed potato	1 meal	430	30.0
Stir fry & cashews	1 meal	340	37.0

(USDA): United States Department of Agriculture
(HEW/FAO):   Health, Education and Welfare/Food and Agriculture
            Organization
* Prepared as Package Directs

Food and Description	Measure or Quantity	Calories	Carbo-hydrates (grams)
Stir fry and garden vegetables	10-oz. entree	250	29.0
Stir fry, sweet & sour	10-oz. entree	300	14.0
Twin pouch			
& broccoli, with rice in cheese sauce	9½-oz. entree	300	26.0
& pea pods in sauce with rice & vegetables	10-oz. entree	300	32.0
(Morton):			
Regular:			
Boneless	10-oz. dinner	230	24.0
Fried	11-oz. dinner	460	49.0
Sliced	5-oz. pkg.	130	7.0
Country Table, fried	15-oz. entree	710	96.0
King Size, fried:			
Dinner	17-oz. dinner	860	91.0
Entree	12-oz. entree	640	59.0
(Stouffer's):			
Regular:			
Cacciatore, with spaghetti	11¼-oz. meal	310	29.0
Divan	8½-oz. serving	335	14.0
Lean Cuisine:			
Glazed with vegetable rice	8½-oz. serving	270	23.0
& vegetables with vermicelli	12¾-oz. serving	260	28.0
(Swanson):			
Regular, in white wine sauce	8¼-oz. dinner	350	8.0
Hungry Man:			
Boneless	19-oz. dinner	680	65.0
Fried:			
Dark portion	14-oz. dinner	840	75.0
White portion	15¼-oz. dinner	950	90.0
White portion with whipped potato	11¾-oz. entree	720	49.0
TV Brand, fried:			
Barbecue	11¼-oz. dinner	570	50.0
Nibbles, with french fries	6-oz. entree	380	30.0
With whipped potatoes	7¼-oz. entree	400	33.0
White portions	11½-oz. dinner	570	48.0

Food and Description	Measure or Quantity	Calories	Carbo-hydrates (grams)
3-course, fried (Weight Watchers):	15-oz. dinner	590	53.0
Cacciatore	10-oz. serving	290	30.1
Oriental style	9½-oz. serving	240	27.5
Parmigiana, 2-compartment meal	7¾-oz. serving	220	11.0
Sliced in celery sauce, 2-compartment meal	8½-oz. serving	230	14.9
Southern fried patty, 2-compartment	9½-oz. serving	260	11.0
Sweet & sour with oriental style vegetables	9-oz. serving	210	26.1
CHICKEN FRICASEE (USDA) home recipe	1 cup (8.5 oz.)	386	7.7
CHICKEN, FRIED, frozen: (Banquet):			
Assorted	2-lb. pkg.	1625	100.0
Bread portion	22-oz. pkg.	1190	70.0
Thigh & drumstick	25-oz. pkg.	1385	80.0
Wings	27-oz. pkg.	1384	84.0
(Morton):			
Assorted	2-lb. pkg.	1500	165.0
Breast portion	22-oz. pkg.	1480	120.0
(Swanson):			
Assorted	3¼-oz. serving	290	11.0
Breast portions	3¼-oz. serving	250	15.0
Nibbles	3¼-oz. serving	300	16.0
Take-out style	3¼-oz. serving	270	10.0
Thighs & drumsticks	3¼-oz. serving	280	17.0
CHICKEN GIZZARD (USDA):			
Raw	4 oz.	128	.8
Simmered	4 oz.	168	.8
CHICKEN & NOODLES, frozen: (Green Giant) twin pouch, with vegetables	9-oz. pkg.	390	38.0

(USDA): United States Department of Agriculture
(HEW/FAO):   Health, Education and Welfare/Food and Agriculture Organization
* Prepared as Package Directs

Food and Description	Measure or Quantity	Calories	Carbo-hydrates (grams)
(Stouffer's):			
Escalloped	5¾-oz. serving	250	13.0
Paprikash	10½-oz. serving	385	32.0
CHICKEN NUGGETS, frozen			
(Banquet)			
breaded & fried	12-oz. pkg.	932	56.0
CHICKEN, PACKAGED:			
(Eckrich) breast	1 slice	20	.5
(Louis Rich) breast, oven			
roasted	1-oz. slice	40	Tr.
CHICKEN PATTY, frozen			
(Banquet)			
breaded & fried	12-oz. pkg.	900	52.0
CHICKEN PIE, frozen:			
(Banquet):			
Regular	8-oz. pie	520	45.0
Supreme	8-oz. pie	430	40.0
(Morton)	8-oz. pie	320	33.0
(Stouffer's)	10-oz. pie	500	40.0
(Swanson):			
Regular	8-oz. pie	420	40.0
Hungry Man	16-oz. pie	730	65.0
(Van de Kamp's)	7½-oz. pie	520	47.0
CHICKEN POTTED (USDA)	1 oz.	70	0.
CHICKEN PUFF, frozen			
(Durkee)	½-oz. piece	49	3.0
CHICKEN SALAD (Carnation)	¼ of 7½-oz. can	120	3.8
CHICKEN SOUP (See SOUP, Chicken)			
CHICKEN SPREAD:			
(Hormel)	1 oz.	60	0.
(Swanson)	1 oz.	60	2.0
(Underwood) chunky	½ of 4¾-oz. can	150	2.7

Food and Description	Measure or Quantity	Calories	Carbo-hydrates (grams)
CHICKEN STEW, canned:			
Regular:			
(Libby's) with dumplings	8 oz.	194	20.2
(Swanson)	7⅜-oz.	170	16.0
Dietetic:			
(Dia-Mel)	8-oz. serving	150	19.0
(Featherweight)	7½-oz. serving	170	21.0
CHICKEN STICKS, frozen			
(Banquet) breaded, fried	12-oz. pkg.	912	60.0
CHICKEN STOCK BASE			
(French's)	1 tsp. (3.2 grams)	8	1.0
CHICK-FIL-A:			
Sandwich	5.4-oz. serving	404	40.2
Soup, hearty, breast of chicken:			
Small	8⅕ oz.	131	11.1
Large	14.3 oz.	230	19.3
CHICK'N QUICK, frozen			
(Tyson):			
Breast fillet	3 oz.	210	12.0
Breast pattie	3 oz.	240	11.0
Chick'N Cheddar	3 oz.	250	12.0
Chunks	1 piece (.5 oz.)	30	2.5
Cordon bleu	5 oz.	300	16.0
Diced	3 oz.	150	0.
Kiev	5 oz.	410	16.0
Sticks	1 piece (1 oz.)	80	5.0
Swiss'N Bacon	3 oz.	260	14.0
Turkey patties	6 oz.	210	11.0
CHICK PEAS OR GARBANZOS (USDA) dry	1 cup (7.1 oz.)	720	122.0

(USDA): United States Department of Agriculture
(HEW/FAO):   Health, Education and Welfare/Food and Agriculture
                          Organization
* Prepared as Package Directs

Food and Description	Measure or Quantity	Calories	Carbo-hydrates (grams)
CHILI OR CHILI CON CARNE:			
Canned, regular pack:			
Beans only:			
(Hormel) in sauce	5oz.	130	19.0
(Van Camp) Mexican style	1 cup	250	43.0
With beans:			
(Hormel):			
Regular	7½-oz. serving	310	23.0
Hot	½-oz. serving	310	24.0
Short Orders	7½-oz. can	300	23.0
(Libby's)	7½-oz. serving	270	25.0
(Swanson)	7¾-oz. serving	310	28.0
Canned, regular pack:			
Without beans:			
(Hormel):			
Regular or hot	7½-oz. serving	370	12.0
Short Orders	7½-oz. can	360	11.0
(Libby's)	7½ oz.	390	11.0
Canned, dietetic pack:			
(Dia-Mel) with beans	8-oz. serving	360	31.0
(Featherweight) with beans	7½-oz.	270	25.0
Frozen, with beans:			
(Stouffer's)	8¾-oz. pkg.	270	26.0
(Weight Watchers)			
one-compartment meal	10-oz. pkg.	295	32.9
CHILI SAUCE:			
(USDA)	½ cup (4.8 oz.)	142	33.8
(Del Monte)	¼ cup (2 oz.)	70	17.0
(Ortega) green	1 oz.	6	1.1
(Featherweight) dietetic	1 T.	8	2.0
CHILI SEASONING MIX:			
*(Durkee)	1 cup	465	31.2
(French's) *Chili-O*	2-oz. pkg.	150	20.0
(McCormick)	1.2-oz. pkg.	106	36.1
CHIVES (USDA) raw	1 T. (3 grams)	1	.2
CHOCO-DILE (Hostess)	2-oz. piece	235	34.1
CHOCOLATE, BAKING:			
(Baker's):			
Bitter or unsweetened	1-oz. square	180	8.6

Food and Description	Measure or Quantity	Calories	Carbo-hydrates (grams)
Semi-sweet:			
Regular	1-oz. square	156	16.8
Chips	¼ cup (1½ oz.)	207	31.7
Sweetened, *German's*	1 oz. square	158	17.3
(Hershey's):			
Bitter or unsweetened	1 oz.	188	6.8
Sweetened:			
Dark chips, regular or mini	1 oz.	151	17.8
Milk, chips	1 oz.	148	18.2
Semi-sweet, chips	1 oz.	150	17.3
(Nestlé):			
Bitter or unsweetened, *Choco-bake*	1-oz. packet	180	8.0
Sweet or semi-sweet, morsels	1 oz.	150	17.0
CHOCOLATE ICE CREAM (See **ICE CREAM,** Chocolate)			
CHOCOLATE SYRUP (See **SYRUP,** Chocolate)			
CHOP SUEY:			
Home recipe (USDA) with meat	1 cup (8.8 oz.)	300	12.8
Frozen:			
(Banquet):			
Buffet Supper	2-lb. pkg.	418	39.1
Dinner	12-oz. dinner	282	38.8
(Stouffer's) beef, with rice	12-oz. pkg.	355	47.7
*CHOP SUEY SEASONING MIX (Durkee)	1¾ cups	557	21.0
CHOWDER (See **SOUP,** Chowder)			
CHOW CHOW (USDA):			
Sour	1 cup (8.5 oz.)	70	9.8
Sweet	1 cup (8.6 oz.)	284	66.2

(USDA): United States Department of Agriculture
(HEW/FAO): Health, Education and Welfare/Food and Agriculture
                    Organization
* Prepared as Package Directs

Food and Description	Measure or Quantity	Calories	Carbo-hydrates (grams)
CHOW MEIN:			
Canned:			
(Hormel) pork, *Short Orders*	7½-oz. can	140	13.0
(La Choy):			
Regular:			
Beef	¾ cup	70	5.0
Beef pepper oriental	¾ cup	90	10.0
Chicken	¾ cup	80	6.0
Meatless	¾ cup	35	5.0
Shrimp	¾ cup	60	4.0
*Bi-pack:			
Beef	¾ cup	60	6.0
Beef pepper oriental or shrimp	¾ cup	70	7.0
Chicken	¾ cup	70	5.0
Pork	¾ cup	90	7.0
Vegetable	¾ cup	60	7.0
Frozen:			
(Banquet):			
Buffet Supper	2-lb. pkg.	345	36.4
Dinner	12-oz. dinner	282	38.8
(Green Giant):			
Beef, twin pouch	10-oz. entree	240	33.0
Chicken, twin pouch	9-oz. entree	220	29.0
(La Choy):			
Chicken:			
Dinner	12-oz. dinner	260	44.0
Entree	12-oz. entree	180	16.0
Shrimp:			
Dinner	12-oz. dinner	220	47.0
Entree	12-oz. entree	120	20.0
(Stouffer's):			
Regular, chicken	8-oz. pkg.	145	10.0
Lean Cuisine, chicken, with rice	11¼-oz. serving	240	36.0
(Van de Kamp's)			
Mandarin:			
Beef	11-oz. serving	370	29.0
Chicken	11-oz. serving	380	31.0
CHOW MEIN SEASONING MIX (Kikkoman)	1⅛-oz. pkg.	98	13.8

Food and Description	Measure or Quantity	Calories	Carbo- hydrates (grams)
CINNAMON, GROUND			
(French's)	1 tsp. (1.7 grams)	6	1.4
CINNAMON SUGAR (French's)	1 tsp. (4.3 grams)	16	4.0
CITRUS COOLER DRINK,			
canned (Hi-C)	6 fl. oz.	93	23.0
CLAM:			
Raw (USDA):			
Hard or round:			
Meat & liq.	1 lb. (weighed in shell)	71	6.1
Meat only	1 cup (8 oz.)	182	13.4
Soft:			
Meat & liq.	1 lb. (weighed in shell)	142	5.3
Meat only	1 cup (8 oz.)	186	3.0
Canned (Doxsee) all kinds:			
Chopped & minced, solids & liq.	4 oz.	59	3.2
Chopped, meat only	4 oz.	111	2.1
Steamed meat & broth	1 pt. (8 fl. oz.)	152	DNA
Steamed, meat only	1 pt. (8 fl. oz.)	66	DNA
Frozen:			
(Howard Johnson's) fried	5-oz. pkg.	395	32.0
(Mrs. Paul's) fried, light	2½-oz. serving	230	20.0
CLAMATO COCKTAIL			
(Mott's)	6 fl. oz.	80	19.0
CLAM JUICE (Snow)	½ cup	15	1.2
CLARET WINE:			
(Gold Seal) 12% alcohol	3 fl. oz.	82	.4
(Taylor) 12.5% alcohol	3 fl. oz.	72	2.4

(USDA): United States Department of Agriculture
(HEW/FAO):   Health, Education and Welfare/Food and Agriculture
Organization
* Prepared as Package Directs

Food and Description	Measure or Quantity	Calories	Carbo-hydrates (grams)
CLORETS, gum or mint	1 piece	6	1.3
COBBLER, frozen (Weight Watchers)	4⅜-oz. serving	160	26.0
COCOA:			
Dry, unsweetened:			
(USDA):			
Low fat	1 T. (5 grams)	10	3.1
High fat	1 T. (5 grams)	14	2.8
(Hershey's) American process	1 T. (5 grams)	29	2.3
Mix, regular:			
(Alba '66) instant, all flavors	1 envelope	60	11.0
(Carnation) all flavors	1-oz. pkg.	110	23.0
(Hershey's):			
Hot	1 oz.	115	21.0
Instant	3 T. (.75 oz.)	76	17.0
(Nestlé) With or without mini marshmallows	1 oz.	120	22.0
(Ovaltine) hot'n rich	1 oz.	120	22.0
*Swiss Miss, regular or with mini marshmallows	6 fl. oz.	110	21.0
Mix, dietetic:			
(Carnation):			
70 Calorie	¾-oz. packet	70	15.0
Sugar free	.5-oz. envelope	50	8.0
*(Estee)	6 fl. oz.	50	9.0
*(Featherweight)	6 fl. oz.	50	8.0
(Ovaltine) reduced calorie	.45-oz. envelope	50	8.0
Swiss Miss, instant, lite	3 T.	70	17.0
COCOA KRISPIES, cereal (Kellogg's)	¾ cup (1 oz.)	110	25.0
COCOA PUFFS, cereal (General Mills)	1 cup (1 oz.)	110	25.0
COCONUT:			
Fresh (USDA):			
Whole	1 lb. (weighed in shell)	816	22.2
Meat only	4 oz.	392	10.7

Food and Description	Measure or Quantity	Calories	Carbo-hydrates (grams)
Grated or shredded, loosely packed	½ cup (1.4 oz.)	225	6.1
Dried, canned or packaged: (Baker's):			
Angel Flake:			
Packaged in bag	⅓ cup (.9 oz.)	118	10.6
Canned	⅓ (.9 oz.)	120	10.4
Cookie cut	⅓ (1.3 oz.)	186	17.1
Premium shred	⅓ cup (1 oz.)	138	12.4
Southern style	⅓ cup (.9 oz.)	118	10.3
(Durkee) shredded	¼ cup	69	2.0
COCO WHEATS, cereal	1 T. (12 grams)	44	9.3
COD:			
(USDA):			
Raw, meat only	4 oz.	88	0.
Broiled	4 oz.	193	0.
Dehydrated, lightly salted	4 oz.	425	0.
Frozen (Van de Kamp's)			
Today's Catch	4-oz. serving	80	0.
COFFEE:			
Regular:			
*Max-Pax; Maxwell House Electra Perk; Yuban, Yuban Electra Matic	6 fl. oz.	2	0.
*Mellow Roast	6 fl. oz.	8	2.0
Decaffeinated:			
*Brim, regular or electric perk	6 fl. oz.	2	0.
*Brim, freeze-dried; Decaf; Nescafe	6 fl. oz.	4	1.0
*Sanka, regular or electric perk	6 fl. oz.	2	0.
Instant:			
*Mellow Roast	6 fl. oz.	8	2.0
*Sunrise	6 fl. oz.	6	1.0

(USDA): United States Department of Agriculture
(HEW/FAO):   Health, Education and Welfare/Food and Agriculture
                        Organization
* Prepared as Package Directs

Food and Description	Measure or Quantity	Calories	Carbo-hydrates (grams)
*Mix (General Foods)			
International Coffee:			
Café Amaretto	6 fl. oz.	59	7.0
Café Français	6 fl. oz.	59	6.6
Café Vienna, Orange			
Capuccino	6 fl. oz.	65	10.3
Irish Mocha Mint	6 fl. oz.	55	7.4
Suisse Mocha	6 fl. oz.	58	7.6
COFFEE CAKE (See **CAKE,** Coffee)	1 fl. oz.	93	12.4
COFFEE LIQUEUR (DeKuyper)	1 fl. oz.	93	12.4
COFFEE SOUTHERN	1 fl. oz.	79	8.8
COLA SOFT DRINK (See **SOFT DRINK,** Cola)			
COLD DUCK WINE (Great Western) pink, 12% alcohol	3 fl. oz.	92	7.7
COLESLAW, solids & liq. (USDA):			
Prepared with commercial French dressing	4-oz. serving	108	8.6
Prepared with homemade French dressing	4-oz. serving	146	5.8
Prepared with mayonnaise	4-oz. serving	163	5.4
Prepared with mayonnaise type salad dressing	1 cup (4.2 oz.)	119	8.5
*****COLESLAW MIX** (Libby's)			
Super Slaw	½ cup	240	11.0
COLLARDS:			
Raw (USDA):			
Leaves, including stems	1 lb.	181	32.7
Leaves only	½ lb.	70	11.6
Boiled (USDA) drained:			
Leaves, cooked in large amount of water	½ cup (3.4 oz.)	29	4.6

Food and Description	Measure or Quantity	Calories	Carbo-hydrates (grams)
Leaves & stems, cooked in small amount of water	½ cup (3.4 oz.)	31	4.8
Canned (Sunshine) chopped, solids & liq.	½ cup (4.1 oz.)	25	3.8
Frozen, chopped:			
(Birds Eye)	⅓ pkg. (3.3 oz.)	31	4.4
(McKenzie)	⅓ pkg. (3.3 oz.)	25	4.0
(Southland)	⅕ of 16-oz. pkg.	30	5.0
COMPLETE CEREAL (Elam's)	1 oz.	109	17.5
CONCORD WINE (Gold Seal) 13–14% alcohol	3 fl. oz.	125	9.8
COOKIE, REGULAR:			
Almond Windmill (Nabisco)	1 piece (.3 oz.)	47	7.0
Animal:			
(USDA)	1 piece (3 grams)	11	2.1
(Dixie Belle)	1 piece (.7 oz.)	8	1.5
(Keebler):			
Regular	1 piece (.1 oz.)	12	1.9
Iced	1 piece	24	3.9
(Nabisco) *Barnum's Animals*	1 piece	12	1.9
(Ralston)	1 piece (2 grams)	8	1.5
Apple (Pepperidge Farm)	1 piece (.4 oz.)	50	7.6
Apple Crisp (Nabisco)	1 piece	50	7.0
Apple Spice (Pepperidge Farm)	1 piece (.4 oz.)	53	7.6
Apricot Raspberry (Pepperidge Farm)	1 piece (.4 oz.)	50	7.6
Assortment:			
(Nabisco) *Mayfair:*			
Crown creme sandwich	1 piece	53	8.0
Fancy shortbread biscuit	1 piece	22	3.3
Filigree creme sandwich	1 piece	60	8.5

(USDA): United States Department of Agriculture
(HEW/FAO):   Health, Education and Welfare/Food and Agriculture Organization
* Prepared as Package Directs

Food and Description	Measure or Quantity	Calories	'Carbo-hydrates (grams)
Mayfair creme sandwich	1 piece	65	9.0
Tea rose creme	1 piece	53	7.7
(Pepperidge Farm):			
Butter	1 piece	55	7.0
Champagne	1 piece	32	4.0
Chocolate lace & Pirouette	1 piece	37	7.0
Marseilles	1 piece	45	6.0
Seville	1 piece	55	6.5
Southport	1 piece	75	9.0
Bordeaux (Pepperidge Farm)	1 piece (7.1 grams)	33	5.3
Brown edge wafer (Nabisco)	1 piece (.2 oz.)	28	4.2
Brownie:			
(Hostess):			
Large	2-oz. piece	251	38.6
Small	1¼-oz. piece	157	24.1
(Pepperidge Farm):			
Chocolate nut	.4-oz. piece	57	6.3
Nut, large	.9-oz. piece	140	15.0
(Sara Lee) frozen	⅛ of 13-oz. pkg.	199	26.1
Brussles (Pepperidge Farm)	1 piece (10 grams)	53	6.6
Brussles Mint			
(Pepperidge Farm)	1 piece (.4 oz.)	67	8.3
Butter flavored (Nabisco)	1 piece (.2 oz.)	23	3.5
Buttercup (Keebler)	1 piece (5.1 grams)	24	3.7
Butterscotch chip (Nabisco)	1 piece (.5 oz.)	80	11.0
Cappucino (Pepperidge Farm)	(9 grams)	53	6.0
Capri (Pepperidge Farm)	1 piece (.5 oz.)	80	10.0
Caramel peanut log (Nabisco)			
Heyday	1 piece (.8 oz.)	120	13.0
Chessman (Pepperidge Farm)	1 piece (.3 oz.)	43	6.0
Chocolate & chocolate-covered:			
(Keebler) fridge covered			
fudge strips	1 piece (.4 oz.)	54	7.0
(Nabisco):			
Famous wafer	1 piece (.2 oz.)	28	4.6
Pinwheel, cake	1 piece (1.1 oz.)	140	21.0
Snap	1 piece (.14 oz.)	16	2.8
Chocolate chip:			
(Keebler):			
C.C. Biggs	1 piece (.4 oz.)	56	7.0
Rich'N Chips	1 piece	81	10.0

Food and Description	Measure or Quantity	Calories	Carbo- hydrates (grams)
(Nabisco):			
Chips Ahoy!	1 piece (.4 oz.)	53	7.0
Chocolate	1 piece (.4 oz.)	53	7.3
Coconut	1 piece (.5 oz.)	75	9.0
Cookie Little	1 piece (.05 oz.)	7	1.0
Snaps	1 piece (.2 oz.)	20	3.3
(Pepperidge Farm):			
Regular:			
Regular size	1 piece (.3 oz.)	50	6.7
Large size	1 piece (.9 oz.)	130	18.0
Chocolate	1 piece (.35 oz.)	53	6.3
Chocolate peanut bar (Nabisco)	1 piece (.6 oz.)	95	10.0
Cinnamon sugar (Pepperidge Farm)	1 piece (.4 oz.)	53	6.6
Cinnamon Treats (Nabisco)	1 piece (.2 oz.)	28	5.0
Coconut:			
(Keebler) chocolate drop	1 piece (.6 oz.)	83	9.4
(Nabisco) bar, *Bakers Bonus*	1 piece (.3 oz.)	43	5.3
Coconut Granola (Pepperidge Farm)	1 piece (.4 oz.)	57	6.7
Creme sticks (Dutch Twin) chocolate coated	1 piece (.3 oz.)	39	5.0
Date Nut Granola (Pepperidge Farm)	1 piece (.4 oz.)	53	6.7
Date Pecan (Pepperidge Farm)	1 piece (.4 oz.)	53	7.3
Devil's food cake (Nabisco)	1 piece (.7 oz.)	70	15.5
Double chip fudge (Nabisco)	1 piece (.5 oz.)	80	11.0
Fig bar:			
(Keebler)	1 piece (20 grams)	74	14.0
(Nabisco):			
Fig Newtons	1 piece (.6 oz.)	60	11.0
Fig Wheats	1 piece (.6 oz.)	60	11.5
Geneva (Pepperidge Farm)	1 piece (.4 oz.)	57	6.3
Gingerman (Pepperidge Farm)	1 piece (.24 oz.)	33	5.0
Gingersnaps (Nabisco) old fashioned	1 piece (.25 oz.)	30	5.5

(USDA): United States Department of Agriculture
(HEW/FAO): Health, Education and Welfare/Food and Agriculture Organization
* Prepared as Package Directs

Food and Description	Measure or Quantity	Calories	Carbo-hydrates (grams)
Granola (Pepperidge Farm) large	1 piece (.9 oz.)	120	16.0
Hazelnut (Pepperidge Farm)	1 piece (.4 oz.)	57	7.5
Ladyfinger (USDA)	3¼" × 1⅜" × 1⅛" (.4 oz.)	40	7.1
Lemon nut (Pepperidge Farm) large	1 piece (.9 oz.)	140	15.0
Lemon nut crunch (Pepperidge Farm)	1 piece (.4 oz.)	57	6.3
Lido (Pepperidge Farm)	1 piece (.6 oz.)	95	10.5
Macaroon (Nabisco) soft	1 piece (.7 oz.)	95	11.5
Marshmallow:			
(Nabisco):			
Mallomars	1 piece (.5 oz.)	60	8.5
Puffs, cocoa covered	1 piece (.7 oz.)	85	14.0
Sandwich	1 piece (.3 oz.)	30	5.7
Twirls cakes	1 piece (1 oz.)	130	20.0
(Planters) banana pie	1 oz.	127	22.0
Milano (Pepperidge Farm)	1 piece (.4 oz.)	60	7.0
Mint Milano			
(Pepperidge Farm)	1 piece (.5 oz.)	76	8.3
Molasses (Nabisco) *Pantry*	1 piece (.4 oz.)	60	9.5
Molasses Crisp			
(Pepperidge Farm)	1 piece (.2 oz.)	33	4.0
Nassau (Pepperidge Farm)	1 piece (.5 oz.)	85	9.0
Nilla wafer (Nabisco)	1 piece (.1 oz.)	19	3.0
Oatmeal:			
(Keebler) old fashioned	1 piece (18 grams)	83	12.0
(Nabisco):			
Bakers Bonus	1 piece (.6 oz.)	80	12.0
Cookie Little	1 piece (.1 oz.)	6	1.0
(Pepperidge Farm):			
Irish	1 piece (.3 oz.)	47	6.7
Large	1 piece (.9 oz.)	120	18.0
Raisin	1 piece (.4 oz.)	57	7.7
Orange Milano			
(Pepperidge Farm)	1 piece (.5 oz.)	76	8.3
Orleans (Pepperidge Farm)	1 piece (.2 oz.)	30	3.6
Orleans Sandwich			
(Pepperidge Farm)	1 piece (.3 oz.)	60	7.0

Food and Description	Measure or Quantity	Calories	Carbo-hydrates (grams)
Peanut & peanut butter:			
(Nabisco):			
Biscos	1 piece (.3 oz.)	47	5.7
Cheese flavored	1 piece (.25 oz.)	35	4.3
Chocolate	1 piece (.4 oz.)	57	7.3
Fudge	1 piece (.4 oz.)	50	6.7
Nutter Butter	1 piece (.5 oz.)	70	9.0
(Pepperidge Farm) chip:			
Regular	1 piece (10 grams)	53	6.3
Large	1 piece (25 grams)	130	16.0
Peanut brittle (Nabisco)	1 piece (.4 oz.)	50	6.3
Pecan Sandies (Keebler)	1 piece (16 grams)	86	9.3
Piccolo (Nabisco)	1 piece (.15 oz.)	22	6.3
Raisin (USDA)	1 oz.	107	22.9
Raisin fruit biscuit (Nabisco)	1 piece (.6 oz.)	60	12.0
Raisin bar (Keebler) iced	1 piece (16 grams)	80	11.0
Raisin Bran (Pepperidge Farm)	1 piece (.4 oz.)	53	6.7
Sandwich:			
(Keebler):			
Chocolate fudge	1 piece (17 grams)	83	12.0
Elfwich	1 piece (11 grams)	55	8.1
Fudge creme	1 piece (12 grams)	55	8.3
Peanut butter	1 piece (13 grams)	64	16.0
Pitter Patter	1 piece (17 grams)	83	11.0
Vanilla creme	1 piece (12 grams)	56	8.5
Vanilla, french	1 piece (17 grams)	83	12.0

(USDA): United States Department of Agriculture
(HEW/FAO): Health, Education and Welfare/Food and Agriculture Organization
* Prepared as Package Directs

Food and Description	Measure or Quantity	Calories	Carbo-hydrates (grams)
(Nabisco):			
Brown edge	1 piece (.6 oz.)	80	10.0
Cameo, creme	1 piece (.5 oz.)	70	10.5
Cheese flavored	1 piece (.2 oz.)	27	3.3
Gaity, fudge	1 piece (.4 oz.)	53	7.0
Mystic mint	1 piece (.6 oz.)	90	11.0
Oreo	1 piece (.4 oz.)	50	7.3
Oreo, double stuf	1 piece (.4 oz.)	70	9.0
Vanilla, *Cookie Break*	1 piece (.4 oz.)	50	7.3
Shortbread or shortcake:			
(Nabisco):			
Cookie Little	1 piece (.1 oz.)	7	1.1
Lorna Doone	1 piece (.3 oz.)	40	5.0
Melt-A-Way	1 piece (.4 oz.)	70	8.0
Pecan	1 piece (.5 oz.)	80	8.5
(Pepperidge Farm)	1 piece (.5 oz.)	75	8.5
Social Tea, biscuit (Nabisco)	1 piece	22	3.5
Spiced wafer (Nabisco)	1 piece (.3 oz.)	33	6.0
Spiced Windmill (Keebler)	1 piece (13 grams)	60	9.2
St. Moritz (Pepperidge Farm)	1 piece (.4 oz.)	57	6.6
Strawberry (Pepperidge Farm)	1 piece (.4 oz.)	50	7.6
Sugar:			
(Nabisco) rings, *Bakers Bonus*	1 piece (.5 oz.)	70	10.5
(Pepperidge Farm):			
Regular	1 piece (.4 oz.)	50	6.7
Large	1 piece (.9 oz.)	120	17.0
Sugar wafer:			
(Dutch Twin) any flavor	1 piece (.3 oz.)	36	4.7
(Keebler) *Krisp Kreem*	1 piece	29	4.2
(Nabisco) *Biscos*	1 piece (.1 oz.)	19	2.6
Sunflower Raisin (Pepperidge Farm)	1 piece (.4 oz.)	53	6.3
Tahiti (Pepperidge Farm)	1 piece (.5 oz.)	85	8.5
Vanilla wafer (Keebler)	1 piece (4 grams)	19	2.6
Waffle creme:			
(Dutch Twin)	1 piece (.3 oz.)	45	5.7
(Nabisco)	1 piece (.3 oz.)	43	6.0
Zanzibar (Pepperidge Farm)	1 piece (.3 oz.)	40	4.3

Food and Description	Measure or Quantity	Calories	Carbo-hydrates (grams)
COOKIE, DIETETIC (Estee):			
Chocolate chip, coconut or oatmeal raisin	1 piece	25	3.0
Sandwich duplex	1 piece (.3 oz.)	45	5.0
Vanilla, thin	1 piece (.2 oz.)	25	3.0
Wafer, chocolate covered	1 piece (.9 oz.)	120	14.0
COOKIE CRISP, cereal, any flavor	1 cup (1 oz.)	110	25.0
***COOKIE DOUGH:**			
Refrigerated (Pillsbury):			
Brownie, fudge	1 cookie	140	22.0
Chocolate chip or sugar	1 cookie	57	7.7
Double chocolate	1 cookie	50	7.7
Peanut butter	1 cookie	50	6.7
Frozen (Rich's):			
Chocolate chip	1 cookie	138	20.3
Oatmeal	1 cookie	125	18.3
Oatmeal & raisins	1 cookie	122	19.1
Peanut butter	1 cookie	128	14.6
Sugar	1 cookie	118	17.4
COOKIE, HOME RECIPE			
(USDA):			
Brownie with nuts	1¾″ × 1¾″ × ⅞″	97	10.2
Chocolate chip	1 oz.	146	17.0
Sugar, soft, thick	1 oz.	126	19.3
COOKIE MIX:			
Regular:			
Brownie:			
*(Betty Crocker):			
Fudge:			
Regular size	¹⁄₁₆ of pan	150	22.0
Family size	¹⁄₂₄ of pan	130	21.0
Supreme	¹⁄₂₄ of pan	120	21.0

(USDA): United States Department of Agriculture
(HEW/FAO):   Health, Education and Welfare/Food and Agriculture
Organization
* Prepared as Package Directs

Food and Description	Measure or Quantity	Calories	Carbo-hydrates (grams)
Walnut:			
Regular	1/16 of pan	160	22.0
Family size	1/24 of pan	130	19.0
(Duncan Hines)	1/24 of pan	129	19.4
(Nestlé)	1/24 of pkg.	150	22.0
(Pillsbury) fudge:			
Regular size	2″ sq. (1/16 pkg.)	150	23.0
Family size	2″ sq. (1/24 pkg.)	150	22.0
Chocolate (Duncan Hines) double	1/36 of pkg.	67	9.2
Chocolate chip:			
*(Betty Crocker)			
Big Batch	1 cookie	60	8.0
(Duncan Hines)	1/36 of pkg.	72	9.1
*(Nestlé)	1 cookie	60	7.5
*(Quaker)	1 cookie	75	8.5
Date bar (Betty Crocker)	1/24 of pkg.	80	10.0
Macaroon, coconut (Betty Crocker)	1/24 of pkg.	80	10.0
Oatmeal:			
*(Betty Crocker)			
Big Batch	1 cookie	65	8.5
(Duncan Hines)	1/36 of pkg.	68	9.1
*(Nestlé)	1 cookie	60	9.0
*(Quaker)	1 cookie	66	9.4
Peanut butter:			
(Duncan Hines)	1/36 pkg.	68	7.5
*(Nestlé)	1 cookie	65	7.5
*(Quaker)	1 cookie	75	8.0
Sugar:			
*(Betty Crocker)			
Big Batch	1 cookie	60	9.0
(Duncan Hines) golden	1/36 of pkg.	59	8.4
*(Nestlé)	1 cookie	65	8.5
*Vienna dream bar (Betty Crocker)	1/24 of pkg.	90	10.0
*Dietetic (Estee) brownie	2″×2″ sq. cookie	45	8.0
COOKING SPRAY, *Mazola No Stick*	2-second spray	8	0.
CORIANDER SEED (French's)	1 tsp. (1.4 grams)	6	.8

Food and Description	Measure or Quantity	Calories	Carbo-hydrates (grams)
CORN:			
Fresh, white or yellow (USDA):			
Raw:			
Untrimmed, on the cob	1 lb. (weighed in husk)	167	36.1
Trimmed, on cob	1 lb. (husk removed)	240	55.1
Boiled:			
Kernels, cut from cob, drained	1 cup (5.8 oz.)	137	31.0
Whole	4.9-oz. ear (5" × 1¾")	70	16.2
Trimmed, on the cob	5" × 1¾" ear	70	16.2
Canned, regular pack:			
(USDA):			
Golden or yellow, whole kernel, solids & liq., vacuum pack	½ cup (3.7 oz.)	87	21.6
Golden or yellow, whole kernel, wet pack	½ cup (4.5 oz.)	84	20.1
Golden or yellow, whole kernel, drained solids, wet pack	½ cup (3 oz.)	72	16.4
White kernel, drained solids	½ cup (2.8 oz.)	70	16.4
White, whole kernel, drained liq., wet pack	4 oz.	29	7.8
Cream style	½ cup (4.4 oz.)	105	25.6
(Del Monte) solids & liq.:			
Cream style, golden,	½ cup (4 oz.)	80	18.0
Cream style, white	½ cup (4 oz.)	90	21.0
Whole kernel, golden or white	½ cup	70	17.0
Whole kernel, vacuum pack	½ cup	90	22.0
(Green Giant) solids & liq.:			
Cream style	4¼ oz.	100	21.0

(USDA): United States Department of Agriculture
(HEW/FAO):   Health, Education and Welfare/Food and Agriculture
                        Organization
* Prepared as Package Directs

Food and Description	Measure or Quantity	Calories	Carbo-hydrates (grams)
Whole kernel or shoe peg, golden	4¼ oz.	90	18.0
Whole kernel, vacuum pack	3½ oz.	90	20.0
Whole kernel, *Mexicorn*	3½ oz.	80	18.0
Whole kernel, white, vacuum pack	4 oz.	105	23.3
(Le Sueur) whole kernel, solids & liq.	4¼ oz.	80	18.0
(Libby's) cream style	½ cup (4.3 oz.)	100	21.2
(Stokely-Van Camp) solids & liq.:			
Cream style, golden	½ cup (4.5 oz.)	105	23.5
Cream style, white	½ cup (4.6 oz.)	110	24.5
Whole kernel, golden	½ cup	90	19.5
Canned, dietetic pack, solids & liq.:			
(Del Monte) No Salt Added:			
Cream style	½ cup	80	20.0
Whole kernel:			
Regular	½ cup (4.3 oz.)	80	18.0
Vacuum pack	½ cup (4 oz.)	90	22.0
(Diet Delight) whole kernel	½ cup	60	15.0
(Featherweight) whole kernel	½ cup (4 oz.)	80	16.0
(S&W) *Nutradiet*, whole kernel, green label	½ cup	100	21.0
Frozen:			
(Birds Eye):			
On the cob:			
Farmside	4.4-oz. ear	140	28.7
Little Ears	2.3-oz. ear	73	15.0
Natural ears	5¾-oz. ear	183	37.6
Whole kernel	⅓ of 10-oz. pkg.	98	17.3
With butter sauce	⅓ of 10-oz. pkg.	98	17.3
(Green Giant):			
On the cob:			
Nibbler	2.7-oz. ear	80	16.0
Niblet Ear	4.9-oz. ear	140	30.0
Cream style	½ cup	120	25.0
Whole kernel, *Niblets*:			
In butter sauce	½ cup	100	18.0
In cream sauce	½ cup	130	18.0

Food and Description	Measure or Quantity	Calories	Carbo-hydrates (grams)
Harvest Fresh	½ cup	100	22.0
Polybag	½ cup	80	16.0
(McKenzie):			
On the cob	5″ ear (4.4 oz.)	120	29.0
Whole kernel	3.3 oz.	80	19.0
(Seabrook Farms):			
On the cob	5″ ear	140	30.0
Whole kernel	⅓ of 10-oz. pkg.	97	19.9

CORNBREAD:
Home recipe (USDA):

Corn pone, prepared with white, whole-ground cornmeal	4 oz.	231	41.1
Johnnycake, prepared with yellow, degermed cornmeal	4 oz.	303	51.6
Southern style, prepared with degermed cornmeal	2½″ × 2½″ × 1⅝″ piece	186	28.8
Southern style, prepared with whole-ground cornmeal	4 oz.	235	33.0
Spoon bread, prepared with white, whole-ground cornmeal	4 oz.	221	19.2
*Mix:			
(Aunt Jemima)	⅙ of pkg.	220	34.0
(Dromedary)	2″ × 2″ piece (1 1/16 of pkg.)	130	19.0
(Pillsbury) *Ballard*	⅛ of recipe	140	25.0

*CORN DOGS, frozen:

(Hormel)	1 piece	220	21.0
(Oscar Mayer)	1 piece (4 oz.)	328	27.9

CORNED BEEF:

Cooked (USDA), boneless, medium fat	4-oz. serving	422	0.

(USDA): United States Department of Agriculture
(HEW/FAO): Health, Education and Welfare/Food and Agriculture Organization
* Prepared as Package Directs

Food and Description	Measure or Quantity	Calories	Carbo-hydrates (grams)
Canned, regular pack:			
Dinty Moore (Hormel)	2-oz. serving	130	0.
(Libby's)	⅓ of 7-oz. can	160	2.0
Canned, dietetic			
(Featherweight) loaf	2½-oz. serving	90	0.
Packaged (Eckrich) sliced	1-oz. slice	40	1.0
CORNED BEEF HASH, CANNED:			
(Libby's)	⅓ of 24-oz. can	420	21.0
Mary Kitchen (Hormel):			
Regular	½ of 15-oz. can	360	19.0
Short Orders	7½-oz. can	360	17.0
CORNED BEEF HASH DINNER, frozen (Banquet)	10-oz. dinner	372	421.6
CORNED BEEF SPREAD, canned:			
(Hormel)	1 oz.	70	0.
(Underwood)	½ of 4½-oz. can	120	Tr.
CORN FLAKE CRUMBS (Kellogg's)	¼ cup (1 oz.)	110	25.0
CORN FLAKES, cereal:			
(General Mills) *Country*	1 cup (1 oz.)	110	25.0
(Kellogg's):			
Regular	1 cup (1 oz.)	110	25.0
Banana Frosted Flakes	⅔ cup (1 oz.)	110	25.0
Honey & Nut	¾ cup (1 oz.)	120	24.0
Sugar Frosted Flakes	¾ cup (1 oz.)	110	26.0
(Ralston Purina):			
Regular	1 cup (1 oz.)	110	25.0
Sugar Frosted	¾ cup (1 oz.)	110	26.0
CORNMEAL, WHITE or YELLOW:			
Dry:			
Bolted:			
(USDA)	1 cup (4.3 oz.)	442	90.9
(Aunt Jemima/Quaker)	1 cup (4 oz.)	408	84.8

Food and Description	Measure or Quantity	Calories	Carbo- hydrates (grams)
Degermed:			
(USDA)	1 cup (4.9 oz.)	502	108.2
(Aunt Jemima/Quaker)	1 cup (4 oz.)	404	88.8
Self-rising degermed:			
(USDA)	1 cup (5 oz.)	491	105.9
(Aunt Jemima)	1 cup (6 oz.)	582	126.0
Self-rising, whole ground			
(USDA)	1 cup (5 oz.)	489	101.4
Whole ground, unbolted			
(USDA)	1 cup (4.3 oz.)	433	90.0
Cooked:			
(USDA)	1 cup (8.5 oz.)	120	25.7
(Albers) degermed	1 cup	119	25.5
Mix (Aunt Jemima/Quaker)			
bolted	1 cup (4 oz.)	392	80.4
CORN PUDDING, home recipe			
(USDA)	1 cup (8.6 oz.)	255	31.9
CORNSTARCH (Argo; Kingsford's; Duryea)	1 tsp. (8 grams)	10	8.3
CORN SYRUP (See **SYRUP,** Corn)			
COTTAGE PUDDING, home recipe (USDA):			
Without sauce	2 oz.	195	30.8
With chocolate sauce	2 oz.	180	32.1
With strawberry sauce	2 oz.	166	27.4
COUGH DROP:			
(Beech-Nut)	1 drop	10	2.5
(Pine Bros.)	1 drop	8	2.0
COUNT CHOCULA, cereal			
(General Mills)	1 oz. (1 cup)	110	24.0

(USDA): United States Department of Agriculture
(HEW/FAO):   Health, Education and Welfare/Food and Agriculture
                        Organization
* Prepared as Package Directs

Food and Description	Measure or Quantity	Calories	Carbo-hydrates (grams)
COWPEA (USDA):			
Immature seeds:			
Raw, whole	1 lb. (weighed in pods)	317	54.4
Raw, shelled	½ cup (2.5 oz.)	92	15.8
Boiled, drained solids	½ cup (2.9 oz.)	89	15.0
Canned, solids & liq.	4 oz.	79	14.1
Frozen, (See **BLACK-EYED PEAS,** frozen)			
Young pods with seeds:			
Raw, whole	1 lb. (weighed untrimmed)	182	39.2
Boiled, drained solids	4 oz.	39	7.9
Mature seeds, dry:			
Raw	1 lb.	1556	279.9
Raw	½ cup (3 oz.)	292	52.4
Boiled	½ cup (4.4 oz.)	95	17.2
CRAB:			
Fresh, steamed (USDA):			
Whole	½ lb. (weighed in shell)	202	1.1
Meat only	4 oz.	105	.6
Canned, drained (USDA)	4 oz.	115	1.2
Frozen (Wakefield's)	4 oz.	86	.7
CRAB APPLE, flesh only (USDA)	¼ lb.	71	20.2
CRAB APPLE JELLY (Smucker's)	1 T. (.7 oz.)	53	13.5
CRAB, DEVILED:			
frozen (Mrs. Paul's) breaded & fried	½ of 6-oz. pkg.	170	20.0
Home recipe (USDA)	4 oz.	213	15.1
CRAB IMPERIAL, home recipe (USDA)	1 cup (7.8 oz.)	323	8.6
CRACKER, PUFFS & CHIPS:			
American Harvest (Nabisco)	1 piece (3.2 grams)	16	2.0

Food and Description	Measure or Quantity	Calories	Carbo-hydrates (grams)
Arrowroot biscuit (Nabisco)	1 piece (.2 oz.)	20	3.5
Bacon'n Dip (Nabisco)	1 piece (.1 oz.)	9	.9
Bacon-flavored thins (Nabisco)	1 piece (.1 oz.)	11	1.2
Bacon Nips	1 oz.	147	15.6
Bacon toast (Keebler)	1 piece (3.2 grams)	16	2.0
Biscos (Nabisco)	1 piece (.13. oz.)	19	2.6
Bran wafer (Featherweight)	1 piece	13	2.0
Bugles (General Mills)	1 oz.	150	18.0
Cheese flavored:			
Bops (Nally's)	1 oz.	147	13.6
Cheddar triangles (Nabisco)	1 piece (.1 oz.)	9	.9
Cheese'n Crunch (Nabisco)	1 oz.	160	14.0
Chee-Tos, cruncy or puffy	1 oz.	160	15.0
Cheez Balls (Planters)	1 oz.	160	15.0
Cheez Curls (Planters)	1 oz.	160	15.0
Country cheddar'n sesame (Nabisco)	1 piece (.1 oz.)	9	1.0
Curl (Featherweight)	1 oz.	150	16.0
Dip In A Chip (Nabisco)	1 piece (.1 oz.)	10	1.1
(Dixie Belle)	1 piece	6	.7
Nacho cheese cracker (Keebler)	1 piece (.04 oz.)	11	1.6
Nips (Nabisco)	1 piece (.04 oz.)	5	.7
(Ralston)	1 piece (1.1 grams)	6	.7
Swiss cheese (Nabisco)	1 piece (.1 oz.)	10	1.1
Tid-Bit (Nabisco)	1 piece	5	.5
Chicken in a Biskit (Nabisco)	1 piece (.1 oz.)	11	1.1
Chippers (Nabisco)	1 piece (.1 oz.)	15	1.7
Chipsters (Nabisco)	1 piece (.02 oz.)	2	.3
Club cracker (Keebler)	1 piece (3.2 grams)	15	2.1
Corn chips:			
(Bachman) regular or BBQ	1 oz.	150	15.0
(Featherweight) low sodium	1 oz.	170	15.0
Fritos:			
Regular	1 oz.	160	16.0
Barbecue flavor	1 oz.	150	15.5

(USDA): United States Department of Agriculture
(HEW/FAO):   Health, Education and Welfare/Food and Agriculture
              Organization
* Prepared as Package Directs

Food and Description	Measure or Quantity	Calories	Carbo-hydrates (grams)
Corn & Sesame Chips			
(Nabisco)	1 piece (.1 oz.)	10	.9
Creme Wafer Stick (Nabisco)	1 piece (.3 oz.)	47	6.3
Crown Pilot (Nabisco)	1 piece (.6 oz.)	75	13.0
Diggers (Nabisco)	1 piece (.03 oz.)	4	.5
Dixies (Nabisco)	1 piece	8	.9
Doo Dads (Nabisco)	1 piece	2	.3
English Water Biscuit (Pepperidge Farm)	1 piece (.1 oz.)	17	3.1
Escort (Nabisco)	1 piece (.1 oz.)	21	2.6
Flings (Nabisco)	1 piece (.1 oz.)	10	.9
Goldfish (Pepperidge Farm):			
Thins	1 piece (.1 oz.)	10	1.1
Tiny	1 piece (.02 oz.)	3	.4
Graham:			
(Dixie Belle) sugar-honey coated	1 piece	15	2.6
Flavor Kist (Schulze and Burch) sugar-honey coated	1 double cracker	57	10.0
Honey Maid (Nabisco)	1 piece (.25 oz.)	30	5.5
Party Graham (Nabisco)	1 piece	47	6.0
(Ralston) sugar-honey coated	1 piece	15	2.6
Graham, chocolate or cocoa-covered:			
Fancy Dip (Nabisco)	1 piece	65	8.0
(Keebler) deluxe	1 piece (.3 oz.)	43	5.6
(Nabisco)	1 piece (.4 oz.)	57	7.0
Korkers (Nabisco)	1 piece	8	.8
Meal Mates (Nabisco)	1 piece	22	3.2
Melba Toast (See **MELBA TOAST**)			
Milk Lunch Biscuit (Keebler)	1 piece	27	4.5
Mucho Macho Nacho, Flavor Kist (Schulze and Burch)	1 oz.	121	18.0
Onion:			
(Keebler) toast	1 piece	15	2.1
(Nabisco) french	1 piece	13	
Oyster:			
(Dixie Belle)	1 piece (.03 oz.)	4	.6
(Keebler) *Zesta*	1 piece	2	.3
(Nabisco) *Dandy* or *Oysterettes*	1 piece (.03 oz.)	3	.5

Food and Description	Measure or Quantity	Calories	Carbo-hydrates (grams)
(Ralston)	1 piece	4	.6
Pumpernickel Toast (Keebler)	1 piece	15	2.1
Ritz (Nabisco)	1 piece (.1 oz.)	17	2.0
Rich & Crisp, (Dixie Bell; Ralston)	1 piece	14	1.9
Roman Meal Wafer, boxed	1 piece	11	1.3
Royal Lunch (Nabisco)	1 piece	55	8.0
Rusk, *Holland* (Nabisco)	1 piece (.35 oz.)	40	7.5
Rye toast (Keebler)	1 piece	16	2.1
RyKrisp:			
Natural	1 triple cracker	25	5.0
Seasoned or sesame	1 triple cracker	30	4.5
Saltine:			
(Dixie Belle) regular or unsalted	1 piece (.1 oz.)	12	2.0
Flavor Kist (Schulze and Burch)	1 piece	12	2.0
Premium (Nabisco)	1 piece (.1 oz.)	12	2.0
(Ralston) regular or unsalted	1 piece	12	2.0
Zesta (Keebler)	1 piece	13	2.1
Sea Rounds (Nabisco)	1 piece (.4 oz.)	45	7.5
Sea Toast (Keebler)	1 piece	60	10.0
Sesame:			
Butter flavored (Nabisco)	1 piece	17	1.9
(Pepperidge Farm)	1 piece	23	3.0
Sesame Wheats! (Nabisco)	1 piece	17	1.8
Toast (Keebler)	1 piece	15	2.0
Sesame & poppyseed (Keebler)	1 piece	12	1.5
Shindigs (Keebler)	1 piece	6	.9
Snackers (Dixie Bell; Ralston)	1 piece	17	2.2
Snackin' Crisp (Durkee)			
O & C	1 oz.	155	15.0
Snacks Ahoy (Nabisco)	1 piece (.1 oz.)	9	1.1
Snacks Sticks (Pepperidge Farm):			
Cheese	1 piece	17	2.3
Lightly salted, pumpernickel, rye & sesame	1 piece	16	2.5
Parmesan pretzel	1 piece	15	2.6

(USDA): United States Department of Agriculture
(HEW/FAO): Health, Education and Welfare/Food and Agriculture Organization
* Prepared as Package Directs

Food and Description	Measure or Quantity	Calories	Carbo-hydrates (grams)
Sociables (Nabisco)	1 piece	11	1.3
Soda (Nabisco) *Gitana*	1 piece	15	2.5
Table Water Cracker (Carr's):			
Small	1 piece (.12 oz.)	15	2.6
Large	1 piece (3 oz.)	32	5.9
Tortillo chips:			
(Bachman) nacho, taco flavor or toasted	1 oz.	140	17.0
Buenos (Nabisco)	1 piece	11	1.2
Doritos, nacho or taco	1 oz.	140	18.0
(Nabisco) regular and nacho	1 piece	11	1.3
Town House Cracker (Keebler)	1 piece (3.1 grams)	16	1.8
Triscuit (Nabisco)	1 piece (.2 oz.)	20	3.0
Twiddle Sticks (Nabisco)	1 piece	53	7.0
Twigs (Nabisco)	1 piece (.1 oz.)	14	1.6
Uneeda Biscuit (Nabisco)	1 piece	22	3.7
Unsalted:			
(Estee)	1 piece (.1 oz.)	15	2.5
(Featherweight)	2 sections (½ cracker)	30	5.0
Vegetable thins (Nabisco)	1 piece	12	1.3
Waldorf (Keebler)	1 piece	14	2.3
Waverly Wafer (Nabisco)	1 piece	18	2.6
Wheat (Pepperidge Farm) cracked or hearty	1 piece (.2 oz.)	28	3.6
Wheat Chips (Nabisco)	1 piece (.3 oz.)	4	.5
Wheat Crisps (Keebler)	1 piece (3 grams)	13	1.7
Wheatmeal Biscuit (Carr's):			
Small	1 piece (.03 oz.)	42	5.9
Large	1 piece (.5 oz.)	66	8.4
Wheat Snack (Dixie Belle)	1 piece	9	1.2
Wheatsworth (Nabisco)	1 piece	14	1.8
Wheat Thins (Nabisco)	1 piece (.1 oz.)	10	1.2
Wheat Toast (Keebler)	1 piece (3.2 grams)	15	2.0
Wheat wafer:			
(Estee) 6 *Calories*	1 piece	6	1.0
(Featherweight) unsalted	1 piece	13	2.3
CRACKER CRUMBS, graham (Nabisco)	⅛ of 9″ pie shell	70	12.0

Food and Description	Measure or Quantity	Calories	Carbo-hydrates (grams)
CRACKER MEAL (USDA)	3 oz.	373	60.0
CRANAPPLE JUICE (Ocean Spray) canned:			
Regular	6 fl. oz.	129	32.1
Dietetic	6 fl. oz.	32	7.4
CRANBERRY, fresh (Ocean Spray)	½ cup (2 oz.)	26	6.1
CRANBERRY JUICE COCKTAIL: Canned (Ocean Spray):			
Regular	6 fl. oz. (6.5 oz.)	106	26.4
Dietetic	6 fl. oz. (6.3 oz.)	36	8.3
*Frozen (Welch's)	6 fl. oz.	100	26.0
CRANBERRY-ORANGE RELISH (Ocean Spray)	2 oz.	104	25.8
CRANBERRY-RASPBERRY SAUCE (Ocean Spray) jellied	2 oz.	89	20.8
CRANBERRY SAUCE: Home recipe (USDA)			
sweetened, unstrained	4 oz.	202	51.6
Canned (Ocean Spray):			
Jellied	2 oz.	88	21.7
Whole berry	2 oz.	89	22.0
CRANGRAPE (Ocean Spray)	6 fl. oz.	108	26.2
CRANICOT (Ocean Spray)	6 fl. oz.	120	30.0
CRANTASTIC JUICE DRINK, canned (Ocean Spray)	6 fl. oz.	110	27.0

(USDA): United States Department of Agriculture
(HEW/FAO): Health, Education and Welfare/Food and Agriculture Organization
* Prepared as Package Directs

Food and Description	Measure or Quantity	Calories	Carbo-hydrates (grams)
CRAZY COW, cereal			
(General Mills)	1 cup (1 oz.)	110	25.0
CREAM:			
Half & Half (Dairylea)	1 fl. oz.	40	1.0
Light, table or coffee (Sealtest)			
16% fat	1 T.	26	.6
Light, whipping, 30% fat			
(Sealtest)	1 T. (.5 oz.)	45	1.0
Heavy whipping (Dairylea)	1 fl. oz.	60	1.0
Sour (Dairylea)	1 fl. oz.	60	1.0
Sour, imitation (Pet)	1 T. (.5 oz.)	25	1.0
Substitute (See **CREAM SUBSTITUTE)**			
CREAM PUFFS:			
Home recipe (USDA) custard filling	3½″ × 2″ piece	303	26.7
Frozen (Rich's):			
Bavarian	1⅓-oz. piece	145	17.4
Chocolate	1⅓-oz. piece	146	16.9
CREAMSICLE (Popsicle Industries)	2½-fl.-oz. piece	80	13.0
CREAM SUBSTITUTE:			
Coffee Mate (Carnation)	1 tsp.	11	1.1
Coffee Rich (Rich's)	½ oz.	22	2.1
Dairy Light (Alba)	2.8-oz. envelope	10	1.0
N-Rich	3-gram packet	16	1.6
(Pet)	1 tsp.	10	1.0
CREAM, OF WHEAT, cereal:			
Regular	1 T.	40	8.8
Instant	1 T.	40	8.8
*Mix'n Eat:			
Regular	1-oz. packet	140	24.0
Baked apple & cinnamon	1.25-oz. packet	170	32.0
Banana & spice	1.25-oz. packet	170	32.0
Maple & brown sugar	1.25-oz. packet	170	32.0
Quick	1 T.	40	8.8

Food and Description	Measure or Quantity	Calories	Carbo-hydrates (grams)
CREME DE BANANA			
LIQUEUR (Mr. Boston) 27% alcohol	1 fl. oz.	93	12.0
CREME DE CACAO:			
(Hiram Walker) (54 proof)	1 fl. oz.	104	15.0
(Mr. Boston) 27% alcohol:			
Brown	1 fl. oz.	102	14.3
White	1 fl. oz.	93	12.0
CREME DE CASSIS			
(Mr. Boston) 17½% alcohol	1 fl. oz.	85	14.1
CREME DE MENTHE:			
(De Kuyper)	1 fl. oz.	94	11.3
(Mr. Boston) 27% alcohol:			
Green	1 fl. oz.	109	16.0
White	1 fl. oz.	97	13.0
CREME DE NOYAUX			
(Mr. Boston) 27% alcohol	1 fl. oz.	99	13.5
CREPE, frozen:			
(Mrs. Paul's):			
Crab	5½-oz. pkg.	248	24.6
Shrimp	5½-oz. pkg.	252	23.8
(Stouffer's):			
Chicken with mushroom sauce	8¼-oz. pkg.	390	19.0
Ham & asparagus	6¼-oz. pkg.	325	21.0
Ham & swiss cheese with cheddar cheese sauce	7½-oz. pkg.	410	23.0
Spinach with cheddar cheese sauce	9½-oz. pkg.	415	30.0
CRISP RICE CEREAL:			
(Featherweight) low sodium	1 cup (1 oz.)	110	26.0
(Ralston Purina)	1 cup (1 oz.)	110	25.0

(USDA): United States Department of Agriculture
(HEW/FAO):   Health, Education and Welfare/Food and Agriculture
                        Organization
* Prepared as Package Directs

Food and Description	Measure or Quantity	Calories	Carbo-hydrates (grams)
CRISPY WHEATS'N RAISINS, cereal (General Mills)	¾ cup (1 oz.)	110	23.0
CROAKER (USDA):			
Atlantic:			
Raw, whole	1 lb. (weighed whole)	148	0.
Raw, meat only	4 oz.	109	0.
Baked	4 oz.	151	0.
White, raw meat only	4 oz.	95	0.
Yellowfin, raw, meat only	4 oz.	101	0.
CROUTON:			
(Arnold):			
Bavarian or English style	½ oz.	65	9.5
French, Italian or Mexican style	½ oz.	66	8.7
(Kellogg's) *Croutettes*	⅔ cup (.7 oz.)	70	14.0
(Pepperidge Farm):			
Cheddar & romano	.5 oz.	60	10.0
Cheese & garlic, onion & garlic, seasoned or sour cream & chive	.5 oz.	70	9.0
C-3PO'S, cereal (Kellogg's)	¾ cup (1 oz.)	110	24.0
CUCUMBER (USDA):			
Eaten with skin	8-oz. cucumber (weighed whole)	32	7.4
Pared	7½″ × 2″ pared (7.3 oz.)	29	6.6
Pared	3 slices (.9 oz.)	4	.5
CUMIN SEED (French's)	1 tsp.	7	.7
CUPCAKE:			
Home recipe (USDA):			
Without icing	1.4-oz. cupcake	146	22.4
With chocolate icing	1.8-oz. cupcake	184	29.7
With boiled white icing	1.8-oz. cupcake	176	30.9
With uncooked white icing	1.8-oz. cupcake	184	31.6

Food and Description	Measure or Quantity	Calories	Carbo-hydrates (grams)
Regular (Hostess):			
Chocolate	1 cupcake (1¾ oz.)	166	29.8
Orange	1 cupcake (1½ oz.)	151	26.8
Frozen (Sara Lee) yellow	1 cupcake (1¾ oz.)	190	31.5
*CUPCAKE MIX (Flako)	1 cupcake	150	25.0
CUP O'NOODLES (Nissin Foods):			
Beef	2½-oz. serving	343	39.2
Beef, twin pack	1.2-oz. serving	151	18.2
Beef onion	2½-oz. serving	323	36.8
Beef onion, twin pack	1.2-oz. serving	158	19.4
Chicken	2½-oz. serving	343	40.0
Chicken, twin pack	1.2-oz. serving	155	18.6
Pork	2½-oz. serving	331	40.7
Shrimp	2½-oz. serving	336	40.0
CURACAO LIQUEUR:			
(Bols)	1 fl. oz.	105	10.3
(Hiram Walker)	1 fl. oz.	96	11.8
CURRANT:			
Fresh (USDA):			
Black European:			
Whole	1 lb. (weighed with stems)	240	58.2
Stems removed	4 oz.	61	14.9
Red and white:			
Whole	1 lb. (weighed with stems)	220	53.2
Stems removed	1 cup (3.9 oz.)	55	13.3
Dried:			
(Del Monte) Zante	½ cup (2.4 oz.)	200	53.0
(Sun-Maid)	½ cup	220	53.0

(USDA): United States Department of Agriculture
(HEW/FAO): Health, Education and Welfare/Food and Agriculture Organization
* Prepared as Package Directs

Food and Description	Measure or Quantity	Calories	Carbo-hydrates (grams)
CUSTARD:			
Home recipe (USDA)	½ cup (4.7 oz.)	152	14.7
Chilled, *Swiss Miss,* chocolate or egg flavor	4-oz. container	150	22.0
*Mix, dietetic (Featherweight)	½ cup	80	15.0
C.W. Post, cereal:			
Plain	¼ cup (1 oz.)	131	20.3
With raisins	¼ cup	128	20.4

Food and Description	Measure or Quantity	Calories	Carbo-hydrates (grams)

D

DAIRY QUEEN/BRAZIER:

Food and Description	Measure or Quantity	Calories	Carbo-hydrates (grams)
Banana split	13.5-oz. serving	540	103.0
Brownie Delight, hot fudge	9.4-oz. serving	600	85.0
Buster Bar	5¼-oz. piece	460	41.0
Chicken sandwich	7.8-oz. sandwich	670	46.0
Cone:			
Plain, any flavor:			
Small	3-oz. cone	140	22.0
Regular	5-oz. cone	240	38.0
Large	7½-oz. cone	340	57.0
Dipped, chocolate:			
Small	3¼-oz. cone	190	25.0
Regular	5½-oz. cone	340	42.0
Large	8¼-oz. cone	510	64.0
Dilly Bar	3-oz. piece	210	21.0
Double Delight	9-oz. serving	490	69.0
DQ Sandwich	2.1-oz. sandwich	140	24.0
Fish sandwich:			
Plain	6-oz. sandwich	400	41.0
With cheese	6¼-oz. sandwich	440	39.0
Float	14-oz. serving	410	82.0
Freeze, vanilla	12-oz. serving	500	89.0
French fries:			
Regular	2½-oz. serving	200	25.0
Large	4-oz. serving	320	40.0
Frozen desert	4-oz. serving	180	27.0
Hamburger:			
Plain:			
Single	5.2-oz. burger	360	33.0
Double	7.4-oz. burger	530	33.0
Triple	9.6-oz. burger	710	33.0

(USDA): United States Department of Agriculture
(HEW/FAO):   Health, Education and Welfare/Food and Agriculture
                        Organization
* Prepared as Package Directs

Food and Description	Measure or Quantity	Calories	Carbo-hydrates (grams)
With cheese:			
Single	5.7-oz. burger	410	33.0
Double	8.4-oz. burger	650	34.0
Triple	10.63-oz. burger	820	34.0
Hot dog:			
Regular:			
Plain	3.5-oz. serving	280	21.0
With cheese	4-oz. serving	330	21.0
With chili	4½-oz. serving	320	23.0
Super:			
Plain	6.2-oz. serving	520	44.0
With cheese	6.9-oz. serving	580	45.0
With chili	7.7-oz. serving	570	47.0
Malt, chocolate:			
Small	10¼-oz. serving	520	91.0
Regular	14¾-oz. serving	760	134.0
Large	20¾-oz. serving	1060	187.0
Mr. Misty:			
Plain:			
Small	8¼-oz. serving	190	48.0
Regular	11.64-oz. serving	250	63.0
Large	15½-oz. serving	340	84.0
Kiss	3.14-oz. serving	70	17.0
Float	14.5-oz. serving	390	74.0
Freeze	14.5-oz. serving	500	94.0
Onion rings	3-oz. serving	280	31.0
Parfait	10-oz. serving	430	76.0
Peanut Butter Parfait	10¾-oz. serving	750	94.0
Shake, chocolate:			
Small	10¼-oz. serving	490	82.0
Regular	14¾-oz. serving	710	120.0
Large	20¾-oz. serving	990	168.0
Strawberry shortcake	11-oz. serving	540	100.0
Sundae, chocolate:			
Small	3¾-oz. serving	190	33.0
Regular	6¼-oz. serving	310	56.0
Large	8¾-oz. serving	440	78.0
Tomato	½ oz.	4	1.0
DAIQUIRI COCKTAIL			
(Mr. Boston):			
Regular, 12% alcohol	3 fl. oz.	99	9.0
Strawberry, 12½% alcohol	3 fl. oz.	111	12.0

Food and Description	Measure or Quantity	Calories	Carbo-hydrates (grams)
DAMSON PLUM (See **PLUM**)			
DANDELION GREENS, raw (USDA):			
Trimmed	1 lb.	204	41.7
Boiled, drained	½ cup (3.2 oz.)	30	5.8
DATE, dry:			
Domestic:			
(USDA):			
With Pits	1 lb. (weighed with pits)	1081	287.7
Without pits	4 oz.	311	82.7
Without pits chopped	1 cup (6.1 oz.)	477	126.8
(Dromedary):			
Without pits	1 date	20	4.6
Without pits, chopped	¼ cup (1¼ oz.)	130	31.0
Imported (Bordo) Iraq:			
With pits	4 average dates (.9 oz.)	73	18.2
Without pits, chopped	½ cup (2 oz.)	159	39.8
DE CHAUNAC WINE			
(Great Western) 12% alcohol	3 fl. oz.	71	2.4
DELI'S, frozen			
(Pepperidge Farm):			
Beef with barbecue sauce	4-oz. piece	270	30.0
Mexican style	4-oz. piece	280	27.0
Pizza style	4-oz. piece	290	29.0
Reuben in rye pastry	4-oz. piece	360	25.0
Savory chicken salad	4-oz. piece	340	26.0
Scrambled eggs, bacon & cheese	3½-oz. piece	290	25.0
Sliced beef with brown sauce	4-oz. piece	270	27.0
Turkey, ham & cheese	4-oz. piece	270	24.0
Western style omelet	4-oz. piece	290	27.0

(USDA): United States Department of Agriculture
(HEW/FAO):   Health, Education and Welfare/Food and Agriculture
                       Organization
* Prepared as Package Directs

Food and Description	Measure or Quantity	Calories	Carbo-hydrates (grams)
DESSERT CUPS (Hostess)	¾-oz. piece	62	13.8
DILL SEED (French's)	1 tsp. (2.1 grams)	9	1.2
DING DONG (Hostess)	1 cake (1⅓ oz.)	172	21.5
DINNER, FROZEN (See individual listings such as BEEF, CHICKEN, TURKEY, etc.)			
DIP:			
Avocado (Nalley's)	1 oz.	114	.9
Barbecue (Nalley's)	1 oz.	114	1.1
Blue cheese:			
(Dean) tang	1 oz.	61	2.3
(Nalley's)	1 oz.	110	.9
Clam (Nalley's)	1 oz.	101	1.1
Endhilada, *Fritos*	1 oz.	37	3.9
Guacamole (Nalley's)	1 oz.	114	.9
Jalapeno:			
Fritos	1 oz.	34	3.7
(Hain) natural	1 oz.	40	2.5
Onion bean (Hain) natural	1 oz.	41	3.6
DISTILLED LIQUOR, any brand:			
80 proof	1 fl. oz.	65	Tr.
86 proof	1 fl. oz.	70	Tr.
90 proof	1 fl. oz.	74	Tr.
94 proof	1 fl. oz.	77	Tr.
100 proof	1 fl. oz.	83	Tr.
DONUTZ, cereal (General Mills):			
Chocolate flavor	1 cup (1 oz.)	120	23.0
Powdered sugar	1 cup (1 oz.)	120	22.0
DOUGHNUT (See also *WINCHELL'S*): (USDA):			
Cake type	1.1-oz. piece	125	16.4
Yeast leavened	2-oz. piece	235	21.4

Food and Description	Measure or Quantity	Calories	Carbo-hydrates (grams)
Regular (Hostess):			
Chocolate coated	1-oz. piece	137	13.6
Cinnamon	1-oz. piece	114	14.5
Donettes:			
Frosted	1 piece	58	6.0
Powdered	1 piece	39	5.0
Krunch	1-oz. piece	103	15.6
Old fashioned:			
Plain	1.5-oz. piece	179	23.0
Glazed	2-oz. piece	239	30.7
Plain	1-oz. piece	120	12.8
Powdered	1-oz. piece	120	15.1
Frozen (Morton):			
Regular:			
Bavarian creme	2-oz. piece	180	22.0
Boston creme	2⅓-oz. piece	210	28.0
Chocolate iced	1.5-oz. piece	150	20.0
Glazed	1.5-oz. piece	150	19.0
Jelly	1.8-oz. piece	180	23.0
Mini	1.1-oz. piece	120	16.0
Donut Holes	⅕ of 7¾-oz. pkg.	160	21.0
Morning Light:			
Chocolate	2-oz. piece	200	26.0
Glazed	2-oz. piece	200	26.0
Jelly	2.6-oz. piece	250	33.0
DRAMBUIE (Hiram Walker) (80 proof)	1 fl. oz.	110	11.0
DRUMSTICK, frozen:			
Ice Cream, in a cone:			
Topped with peanuts	1 piece	181	22.7
Topped with peanuts & cone bisque	1 piece	168	23.6
Ice Milk, in a cone:			
Topped with peanuts	1 piece	163	24.3
Topped with peanuts & cone bisque	1 piece	150	25.2

(USDA): United States Department of Agriculture
(HEW/FAO):   Health, Education and Welfare/Food and Agriculture
                        Organization
* Prepared as Package Directs

Food and Description	Measure or Quantity	Calories	Carbo-hydrates (grams)
DUCK, raw (USDA):			
Domesticated:			
Ready-to-cook	1 lb. (weighed with bone)	1213	0.
Meat only	4 oz.	187	0.
Wild:			
Dressed	1 lb. (weighed dressed)	613	0.
Meat only	4 oz.	156	0.
DUMPLINGS, stuffed, canned, dietetic:			
(Dia-Mel)	8 oz. serving	160	15.0
(Featherweight)	7½-oz. serving	160	18.0

Food and Description	Measure or Quantity	Calories	Carbo-hydrates (grams)

E

ECLAIR:

Home recipe (USDA), with custard filling and chocolate

icing	4-oz. piece	271	26.3
Frozen (Rich's) chocolate	1 piece (2.6 oz.)	234	30.0

EEL (USDA):

Raw, meat only	4 oz.	264	0.
Smoked, meat only	4 oz.	374	0.

EGG (USDA) (See also **EGG SUBSTITUTE**):

Chicken:

Raw:

White only	1 large egg (1.2 oz.)	17	.3
White only	1 cup (9 oz.)	130	2.0
Yolk only	1 large egg (.6 oz.)	59	.1
Yolk only	1 cup (8.5 oz.)	835	1.4
Whole, small	1 egg (1.3 oz.)	60	.3
Whole, medium	1 egg (1.5 oz.)	71	.4
Whole, large	1 egg (1.8 oz.)	81	.4
Whole	1 cup (8.8 oz.)	409	2.3
Whole, extra large	1 egg (2. oz.)	94	.5
Whole, jumbo	1 egg (2.3 oz.)	105	.6

Cooked:

Boiled	1 large egg (1.8 oz.)	81	.4
Fried in butter	1 large egg	99	.1

(USDA): United States Department of Agriculture

(HEW/FAO):   Health, Education and Welfare/Food and Agriculture Organization

* Prepared as Package Directs

Food and Description	Measure or Quantity	Calories	Carbo-hydrates (grams)
Omelet, mixed with milk and cooked in fat	1 large egg	107	1.5
Poached	1 large egg	78	.4
Scrambled, mixed with milk & cooked in fat	1 large egg	111	1.5
Scrambled, mixed with milk & cooked in fat	1 cup (7.8 oz.)	381	5.3
Dried:			
Whole	1 cup (3.8 oz.)	639	4.4
White, powder	1 oz.	105	1.6
Yolk	1 cup (3.4 oz.)	637	2.4
Duck, raw	1 egg (2.8 oz.)	153	.6
Goose, raw	1 egg (5.8 oz.)	303	2.1
Turkey, raw	1 egg (3.1 oz.)	150	1.5
EGG MIX (Durkee):			
Omelet:			
*With bacon	½ of pkg.	310	10.0
*Puffy	½ of pkg.	302	10.5
Scrambled:			
Plain	.8-oz. pkg.	124	4.0
With bacon	1.3-oz. pkg.	181	6.0
EGG NOG, dairy (Meadow Gold) 6% fat	½ cup	164	25.5
EGG NOG COCKTAIL (Mr. Boston) 15% alcohol	3 fl. oz.	180	18.9
EGGPLANT:			
Raw (USDA) whole	1 lb. (weighed whole)	92	20.6
Boiled (USDA) drained, diced	1 cup (7.1 oz.)	38	8.2
Frozen:			
(Mrs. Paul's):			
Parmesan	5½-oz. serving	270	20.0
Sticks, breaded & fried	3½-oz. serving	262	27.3
(Weight Watchers) parmigiana	13-oz. pkg.	285	25.0
EGG ROLL, frozen (La Choy):			
Chicken	.4-oz. roll	30	4.0

Food and Description	Measure or Quantity	Calories	Carbo- hydrates (grams)
Lobster	.4-oz. roll	27	4.3
Meat & shrimp	.25-oz. roll	7	2.5
Meat & shrimp	.4-oz. roll	27	4.0
Shrimp	.4-oz. roll	27	4.3
Shrimp	3-oz. roll	160	24.0
EGG ROLL DINNER, frozen (Van de Kamp's) Cantonese	10½-oz. serving	550	64.0
EGG, SCRAMBLED, FROZEN (Swanson) and sausage, with hashed brown potatoes, *TV Brand*	6½-oz. entree	430	17.0
EGG SUBSTITUTE:			
Egg Magic (Featherweight)	½ of envelope	60	1.0
Scramblers (Morningstar Farms)	1 egg substitute	35	1.5
Second Nature (Avoset)	3 T.	42	2.0
ELDERBERRY, fresh (USDA):			
Whole	1 lb. (weighed with stems)	307	69.9
Stems removed	4 oz.	82	18.6
ENCHILADA OR ENCHILADA DINNER, frozen:			
Beef:			
(Banquet):			
Buffet Supper	2-lb. pkg.	1056	148.0
Cookin' Bag	6-oz. pkg.	215	34.0
Dinner, International Favorites	12-oz. dinner	497	72.0
(Green Giant) Sonora style	12-oz. entree	700	48.0
(Hormel)	1 enchilada	140	17.0
(Morton)	11-oz. dinner	280	44.0

(USDA): United States Department of Agriculture
(HEW/FAO): Health, Education and Welfare/Food and Agriculture
Organization
* Prepared as Package Directs

Food and Description	Measure or Quantity	Calories	Carbo-hydrates (grams)
(Swanson) *TV Brand*	15-oz. dinner	570	72.0
(Van de Kamp's) dinner	12-oz. dinner	390	45.0
Cheese:			
(Banquet):			
Extra Helping	21¼-oz. dinner	777	105.0
International Favorites	12-oz. dinner	543	71.0
(Hormel)	1 enchilada	151	18.0
(Van de Kamp's):			
Dinner	12-oz. dinner	450	44.0
Entree	7½-oz. pkg.	270	23.0
Entree, Ranchero	5½-oz. serving	252	22.0
Chicken (Van de Kamp's):			
Regular	7½-oz. pkg.	250	24.0
Suiza	5½-oz. serving	230	21.0
ENCHILADA SAUCE:			
Canned:			
(Del Monte) hot or mild	½ cup (4 oz.)	45	11.0
Old El Paso:			
Green chili	1 oz.	7	1.7
Hot	1 oz.	14	2.0
Mild	1 oz.	13	1.7
Mix:			
*(Durkee)	½ cup	29	6.2
(French's)	1⅜-oz. pkg.	120	20.0
ENDIVE, CURLY raw (USDA):			
Untrimmed	1 lb. (weighed untrimmed)	80	16.4
Trimmed	½ lb.	45	9.3
Cut up or shredded	1 cup (2.5 oz.)	14	2.9
ESCAROLE, raw (USDA):			
Untrimmed	1 lb. (weighed untrimmed)	80	16.4
Trimmed	½ lb.	46	9.2
Cut up or shredded	1 cup (2.5 oz.)	14	2.9
EULACHON or SMELT, raw (USDA) meat only	4 oz.	134	0.

Food and Description	Measure or Quantity	Calories	Carbo-hydrates (grams)
EXPRESSO COFFEE LIQUEUR (Mr. Boston) 26½% alcohol	1 fl. oz.	104	15.0

(USDA): United States Department of Agriculture
(HEW/FAO):   Health, Education and Welfare/Food and Agriculture
                          Organization
* Prepared as Package Directs

Food and Description	Measure or Quantity	Calories	Carbo-hydrates (grams)

F

FARINA:
(H-O) dry, regular	1 T. (.4 oz.)	40	8.5
Malt-O-Meal, dry:			
Regular	1 oz.	96	21.0
Quick cooking	1 oz.	100	22.2
*(Pillsbury) made with water and salt	⅔ cup	80	17.0

FAT, COOKING:
(USDA):			
Lard	1 T. (.5 oz.)	115	0.
Vegetable oil	1 T. (1.4 oz.)	106	0.
Crisco:			
Regular	1 T. (.4 oz.)	110	0.
Butter flavor	1 T. (.5 oz.)	126	0.
(Mrs. Tucker's)	1 T.	120	0.
Spry	1 T. (.4 oz.)	94	0.

FENNEL SEED (French's)
	1 tsp. (2.1 grams)	8	1.3

FETTUCINI ALFREDO, frozen
(Stouffer's)	½ of 10 oz. pkg.	270	19.0

FIG:
Fresh (USDA):			
Regular size	1 lb.	363	92.1
Small	1.3-oz. fig (1½″ dia.)	30	7.7
Candied (Bama)	1 T. (.7 oz.)	37	9.6
Canned, regular pack, solids & liq.:			
(USDA):			
Light syrup	4 oz.	74	19.1
Heavy Syrup	3 figs & 2 T. syrup (4 oz.)	96	24.9

Food and Description	Measure or Quantity	Calories	Carbo-hydrates (grams)
Heavy syrup	½ cup (4.4 oz.)	106	27.5
Extra heavy syrup	4 oz.	117	30.3
(Del Monte) whole	½ cup (4.3 oz.)	100	28.0
Canned, unsweetened or dietetic, solids & liq.:			
(USDA) water pack	4 oz.	54	14.1
(Diet Delight) Kadota	½ cup (4.4 oz.)	76	18.2
(Featherweight) Kadota water pack	½ cup	60	15.0
Dried (Sun-Maid):			
Calimyrna	½ cup (3.5 oz.)	250	58.0
Mission, regular or figlets	½ cup (3 oz.)	210	50.0
FIG JUICE (Sunsweet)	6 fl. oz.	120	30.0
FIGURINES (Pillsbury) all flavors	1 bar	138	10.5
FILBERT:			
(USDA):			
Whole	1 lb. (weighed in shell)	1323	34.9
Shelled	1 oz.	180	4.7
(Fisher) oil dipped, salted	½ cup (2 oz.)	360	5.4
FISH CAKE:			
Home recipe (USDA)	2 oz.	98	5.3
Frozen (Mrs. Paul's):			
Breaded & fried	2-oz. piece	110	12.0
Beach Hanen	2-oz. piece	115	12.0
Thins, breaded & fried	½ of 10-oz. pkg.	300	25.0
FISH & CHIPS, frozen:			
(Banquet) *Man-Pleaser*	14-oz. dinner	769	97.0
(Mrs. Paul's) batter fried	½ of 14-oz. pkg.	366	43.3
(Swanson):			
Hungry Man	15¾-oz. dinner	820	87.0

(USDA): United States Department of Agriculture
(HEW/FAO):   Health, Education and Welfare/Food and Agriculture
                        Organization
* Prepared as Package Directs

Food and Description	Measure or Quantity	Calories	Carbo-hydrates (grams)
TV Brand:			
Dinner	10¼-oz. dinner	460	43.0
Entree	5-oz. entree	300	30.0
(Van de Kamp's) batter dipped, french fried	8-oz. pkg.	500	45.0
FISH DINNER, frozen:			
(Banquet)	8¾-oz. dinner	553	45.0
(Morton)	9-oz. dinner	260	22.0
(Mrs. Paul's) parmesan	½ of 10-oz. pkg.	220	16.0
(Stouffer's) *Lean Cuisine:*			
Filet, divan	12⅜-oz. pkg.	270	16.0
Florentine	9-oz. pkg.	230	13.0
(Weight Watchers):			
Au gratin, 2-compartment meal	9¼-oz. meal	200	14.0
Italian style, 2-compartment meal	9 oz. meal	180	6.0
Oven fried, 2-compartment meal	6¾-oz. meal	220	8.0
FISH FILLET, frozen:			
(Mrs. Paul's):			
Batter fried, light:			
Crunchy	2¼-oz. piece	155	13.5
Supreme	3⅝-oz. piece	220	19.0
Breaded & fried:			
Crispy, crunchy	2.1-oz. piece	145	11.0
Light & natural	6-oz. serving	290	21.0
Buttered	2½-oz. serving	105	0.
(Van de Kamp's):			
Batter dipped, french fried:			
Regular	3-oz. piece	220	12.5
Country seasoned	2.4-oz. piece	180	10.5
Light & crispy	¾-oz. piece	58	4.2
Today's Catch	4-oz. serving	90	0.
FISH KABOBS, frozen:			
(Mrs. Paul's) batter fried, supreme light	⅓ of 10-oz. pkg.	200	17.7
(Van de Kamp's) batter dipped, french fried	.4-oz. piece	26	1.6

Food and Description	Measure or Quantity	Calories	Carbo-hydrates (grams)
FISH LOAF, Home recipe (USDA)	4 oz.	141	8.3
FISH SEASONING (Featherweight) dietetic	¼ tsp.	Tr.	Tr.
FISH STICK, frozen:			
(Mrs. Paul's):			
Batter fried, light & crunchy	1 piece (.9 oz.)	60	5.3
Breaded & fried, crispy	1 piece (¾ oz.)	50	4.2
(Van de Kamp's) batter dipped, french fried:			
Regular	1-oz. piece	58	5.2
Light & crispy	¾-oz. piece	57	4.2
FIT'N FROSTY (Alba '77):			
Chocolate	¾-oz. envelope	74	11.5
Chocolate & marshmallow	1 envelope	70	11.05
Strawberry	¾-oz. envelope	74	12.0
Vanilla	¾-oz. envelope	69	11.3
FIVE ALIVE (Snow Crop)	6 fl. oz.	85	20.8
FLOUNDER:			
Raw (USDA):			
Whole	1 lb. (weighed whole)	118	0.
Meat only	4 oz.	90	0.
Baked (USDA)	4 oz.	229	0.
Frozen:			
(Mrs. Paul's) fillets:			
Breaded & fried	3-oz. piece	140	9.5
Batter fried, crunchy, light	2¼-oz. piece	155	13.0
(Van de Kamp's) _Today's Catch_	4 oz.	80	0.
(Weight Watchers) with lemon flavored bread crumbs	6½-oz. serving	134	12.0

(USDA): United States Department of Agriculture
(HEW/FAO):   Health, Education and Welfare/Food and Agriculture
            Organization
* Prepared as Package Directs

Food and Description	Measure or Quantity	Calories	Carbo-hydrates (grams)
FLOUR:			
(USDA)			
Buckwheat, dark, sifted	1 cup (3.5 oz.)	326	70.6
Buckwheat, light sifted	1 cup (3.5 oz.)	340	77.9
Cake:			
Unsifted, dipped	1 cup (4.2 oz.)	433	94.5
Unsifted, spooned	1 cup (3.9 oz.)	404	88.1
Carob or St. John's bread	1 oz.	51	22.9
Chestnut	1 oz.	103	21.6
Corn	1 cup (3.9)	405	84.5
Cottonseed	1 oz.	101	9.4
Fish, from whole fish	1 oz.	95	0.
Lima bean	1 oz.	95	17.9
Potato	1 oz.	100	22.7
Rice, stirred spooned	1 cup (5.6 oz.)	574	125.6
Rye:			
Light:			
Unsifted, spooned	1 cup (3.6 oz.)	361	78.7
Sifted, spooned	1 cup (3.1 oz.)	314	68.6
Medium:	1 oz.	99	21.1
Dark:			
Unstirred	1 cup (4.5 oz.)	419	87.2
Stirred	1 cup (4.5 oz.)	415	86.5
Soybean, defatted, stirred	1 cup (3.6 oz.)	329	38.5
Soybean, high fat	1 oz.	108	9.4
Sunflower seed, partially defatted	1 oz.	96	10.7
Wheat:			
All-purpose:			
Unsifted, dipped	1 cup (5 oz.)	521	108.8
Unsifted, spooned	1 cup (4.4 oz.)	459	95.9
Sifted, spooned	1 cup (4.1 oz.)	422	88.3
Bread:			
Unsifted, dipped	1 cup (4.8 oz.)	496	101.6
Unsifted, spooned	1 cup (4.3 oz.)	449	91.9
Sifted, spooned	1 cup (4.1 oz.)	427	87.4
Gluten:			
Unsifted, dipped	1 cup (5 oz.)	537	67.0
Sifted, spooned	1 cup (4.8 oz.)	514	64.2
Self-rising:			
Unsifted, dipped	1 cup (4.6 oz.)	458	96.5
Sifted, spooned	1 cup (3.7 oz.)	373	78.7

Food and Description	Measure or Quantity	Calories	Carbo-hydrates (grams)
Whole wheat	1 oz.	94	20.1
(Aunt Jemima) self-rising	¼ cup (1 oz.)	109	23.6
Ballard:			
Self-rising	¼ cup	91	23.6
All-purpose	¼ cup (1 oz.)	100	21.8
Bisquick (Betty Crocker)	¼ cup (1 oz.)	120	19.0
(Drifted Snow)	¼ cup	100	21.8
(Elam's):			
Brown rice, whole grain, sodium & gluton free	¼ cup (1.2 oz.)	125	.2
Buckwheat, pure	¼ cup (¼ oz.)	131	27.2
Pastry, whole wheat	¼ cup (1.2 oz.)	122	24.9
Rye, whole grain	¼ cup	118	24.2
Soy, roasted, defatted	¼ cup (1.1 oz.)	108	9.8
3-in-1 mix	1 oz.	99	20.0
White, with wheat germ	¼ cup (1 oz.)	101	20.7
Whole wheat	¼ cup (1.1 oz.)	111	21.7
(Featherweight):			
Gluton	¼ cup	105	13.7
Soy	¼ cup	117	8.4
Gold Medal (Betty Crocker):			
All purpose or unbleached	¼ cup (1 oz.)	100	21.8
Better For Bread	¼ cup	100	20.7
Self-rising	¼ cup	95	20.8
Whole wheat	¼ cup	98	19.5
La Pina	¼ cup	100	21.8
Pillsbury's Best:			
All-purpose or rye and wheat Bohemian style	¼ cup	100	21.5
Bread or rye, medium	1.4 cup	100	20.8
Sauce & gravy	2 T.	50	11.0
Self-rising	¼ cup	95	21.0
Whole wheat	¼ cup	100	21.0
Presto, self-rising	¼ cup (1 oz.)	98	21.6
Red Band:			
All purpose or unbleached	¼ cup	100	21.8
Self-rising	¼ cup	95	20.8
Wondra	¼ cup	100	21.8

(USDA): United States Department of Agriculture
(HEW/FAO): Health, Education and Welfare/Food and Agriculture Organization
* Prepared as Package Directs

Food and Description	Measure or Quantity	Calories	Carbo-hydrates (grams)
FOLLE BLANC WINE (Louis M. Martini) 12.5% alcohol	3 fl. oz.	63	.2
FOOD STICKS (Pillsbury) chocolate	1 piece	45	
FRANKEN*BERRY, cereal (General Mills)	1 cup (1 oz.)	110	24.0
FRANKFURTER, raw or cooked: (USDA): Raw:			
All kinds	1 frankfurter (10 per lb.)	140	.8
Meat	1 frankfurter (10 per lb.)	134	1.1
With cereal	1 frankfurter (10 per lb.)	112	<.1
Cooked, all kinds	1 frankfurter (10 per lb.)	136	.7
(Eckrich): Beef	1.2-oz. frankfurter	110	2.0
Beef	1.6-oz. frankfurter	150	3.0
Beef	2-oz. frankfurter	190	3.0
Cheese	2-oz. frankfurter	190	3.0
Meat	1.2-oz. frankfurter	120	2.0
Meat	1.6-oz. frankfurter	150	3.0
Meat	2.-oz. frankfurter	190	3.0
(Hormel): Beef	1 frankfurter (12-oz. pkg.)	100	1.0
Beef	1 frankfurter (1 lb. pkg.)	140	1.0
Meat	1 frankfurter (12-oz. pkg.)	110	1.0
Meat	1 frankfurter (1-lb. pkg.)	140	1.0

Food and Description	Measure or Quantity	Calories	Carbo-hydrates (grams)
Range Brand Wrangler, smoked:	1 frankfurter	170	1.0
Beef	1 frankfurter	170	2.0
Cheese	1 frankfurter	180	1.0
(Hygrade) beef, Ball Park	2-oz. frankfurter	169	Tr.
(Louis Rich):			
Turkey	1.5-oz. frankfurter	95	1.0
Turkey	1.6-oz. frankfurter	100	1.0
Turkey	2.-oz. frankfurter	125	1.0
(Oscar Mayer):			
Beef:			
Regular	1.6-oz. frankfurter	145	.9
Jumbo	2-oz. frankfurter	183	1.2
Big One	4-oz. frankfurter	366	2.4
Little Wiener	2″ frankfurter	30	.2
Wiener	1.2-oz. frankfurter	109	.6
Wiener	1.6-oz. frankfurter	145	.8
Wiener	2-oz. frankfurter	183	1.0
Wiener	2.7-oz. frankfurter	244	1.4
Wiener	4-oz. frankfurter	363	2.0
Wiener, with cheese	1.6-oz. frankfurter	146	.7
(Swift)	1.6-oz. frankfurter	150	1.2
FRANKS-N-BLANKETS, frozen (Durkee)	1 piece	45	1.0
FRENCH TOAST, frozen:			
(Aunt Jemima):			
Regular	1 slice (1½ oz.)	85	13.2
Cinnamon swirl	1 slice (1½ oz.)	97	13.6

(USDA): United States Department of Agriculture
(HEW/FAO):   Health, Education and Welfare/Food and Agriculture
                      Organization
* Prepared as Package Directs

Food and Description	Measure or Quantity	Calories	Carbohydrates (grams)
(Swanson) with sausage, TV Brand	4½-oz. pkg.	270	28.0
FRITTERS:			
Home recipe (USDA):			
Clam	2″ × 1¾″ (1.4 oz.)	124	12.4
Corn	2″ × 1½″ (1.2 oz.)	132	13.9
Frozen (Mrs. Paul's):			
Apple	2-oz. piece	140	16.5
Corn	2-oz. piece	125	15.0
FROG LEGS, raw (USDA):			
Bone-in	1 lb. (weighed with bone)	215	0.
Meat only	4 oz.	83	0.
FROOT LOOPS, cereal (Kellogg's)	1 cup (1 oz.)	110	25.0
FROSTED RICE, cereal (Ralston Purina)	1 cup (1 oz.)	110	26.0
FROSTS (Libby's):			
Dry:			
Banana	.5 oz.	50	14.0
Orange, strawberry or pineapple	.5 oz.	60	16.0
Liquid:			
Banana	7 fl. oz.	120	25.0
Orange	8 fl. oz.	120	29.0
Pineapple	6 fl. oz.	110	22.0
Strawberry	8 fl. oz.	120	21.0
FROZEN DESSERT, dietetic:			
(Baskin-Robbins) *Special Diet:*			
Mountain Coffee	1 scoop (2½ fl. oz.)	90	16.8
Sunny Orange	1 scoop (2½ fl. oz.)	90	16.4
Wild Strawberry	1 scoop (2½ fl. oz.)	83	16.0

Food and Description	Measure or Quantity	Calories	Carbo-hydrates (grams)
Good Humor:			
Bar, vanilla, with chocolate icing	2½-fl.-oz. bar	90	12.0
Cup, vanilla & chocolate (SugarLo) ice cream or ice milk, all flavors	5-fl.-oz. cup	100	17.0
	¼ pt. (2.6 fl. oz.)	135	14.0
FRUIT BITS, dried (Sun-Maid)	1 oz.	90	21.0
FRUIT COCKTAIL:			
Canned, regular pack, solids & liq.: (USDA):			
Light syrup	4 oz.	68	17.8
Heavy syrup	½ cup (4.5 oz.)	97	25.2
Extra syrup	4 oz.	104	26.9
(Del Monte) regular or chunky	½ cup (4½ oz.)	80	23.0
(Libby's) heavy syrup	½ cup (4½ oz.)	101	24.7
(Stokely-Van Camp)	½ cup (4½ oz.)	95	23.0
Canned, dietetic or low calorie, solids & liq.:			
(Del Monte) Lite, syrup pack, regular or chunky	½ cup (4¼ oz.)	50	14.0
(Diet Delight):			
Juice pack	½ cup (4.4 oz.)	50	14.0
Water pack	½ cup (4.3 oz.)	40	10.0
(Featherweight):			
Juice pack	½ cup (4 oz.)	50	12.0
Water pack	½ cup (4 oz.)	40	10.0
(Libby's) Lite water pack	½ cup (4.4 oz.)	50	13.0
(S&W) *Nutradiet* white or blue label	½ cup	40	10.0
***FRUIT COUNTRY** (Comstock):*			
Apple	¼ of pkg.	160	36.0

(USDA): United States Department of Agriculture
(HEW/FAO):   Health, Education and Welfare/Food and Agriculture
        Organization
* Prepared as Package Directs

Food and Description	Measure or Quantity	Calories	Carbo-hydrates (grams)
Blueberry	¼ of pkg.	160	33.0
Cherry	¼ of pkg.	180	38.0
Peach	¼ of pkg.	130	28.0
FRUIT CUP (Del Monte) solids & liq.:			
Mixed fruits	5-oz. container	110	26.7
Peach cling, diced	5-oz. container	116	27.8
FRUIT & FIBER CEREAL (Post)	½ cup (1 oz.)	103	22.3
FRUIT JUICE, canned (Sun-Maid):			
Golden	6 fl. oz.	100	23.0
Purple	6 fl. oz.	100	25.0
Red	6 fl. oz.	100	24.0
FRUIT, MIXED:			
Canned, solids & liq.:			
(Del Monte) Lite, chunky	½ cup	58	14.0
(Libby's) Lite, chunky	½ cup (4.4 oz.)	50	13.0
Dried:			
(Del Monte)	2 oz.	130	34.0
(Sun-Maid/Sunsweet)	2 oz.	150	39.0
Frozen (Birds Eye) quick thaw	5-oz. serving	150	35.8
FRUIT PUNCH:			
Canned:			
Capri Sun, natural	6¾ fl. oz.	102	25.9
(Hi-C)	6 fl. oz.	93	23.0
(Lincoln) party	6 fl. oz.	100	25.0
Chilled:			
Five Alive (Snow Crop)	6 fl. oz.	87	22.7
(Minute Maid)	6 fl. oz.	93	23.0
*Frozen, *Five Alive* (Snow Crop)	6 fl. oz.	87	22.7
*Mix:			
Regular (Hi-C)	6 fl. oz.	72	18.0
Dietetic, *Crystal Light*	6 fl. oz. (6.3 oz.)	2	.1
FRUIT ROLL, frozen (La Choy)	.5-oz. roll	38	6.4

Food and Description	Measure or Quantity	Calories	Carbo- hydrates (grams)
FRUIT ROLL-UPS			
(Betty Crocker)	1 piece (.5 oz.)	50	12.0
FRUIT SALAD:			
Canned, regular pack, solids & liq.:			
(USDA):			
Light syrup	4 oz.	67	17.6
Heavy syrup	½ cup (4.3 oz.)	85	22.0
Extra heavy syrup	4 oz.	102	26.5
(Del Monte) fruits for salad:			
Regular	½ cup (4¼ oz.)	90	22.0
Tropical	½ cup (4 oz.)	90	26.0
(Libby's) heavy syrup	½ cup (4.4 oz.)	99	24.0
Canned, dietetic or low calorie, solids & liq.:			
(Diet Delight) juice pack	½ cup (4.4 oz.)	60	16.0
(S&W) *Nutradiet:*			
Juice pack, white label	½ cup	50	11.0
Water pack, blue label	½ cup	35	10.0
FRUIT SQUARES, frozen			
(Pepperidge Farm):			
Apple	2½-oz. piece	230	27.0
Blueberry or cherry	2½-oz. piece	230	29.0
***FUDGE JUMBLES** (Pillsbury):			
Brown sugar oatmeal	1 bar	100	15.0
Chocolate chip oatmeal, coconut oatmeal or peanut butter oatmeal	1 bar	100	15.0
FUDGSICLE (Popsicle Industries)	2½-fl.-oz. bar	100	23.0

(USDA): United States Department of Agriculture
(HEW/FAO):   Health, Education and Welfare/Food and Agriculture
                      Organization
* Prepared as Package Directs

Food and Description	Measure or Quantity	Calories	Carbo-hydrates (grams)

G

GARLIC:
  Raw (USDA):

Whole	2 oz. (weighed with skin)	68	15.4
Peeled	1 oz.	39	8.7
Flakes (Gilroy)	1 tsp.	13	2.6
Powder (French's)	1 tsp.	10	2.0
Salt (French's)	1 tsp.	4	1.0

GEFILTE FISH, canned:
  (Mother's):

Jellied, old world	4-oz. serving	70	7.0
Jellied, white fish & pike	4-oz. serving	60	4.0
In liquid broth	4-oz. serving	70	7.0
(Rokeach):			
Jelled	4-oz. serving	60	4.0
Jelled, whitefish & pike	4-oz. serving	50	4.0
Natural broth	4-oz. serving	60	4.0
Old Vienna	4-oz. serving	70	8.0

GELATIN, unflavored dry:

(USDA)	7-gram envelope	23	0.
Carmel Kosher	7-gram envelope	30	0.
(Knox)	1 envelope	25	0.

GELATIN DESSERT:

Canned, dietetic (Dia-Mel; Louis Sherry)	4-oz. container	2	Tr.
*Powder:			
Regular:			
Carmel Kosher, all flavors	½ cup (4 oz.)	80	20.0
(Jell-O) all flavors	½ cup (4.9 oz.)	83	18.6
(Royal) all flavors	½ cup (4.9 oz.)	80	19.0
Dietetic:			
Carmel Kosher, all flavors	½ cup	8	0.
(Dia-Mel) all flavors	½ cup (4.2 oz.)	8	Tr.

Food and Description	Measure or Quantity	Calories	Carbo-hydrates (grams)
(D-Zerta) all flavors	½ cup (4.3 oz.)	7	.1
(Estee) all flavors	½ cup	8	Tr.
(Featherweight):			
Regular	½ cup	10	1.0
Artificially sweetened	½ cup	10	0.
(Jell-O) sugar free:			
Cherry	½ cup (4.3 oz.)	12	.1
Lime	½ cup	9	.1
Orange, raspberry or			
strawberry	½ cup	8	.1
(Louis Sherry)	½ cup	8	Tr.
GELATIN, DRINKING			
(Knox) orange	1 envelope	70	10.0
GERMAN STYLE DINNER,			
frozen (Swanson) *TV Brand*	11¾-oz. dinner	370	36.0
GIN, unflavored (See			
DISTILLED LIQUOR)			
GIN, SLOE:			
(DeKuyper)	1 fl. oz.	70	5.2
(Mr. Boston)	1 fl. oz.	68	4.7
GINGER, powder (French's)	1 tsp.	6	1.2
GINGERBREAD MIX:			
(Betty Crocker)	⅑ of cake	210	35.0
(Dromedary)	2″ × 2″ square (¹⁄₁₆ of pkg.)	100	20.0
(Pillsbury)	3″ square (⅑ of cake)	190	36.0
GOLDEN GRAHAMS, cereal			
(General Mills)	¾ cup (1 oz.)	110	24.0

(USDA): United States Department of Agriculture
(HEW/FAO):   Health, Education and Welfare/Food and Agriculture
            Organization
* Prepared as Package Directs

Food and Description	Measure or Quantity	Calories	Carbo-hydrates (grams)
GOOBER GRAPE (Smucker's)	1 oz.	125	14.0
GOOD HUMOR (See **ICE CREAM**)			
GOOD N' PUDDIN (Popsicle Industries) all flavors	2 ⅓-fl.-oz. bar	170	27.0
GOOSE, domesticates (USDA):			
Raw	1 lb. (weighed ready-to-cook)	1172	0.
Roasted:			
Meat & skin	4 oz.	500	0.
Meat only	4 oz.	264	0.
GOOSEBERRY (USDA):			
Fresh	1 lb.	177	44.0
Fresh	1 cup (5.3 oz.)	58	14.6
Canned, water pack, solids & liq.	4 oz.	29	7.5
GOOSE GIZZARD, raw (USDA)	4 oz.	158	0.
GRAHAM CRACKER (See **CRACKER**)			
GRAHAM CRACKOS, cereal (Kellogg's)	1 cup (1 oz.)	110	24.0
GRANOLA BARS, *Nature Valley:*			
Regular:			
Almond, cinnamon or oats'n honey	1 bar (.8 oz.)	110	16.0
Coconut or peanut	1 bar (.8 oz.)	120	15.0
Peanut butter	1 bar (.8 oz.)	140	16.0
Chewy:			
Apple or raisin	1 bar	130	19.0
Chocolate chip or peanut butter	1 bar	140	19.0

Food and Description	Measure or Quantity	Calories	Carbo-hydrates (grams)
*GRANOLA BAR MIX, chewy, *Nature Valley, Bake-A-Bar:* Chocolate chip, oats & honey			
or raisins & spice	¼₄ of pkg.	100	16.0
Peanut butter	¼₄ of pkg.	100	15.0
GRANOLA CEREAL: *Nature Valley:* Cinnamon & raisin, fruit &			
nut or toasted oat	⅓ cup (1 oz.)	130	19.0
Coconut & honey	⅓ cup (1 oz.)	150	18.0
Sun Country (Kretschmer):			
With almonds	½ cup (2 oz.)	253	34.1
With raisins	½ cup (2 oz.)	241	36.9
GRANOLA CLUSTERS, *Nature Valley:*			
Almond	1 piece (1.2 oz.)	140	27.0
Apple-cinnamon	1 piece (1.2 oz.)	140	25.0
Caramel or raisin	1 piece (1.2 oz.)	150	28.0
Chocolate chip	1 piece (1.2 oz.)	150	26.0
GRANOLA & FRUIT BAR, *Nature Valley*	1 bar	150	25.0
GRANOLA SNACK, *Nature Valley:*			
Cinnamon or honey nut	1 pouch	140	19.0
Oats & honey	1 pouch	140	18.0
Peanut butter	1 pouch	140	17.0
GRAPE: Fresh: American type (slip skin), Concord, Delaware, Niagara, Catawba and Scuppernong:			

Food and Description	Measure or Quantity	Calories	Carbo-hydrates (grams)
(USDA)	½ lb. (weighed with stem, skin & seeds)	98	22.4
(USDA)	½ cup (2.7 oz.)	33	7.5
(USDA)	3½" × 3" bunch (3.5 oz.)	43	9.9
European type (adherent skin, Malaga, Muscat, Tompson seedless, Emperor & Flame Tokay:			
(USDA)	½ lb. (weighed with stem & seeds)	139	34.9
(USDA) whole	20 grapes (¾" dia.)	52	13.5
(USDA) whole	½ cup (.3 oz.)	56	14.5
(USDA) halves	½ cup (.3 oz.)	56	14.4
Canned, solids & liq., (USDA) Thompson, seedless, heavy syrup	4 oz.	87	22.7
Canned, dietetic pack, solids & liq.:			
(USDA) Thompson, seedless, water pack	4 oz.	58	15.4
(Featherweight) water pack, seedless	½ cup	60	13.0
GRAPE DRINK:			
Canned:			
Capri Sun	6¾ fl. oz.	104	26.3
(Hi-C)	6 fl. oz.	89	22.0
(Lincoln)	6 fl. oz.	96	23.9
(Welchade)	6 fl. oz.	90	23.0
*Frozen (Welchade)	6 fl. oz.	90	23.0
*Mix (Hi-C)	6 fl. oz.	68	17.0
GRAPEFRUIT:			
Fresh (USDA):			
White:			
Seeded type	1 lb. (weighed with seeds & skin)	86	22.4

Food and Description	Measure or Quantity	Calories	Carbo-hydrates (grams)
Seedless type	1 lb. (weighed with skin)	87	22.6
Seeded type	½ med. grapefruit (3¾" dia., 8.5 oz.)	54	14.1
Pink and red:			
Seeded type	1 lb. (weighed with seeds & skin)	87	22.6
Seedless type	1 lb. (weighed with skin)	93	24.1
Seeded type	½ med. grapefruit (3¾" dia., 8.5 oz.)	46	12.0
Canned, syrup pack (Del Monte) solids & liq.	½ cup	74	17.5
Canned, unsweetened or dietetic pack, solids & liq. (USDA) water pack	½ cup (4.2 oz.)	36	9.1
(Del Monte) sections	½ cup	46	10.5
(Diet Delight) sections, juice pack	½ cup (4.3 oz.)	45	11.0
(Featherweight) sections, juice pack	½ of 8-oz. can	40	9.0
(S&W) Nutradiet, sections	½ cup	40	9.0
GRAPEFRUIT DRINK, canned (Lincoln)	6 fl. oz.	100	25.0
GRAPEFRUIT JUICE:			
Fresh (USDA) pink, red or white	½ cup (4.3 oz.)	46	11.3
Canned, sweetened:			
(Del Monte)	6 fl. oz.(6.6 oz.)	89	20.8
(Texsun)	6 fl. oz.	77	18.0
Canned, unsweetened:			
(Del Monte)	6 fl. oz. (6.5 oz.)	70	17.0

(USDA): United States Department of Agriculture
(HEW/FAO):   Health, Education and Welfare/Food and Agriculture
                      Organization
* Prepared as Package Directs

Food and Description	Measure or Quantity	Calories	Carbo-hydrates (grams)
(Libby's)	6 fl. oz.	75	18.0
(Ocean Spray)	6 fl. oz.	71	16.2
Chilled (Minute Maid)	6 fl. oz.	75	18.1
*Frozen (Minute Maid)	6 fl. oz.	75	18.3
GRAPEFRUIT JUICE COCKTAIL, canned (Ocean Spray) pink	6 fl. oz.	80	20.0
GRAPEFRUIT-ORANGE JUICE COCKTAIL, canned, *Musselman's*	6 fl. oz.	67	17.2
GRAPEFRUIT PEEL, CANDIED (USDA)	1 oz.	90	22.9
GRAPE JAM (Smucker's)	1 T. (.7 oz.)	53	13.7
GRAPE JELLY:			
Sweetened:			
(Smucker's)	1 T. (.5 oz.)	53	13.5
(Welch's)	1 T.	52	13.5
Dietetic:			
(Dia-Mel)	1 T. (.6 oz.)	6	0.
(Diet Delight)	1 T. (.6 oz.)	12	3.0
(Estee)	1 T.	6	1.6
(Featherweight) calorie reduced	1 T.	16	4.0
(Louis Sherry)	1 T. (.6 oz.)	6	0.
(S&W) Nutradiet, red label	1 T.	12	3.0
(Welch's) lite	1 T.	30	6.2
GRAPE JUICE:			
Canned, unsweetened:			
(USDA)	½ cup (4.4 oz.)	83	20.9
(Seneca Foods)	6 fl. oz.	118	30.0
(Welch's)	6 fl. oz.	120	30.0
*Frozen:			
(Minute Maid)	6 fl. oz.	99	13.3
(Welch's)	6 fl. oz.	100	25.0
GRAPE JUICE DRINK, chilled (Welch's)	6 fl. oz.	110	27.0

Food and Description	Measure or Quantity	Calories	Carbo-hydrates (grams)
GRAPE NUTS, cereal (Post):			
Regular	¼ cup (1 oz.)	108	23.3
Flakes	⅞ cup (1 oz.)	108	23.2
Raisin	¼ cup (1 oz.)	103	23.0
GRAPE PRESERVE OR JAM,			
sweetened (Welch's)	1 T.	52	13.5
GRAVY, CANNED:			
Au jus (Franco-American)	2-oz. serving	10	2.0
Beef (Franco-American)	2-oz. serving	25	3.0
Brown:			
(Franco-American) with			
onion	2-oz. serving	25	4.0
(Howard Johnson's)	½ cup	51	4.9
Ready Gravy	¼ cup (2.2 oz.)	44	7.5
Chicken:			
(Franco-American):			
Regular	2-oz. serving	50	3.0
Giblet	2-oz. serving	30	3.0
Mushroom (Franco-American)	2-oz. serving	25	3.0
Turkey:			
(Franco-American)	2-oz. serving	30	3.0
(Howard Johnson's) giblet	½ cup	55	5.5
GRAVYMASTER	1 tsp. (.2 oz.)	12	2.4
GRAVY WITH MEAT OR			
TURKEY, frozen:			
(Banquet):			
Buffet Supper:			
& sliced beef	2-lb. pkg.	1376	24.0
& sliced turkey	2-lb. pkg.	804	24.0
Cookin Bag:			
Giblet gravy & turkey	5-oz. pkg.	137	4.0
& sliced beef	4-oz. pkg.	136	4.0

(USDA): United States Department of Agriculture
(HEW/FAO):   Health, Education and Welfare/Food and Agriculture
                    Organization
* Prepared as Package Directs

Food and Description	Measure or Quantity	Calories	Carbohydrates (grams)
(Morton) Family Meal:			
Gravy, mushroom, & beef patty	2-lb. pkg.	300	12.0
Gravy, onion, & beef	2-lb. pkg.	300	14.0
& beef, sliced	2-lb. pkg.	210	7.0
(Swanson) sliced beef with whipped potatoes, *TV Brand*	8-oz. entree	200	19.0
GRAVY MIX:			
Regular:			
Au jus:			
(Durkee):			
*Regular	½ cup	15	3.2
Roastin' Bag	1-oz. pkg.	64	14.0
*(French's) *Gravy Makins*	½ cup	16	4.0
Brown:			
*(Durkee):			
Regular	½ cup	29	5.0
With mushroom	½ cup	29	5.5
With onion	½ cup	33	6.5
*(French's) *Gravy Makins*	½ cup	40	6.0
(McCormick)	.85-oz. pkg.	87	12.8
*(Pillsbury)	½ cup	30	6.0
*(Spatini)	1 oz.	8	2.0
Chicken:			
(Durkee):			
*Regular	½ cup	43	7.0
*Creamy	½ cup	78	7.0
Roastin' Bag:			
Regular	1.5-oz. pkg.	122	24.0
Creamy	2-oz. pkg.	242	22.0
Italian Style	1.5-oz. pkg.	144	31.0
*(French's) *Gravy Makins*	½ cup	50	8.0
(McCormick)	.85-oz. pkg.	82	13.4
*(Pillsbury)	½ cup	50	8.0
Homestyle:			
*(Durkee)	½ cup	35	5.5
*(French's) *Gravy Makins*	½ cup	50	8.0
*(Pillsbury)	½ cup	30	6.0
Meatloaf (Durkee) *Roastin' Bag*	1.5-oz. pkg.	129	18.0

Food and Description	Measure or Quantity	Calories	Carbo- hydrates (grams)
Mushroom:			
*(Durkee)	½ cup	30	22.0
*(French's) *Gravy Makins*	½ cup	40	6.0
Onion:			
*(Durkee)	½ cup	42	7.5
*(French's) *Gravy Makins*	½ cup	50	8.0
*(McCormick)	.85-oz. pkg.	72	9.8
Pork:			
(Durkee):			
*Regular	½ cup	35	7.0
Roastin' Bag	1.5-oz. pkg.	130	26.0
*(French's) *Gravy Makins*	½ cup	40	6.0
Pot roast (Durkee) *Roastin' Bag,* regular or onion	1.5-oz. pkg.	125	25.0
*Swiss steak (Durkee)	½ cup	22	5.4
Turkey:			
*(Durkee)	½ cup	47	7.0
*(French's) *Gravy Makins*	½ cup	50	8.0
*Dietetic (Weight Watchers):			
Brown	½ cup	16	2.0
Brown, with mushroom	½ cup	24	4.0
Brown, with onion	½ cup	26	4.0
Chicken	½ cup	20	4.0
GREENS, MIXED, canned (Sunshine) solids & liq.	½ cup (4.1 oz.)	20	2.7
GRENADINE (Garnier) non-alcoholic	1 fl. oz.	103	26.0
GROUPER, raw (USDA):			
Whole	1 lb. (weighed whole)	170	0.
Meat only	4 oz.	99	0.

(USDA): United States Department of Agriculture
(HEW/FAO): Health, Education and Welfare/Food and Agriculture Organization
* Prepared as Package Directs

Food and Description	Measure or Quantity	Calories	Carbo-hydrates (grams)
GUAVA, COMMON, fresh (USDA):			
Whole	1 lb. (weighed untrimmed)	273	66.0
Whole	1 guava (2.8 oz.)	48	11.7
Flesh only	4 oz.	70	17.0
GUAVA JAM (Smucker's)	1 T.	53	13.5
GUAVA JELLY (Smucker's)	1 T.	53	13.5
GUAVA NECTAR (Libby's)	6 fl. oz.	70	17.0
GUAVA, STRAWBERRY, fresh (USDA):			
Whole	1 lb. (weighed untrimmed)	289	70.2
Flesh only	4 oz.	74	17.9
GUINEA HEN, raw (USDA):			
Ready-to-cook	1 lb. (weighed ready-to-cook)	594	0.
Meat & skin	4 oz.	179	0.

Food and Description	Measure or Quantity	Calories	Carbo-hydrates (grams)

H

HADDOCK:

Raw (USDA) meat only	4 oz.	90	0.
Fried, breaded (USDA)	4″ × 3″ × ½″ fillet (3.5 oz.)	165	5.8
Frozen:			
(Banquet)	8¾-oz. dinner	418	45.4
(Mrs. Paul's):			
Batter dipped	2¼-oz. fillet	160	14.0
Breaded & fried	2-oz. fillet	125	10.5
Bread & fried, light	6-oz. serving	300	22.0
(Swanson) filet almondine	7½-oz. entree	370	9.0
(Van de Kamp's) batter dipped, french fried	2-oz. piece	165	8.0
(Weight Watchers) with stuffing, 2-compartment meal	7-oz. pkg.	205	14.1
Smoked (USDA)	4-oz. serving	117	0.

HALIBUT:

Raw (USDA):			
Whole	1 lb. (weighed whole)	144	0.
Meat only	4 oz.	84	0.
Broiled (USDA)	4″ × 3″ × ½″ steak (4.4 oz.)	214	0.
Smoked (USDA)	4 oz.	254	0.
Frozen (Van de Kamp's) batter dipped, french fried	½ of 8-oz. pkg.	270	17.0

HAM, (See also **PORK**):

Canned:			
(Hormel):			
Black Label (3- or 5-lb. size)	4 oz.	140	0.

(USDA): United States Department of Agriculture
(HEW/FAO):   Health, Education and Welfare/Food and Agriculture
                        Organization
* Prepared as Package Directs

Food and Description	Measure or Quantity	Calories	Carbo-hydrates (grams)
Chopped	3 oz. (8-lb. ham)	240	1.0
Chunk	6¾-oz. serving	310	Tr.
Curemaster, smoked	4 oz.	140	1.0
EXL	4 oz.	120	0.
Holiday Glaze	4 oz. (3-lb. ham)	140	2.9
Patties	1 patty	180	0.
(Oscar Mayer) *Jubilee*, extra lean, cooked	1-oz. serving	31	.1
(Swift) *Premium*	1¾-oz. slice	111	.3
Deviled:			
(Hormel)	1 T.	35	0.
(Libby's)	1 T. (.5 oz.)	43	0.
(Underwood)	1 T. (.5 oz.)	49	Tr.
Packaged:			
(Eckrich):			
Chopped	1 oz.	45	1.0
Loaf	1 oz.	70	1.0
Cooked or imported, danish	1.2-oz. slice	30	1.2
(Hormel):			
Black, peppered, cooked, glazed or red peppered or smoked	1 slice	25	0.
Chopped	1 slice	55	0.
(Oscar Mayer):			
Chopped	1-oz. slice	64	.9
Cooked, smoked	1-oz. slice	34	0.
Jubilee boneless:			
Sliced	8-oz. slice	264	0.
Steak, 95% fat free	2-oz. steak	69	0.

HAMBURGER (See *McDonald's, Burger King, Dairy Queen, White Castle,* etc.)

HAMBURGER MIX:
*Hamburger Helper
(General Mills):

Beef noodle	⅕ of pkg.	320	25.0
Beef romanoff	⅕ of pkg.	340	28.0
Cheeseburger Macaroni	⅕ of pkg.	360	28.0

Food and Description	Measure or Quantity	Calories	Carbo-hydrates (grams)
Chili tomato	⅕ of pkg.	320	29.0
Hash	⅕ of pkg.	300	24.0
Lasagna	⅕ of pkg.	330	33.0
Pizza dish	⅕ of pkg.	340	33.0
Potatoes au gratin	⅕ of pkg.	320	27.0
Potato Stroganoff	⅕ of pkg.	320	28.0
Rice oriental	⅕ of pkg.	320	25.0
Spaghetti	⅕ of pkg.	330	31.0
Stew	⅕ of pkg.	290	23.0
Tamale pie	⅕ of pkg.	370	39.0
Make a Better Burger (Lipton) mildly seasoned or onion	⅕ of pkg.	30	5.0
HAMBURGER SEASONING MIX:			
*(Durkee)	1 cup	663	7.5
(French's)	1-oz. pkg.	100	20.0
HAM & CHEESE:			
Canned (Hormel):			
Loaf	3 oz.	260	1.0
Patty	1 patty	190	0.
Packaged:			
(Eckrich) loaf	1-oz. serving	60	1.0
(Hormel) loaf	1-oz. slice	65	0.
(Oscar Mayer) loaf	1-oz. slice	77	.6
HAM DINNER, frozen:			
(Banquet) American Favorites	10-oz. dinner	532	61.0
(Morton)	10-oz. dinner	440	57.0
(Swanson) *TV Brand*	10¼-oz. dinner	320	46.0
HAM SALAD, canned			
(Carnation)	¼ of 7½-oz. can (1.9 oz.)	110	4.0
HAM SALAD SPREAD (Oscar Mayer)	1 oz.	62	3.0

(USDA): United States Department of Agriculture
(HEW/FAO): Health, Education and Welfare/Food and Agriculture Organization
* Prepared as Package Directs

Food and Description	Measure or Quantity	Calories	Carbo-hydrates (grams)
HAWAIIAN PUNCH:			
Canned:			
Cherry	6 fl. oz.	87	22.8
Grape	6 fl. oz.	93	23.4
*Mix, red punch	8 fl. oz.	100	25.0
HAWS, SCARLET, raw (USDA):			
Whole	1 lb. (weighed with core)	316	75.5
Flesh & skin	4 oz.	99	23.6
HEADCHEESE:			
(USDA)	1 oz.	76	.3
(Oscar Mayer)	1 oz.	54	0.
HERRING:			
Raw (USDA):			
Atlantic:			
Whole	1 lb. (weighed whole)	407	0.
Meat only	4 oz.	200	0.
Pacific, meat only	4 oz.	111	0.
Canned:			
(USDA) in tomato sauce, solids & liq.	4-oz. serving	200	4.2
(Vita):			
Bismarck, drained	5-oz. jar	273	6.9
In cream sauce, drained	8-oz. jar	397	18.1
Matjis, drained	8-oz. jar	304	26.2
In wine sauce, drained	8-oz. jar	401	16.6
Pickled (USDA) Bismarck type	4-oz. serving	253	0.
Salted or brined (USDA)	4-oz. serving	247	0.
Smoked (USDA):			
Bloaters	4-oz. serving	222	0.
Hard	4-oz. serving	340	0.
Kippered	4-oz. serving	239	0.
HICKORY NUT (USDA):			
Whole	1 lb. (weighed in shell)	1068	20.3
Shelled	4 oz.	763	14.5

Food and Description	Measure or Quantity	Calories	Carbohydrates (grams)
HO-HO (Hostess)	1-oz. piece	126	17.0
HOMNIY GRITS:			
Dry:			
(USDA):			
Degermed	1 oz.	103	22.1
ʳDegermed	½ cup (2.8 oz.)	282	60.9
(Albers) quick, degermed	1½ oz.	150	33.0
(Aunt Jemima)	3 T. (1 oz.)	101	22.4
(Pocono) creamy	1 oz.	101	23.6
(Quaker):			
Regular or quick	1 T. (.33 oz.)	34	7.5
Instant:			
Regular	.8-oz. packet	79	17.7
With imitation bacon bits	1-oz. packet	101	21.6
With artificial cheese flavor	1-oz. packet	104	21.6
With imitation ham bits	1-oz. packet	99	21.3
(3-Minute Brand) quick, enriched	⅙ cup (1 oz.)	98	22.2
Cooked (USDA) degermed	⅔ cup (5.6 oz.)	84	18.0
HONEY, strained:			
(USDA)	½ cup (5.7 oz.)	494	134.1
(USDA)	1 T. (.7 oz.)	61	16.5
HONEYCOMB, cereal (Post) regular	1⅓ cups (1 oz.)	117	24.5
HONEYDEW, fresh (USDA):			
Whole	1 lb. (weighed whole)	94	22.0
Wedge	2″ × 7″ wedge (5.3 oz.)	31	7.2
Flesh only	4 oz.	37	8.7
Flesh only, diced	1 cup (5.9 oz.)	55	12.9

(USDA): United States Department of Agriculture
(HEW/FAO): Health, Education and Welfare/Food and Agriculture Organization
* Prepared as Package Directs

Food and Description	Measure or Quantity	Calories	Carbo-hydrates (grams)
HONEY SMACKS, cereal (Kellogg's)	¾ cup (1 oz.)	110	25.0
HORSERADISH:			
Raw, pared (USDA)	1 oz.	25	5.6
Prepared (Gold's)	1 tsp.	3	Tr.
HOSTESS O'S (Hostess)	2¼-oz. piece	277	40.5
HYACINTH BEAN (USDA):			
Young bean, raw:			
Whole	1 lb. (weighed untrimmed)	140	29.1
Trimmed	4 oz.	40	8.3
Dry seeds	4 oz.	383	69.2

Food and Description	Measure or Quantity	Calories	Carbo-hydrates (grams)

I

ICE CREAM (Listed by type, such as sandwich or *Whammy*, or by flavor—see also **FROZEN DESSERT**):

Food and Description	Measure or Quantity	Calories	Carbo-hydrates (grams)
Bar (Good Humor) vanilla, chocolate coated	3 fl.-oz. piece	170	12.0
Butter pecan:			
(Breyer's)	¼ pt.	180	15.0
(Good Humor) bulk	4 fl. oz.	150	14.0
Cherry, black (Good Humor) bulk	4 fl. oz.	130	14.0
Chocolate:			
(Baskin-Robbins):			
Regular	1 scoop (2½ fl. oz.)	165	20.4
Fudge	1 scoop (2½ fl. oz.)	178	21.3
(Good Humor) bulk	4 fl. oz.	130	15.0
(Howard Johnson's)	½ cup	221	25.5
(Meadow Gold):			
Regular	½ cup	140	18.0
Old fashioned	½ cup	140	16.0
Chocolate chip (Good Humor)	4 fl. oz.	150	15.0
Chocolate chip cookie (Good Humor)	1 sandwich	480	64.0
Chocolate eclair (Good Humor) bar	3-fl.-oz. piece	220	25.0
Coffee (Breyer's)	¼ pt.	140	15.0
Eskimo Pie, vanilla with chocolate coating	3-fl.-oz. bar	180	15.0
Eskimo Thin Mint, with chocolate coating	2-fl.-oz. bar	140	11.0

(USDA): United States Department of Agriculture
(HEW/FAO): Health, Education and Welfare/Food and Agriculture Organization
* Prepared as Package Directs

Food and Description	Measure or Quantity	Calories	Carbo-hydrates (grams)
Fudge royal (Good Humor)			
bulk	4 fl. oz.	120	14.0
Peach (Breyer's)	¼ pt.	130	18.0
Pralines'N Cream			
(Baskin-Robbins)	1 scoop		
	(2½ fl. oz.)	177	23.7
Sandwich (Good Humor)	2½-oz. piece	200	34.0
Strawberry:			
(Baskin-Robbins)	1 scoop		
	(2½ fl. oz.)	141	15.6
(Good humor) bulk	4 fl. oz.	120	15.0
(Howard Johnson's)	½ cup	187	23.2
Strawberry shortcake			
(Good Humor)	3-fl.-oz. piece	200	21.0
Toasted almond bar			
(Good Humor)	3-fl.-oz. piece	220	21.0
Toffee fudge swirl			
(Good Humor) bulk	4 fl. oz.	130	18.0
Vanilla:			
(Baskin-Robbins):			
Regular	1 scoop		
	(2½ fl. oz.)	147	15.6
French	1 scoop		
	(2½ fl. oz.)	181	15.9
(Good Humor) bulk	4 fl. oz.	140	14.0
(Howard Johnson's)	½ cup	210	21.3
(Meadow Gold)	½ cup	140	16.0
Vanilla-chocolate-strawberry			
(Good Humor)	4 fl. oz.	130	14.0
Vanilla fudge swirl			
(Good Humor) bulk	4 fl. oz.	140	15.0
Whammy (Good Humor):			
Assorted	1.6-oz. piece	100	9.0
Chip crunch bar	1.6-oz. piece	110	10.0
ICE CREAM CONE, cone only			
(Comet):			
Regular	1 piece (.15 oz.)	20	4.0
Rolled sugar	1 piece (.35 oz.)	40	9.0
ICE CREAM CUP, cup only			
(Comet)	1 cup (.15 oz.)	20	4.0

Food and Description	Measure or Quantity	Calories	Carbo-hydrates (grams)
*ICE CREAM MIX (Salada) any flavor	1 cup	310	31.0
ICE MILK:			
(USDA):			
Hardened	1 cup (4.6 oz.)	199	29.3
Soft-serv	1 cup (6.3 oz.)	266	39.2
(Dean):			
Count Calorie, 2.1% fat	1 cup (4.8 oz.)	155	17.1
5% fat	1 cup (4.9 oz.)	227	35.0
(Meadow Gold):			
Chocolate, Viva	1 cup	200	36.0
Vanilla, Viva	1 cup	200	34.0
ICING (See CAKE ICING)			
INSTANT BREAKFAST (See individual brand name or company listings)			
IRISH WHISKEY (See DISTILLED LIQUOR)			
ITALIAN DINNER, frozen (Banquet) International Favorites	12-oz. dinner	597	71.0

Food and Description	Measure or Quantity	Calories	Carbo-hydrates (grams)

J

JACKFRUIT, fresh (USDA):
Whole	1 lb. (weighed with seeds & skin)	124	32.5
Flesh only	4 oz.	111	28.8

JACK MACKERAL, raw (USDA) meat only
	4 oz.	162	.0.

JAM, sweetened (See also individual listings by flavor) (USDA)
	1 T. (.7 oz.)	54	14.0

JELL-O GELATIN POPS:
Cherry, grape, orange, or strawberry	1.7-oz. pop	37	8.5
Raspberry	1.7-oz. pop	34	7.7

JELL-O PUDDING POPS:
Banana, butterscotch or chocolate & vanilla swirl	2-oz. piece	96	15.6
Chocolate or chocolate fudge	2-oz. piece	94	15.5
Chocolate & caramel swirl	2-oz. piece	95	16 1
Vanilla	2-oz. piece	92	15.5

JELLY, sweetened (See also individual flavors) (Crosse & Blackwell) all flavors
	1 T.	51	12.8

JERUSALEM ARTICHOKE (USDA):
Unpared	1 lb. (weighed with skin)	207	52.3
Pared	4 oz.	75	18.9

JOHANNISBERG RIESLING WINE (Louis M. Martini)
	3 fl. oz.	61	.2

Food and Description	Measure or Quantity	Calories	Carbo-hydrates (grams)
JUJUBE OR CHINESE DATE (USDA):			
Fresh, whole	1 lb. (weighed with seeds)	443	116.4
Fresh, flesh only	4 oz.	119	31.3
Dried, whole	1 lb. (weighed with seeds)	1159	297.1
Dried, flesh only	4 oz.	325	83.5

(USDA): United States Department of Agriculture
(HEW/FAO):   Health, Education and Welfare/Food and Agriculture
                      Organization
* Prepared as Package Directs

Food and Description	Measure or Quantity	Calories	Carbo-hydrates (grams)

K

Food and Description	Measure or Quantity	Calories	Carbo-hydrates (grams)
KABOOM, cereal (General Mills)	1 cup (1 oz.)	110	23.0
KALE:			
Raw (USDA) leaves only	1 lb. (weighed untrimmed)	154	26.1
Boiled, leaves only (USDA)	4 oz.	44	6.9
Canned (Sunshine) chopped, solids & liq.	½ cup (4.1 oz.)	21	2.8
Frozen, chopped:			
(Birds Eye)	⅓ of 10-oz. pkg.	31	4.6
(McKenzie)	⅓ of 10-oz. pkg.	25	5.0
(Southland)	⅕ of 16-oz. pkg.	30	5.0
KARO SYRUP (See **SYRUP**)			
KEFIR (Alta-Dena Dairy):			
Plain	1 cup	180	13.0
Flavored	1 cup	190	24.0
KIDNEY (USDA):			
Beef, braised	4 oz.	286	.9
Calf, raw	4 oz.	128	.1
Lamb, raw	4 oz.	119	1.0
KIELBASA (Hormel) Kolbase	2-oz. serving	245	1.2
KINGFISH, raw (USDA):			
Whole	1 lb. (weighed whole)	210	0.
Meat only	4 oz.	119	0.
KING VITAMIN, cereal (Quaker)	1¼ cups	113	23.2
KIX, cereal	1½ cups (1 oz.)	110	24.0

Food and Description	Measure or Quantity	Calories	Carbo-hydrates (grams)
KNOCKWURST (USDA)	1 oz.	79	.6
KOHLRABI (USDA):			
Raw:			
Whole	1 lb. (weighed with skin, without leaves)	96	21.9
Diced	1 cup (4.8 oz.)	40	9.1
Boiled:			
Drained	4 oz.	27	6.0
Drained	1 cup (5.5 oz.)	37	8.2
KOOL-AID (General Foods):			
Unsweetened (sugar to be added)	8 fl. oz. (8.7 oz.)	98	25.0
Pre-sweetened:			
Regular, sugar sweetened:			
Apple or sunshine punch	8 fl. oz.	96	24.5
Cherry or grape	8 fl. oz.	89	22.8
Orange, raspberry or strawberry	8 fl. oz.	88	22.5
Tropical punch	8 fl. oz.	99	25.2
Dietetic, sugar-free:			
Cherry or grape	8 fl. oz.	2	.1
Sunshine punch	8 fl. oz.	4	.3
Tropical punch	8 fl. oz.	3	.3
KUMQUAT, fresh (USDA):			
Whole	1 lb. (weighed with seeds)	274	72.1
Flesh & skin	4 oz.	74	19.4

(USDA): United States Department of Agriculture
(HEW/FAO):   Health, Education and Welfare/Food and Agriculture
              Organization
* Prepared as Package Directs

Food and Description	Measure or Quantity	Calories	Carbo-hydrates (grams)
LAKE COUNTRY WINE (Taylor):			
Gold, 12% alcohol	3 fl. oz.	78	5.4
Red, 12½% alcohol	3 fl. oz.	81	4.8
LAKE HERRING, raw (USDA):			
Whole	1 lb.	226	0.
Meat only	4 oz.	109	0.
LAKE TROUT, raw (USDA):			
Drawn	1 lb. (weighed with head, fins & bones)	282	0.
Meat only	4 oz.	191	0.
LAKE TROUT or SISCOWET, raw (USDA):			
Less than 6.5 lb.:			
Whole	1 lb. (weighed whole)	404	0.
Meat only	4 oz.	273	0.
More than 6.5 lb.:			
Whole	1 lb. (weighed whole)	856	0.
Meat only	4 oz.	594	0.
LAMB, choice grade (USDA):			
Chop, broiled:			
Loin. One 5-oz. chop (weighed before cooking with bone) will give you:			
Lean & fat	2.8 oz.	280	0.
Lean only	2.3 oz.	122	0.
Rib. One 5-oz. chop (weighed before cooking with bone) with give you:			
Lean & fat	2.9 oz.	334	0.

Food and Description	Measure or Quantity	Calories	Carbo-hydrates (grams)
Lean only	2 oz.	118	0.
Fat, separable, cooked	1 oz.	201	0.
Leg:			
Raw, lean & fat	1 lb. (weighed with bone)	845	0.
Roasted, lean & fat	4 oz.	316	0.
Roasted, lean only	4 oz.	211	0.
Shoulder:			
Raw, lean & fat	1 lb. (weighed with bone)	1092	0.
Roasted, lean & fat	4 oz.	383	0.
Roasted, lean only	4 oz.	232	0.
LAMB'S QUARTERS (USDA):			
Raw, trimmed	1 lb.	195	33.1
Boiled, drained	4 oz.	36	5.7
LARD:			
(USDA)	1 cup (6.2 oz.)	1849	0.
(USDA)	1 T. (.5 oz.)	117	0.
LASAGNA:			
Canned (Hormel) *Short Orders*	7½-oz. can	260	25.0
Frozen:			
(Green Giant):			
Bake:			
Regular, with meat sauce	12-oz. entree	490	44.0
Regular, with meat sauce	21-oz. entree	860	90.0
Chicken	12-oz. entree	640	47.0
Spinach	12-oz. entree	540	41.0
Boil'N Bag	9½-oz. entree	290	42.0
(Stouffer's):			
Regular	10½-oz. serving	385	36.0
Lean Cuisine, zucchini	11 oz. serving	240	28.0
(Swanson):			
Regular, with meat	13¼-oz. entree	480	45.0

(USDA): United States Department of Agriculture
(HEW/FAO):   Health, Education and Welfare/Food and Agriculture
              Organization
* Prepared as Package Directs

Food and Description	Measure or Quantity	Calories	Carbo-hydrates (grams)
Hungry Man, with meat:			
Dinner	17¾-oz. dinner	690	90.0
Entree	12¾-oz. entree	460	62.0
TV Brand	13-oz. dinner	420	54.0
(Van de Kamp's):			
Beef & mushroom	11-oz. meal	430	30.0
Creamy spinach	11-oz. meal	400	36.0
Italian sausage	11-oz. meal	440	34.0
(Weight Watchers):			
Regular	12-oz. meal	360	38.0
Italian cheese	11-oz. serving	350	33.0
LEEKS, raw (USDA)			
Whole	1 lb. (weighed untrimmed)	123	26.4
Trimmed	4 oz.	59	12.7
LEMON (USDA):			
Whole	2⅛″ lemon (109 grams)	22	11.7
Peeled	2⅛″ lemon (74 grams)	20	6.1
LEMONADE:			
Canned:			
Capri Sun, natural	6¾ fl. oz.	63	23.3
Country Time	6 fl. oz.	69	17.2
(Hi-C)	6 fl. oz.	68	17.0
Chilled (Minute Maid) regular or pink	6 fl. oz.	79	18.0
*Frozen:			
Country Time, regular or pink	6 fl. oz.	68	18.0
Minute Maid,	6 fl. oz.	74	19.6
(Sunkist)	6 fl. oz.	81	21.1
*Mix:			
Regular:			
Country Time, regular or pink	6 fl. oz.	68	20.6
(Hi-C)	6 fl. oz.	76	19.0
Kool-Aid, regular or pink:			

Food and Description	Measure or Quantity	Calories	Carbo- hydrates (grams)
Sugar to be added	6 fl. oz.	73	18.8
Pre-sweetened with sugar	6 fl. oz.	65	16.3
Lemon Tree (Lipton)	6 fl. oz.	68	16.5
(Minute Maid)	6 fl. oz.	80	20.0
Dietetic:			
Crystal Light	6 fl. oz.	4	.2
Kool-Aid	6 fl. oz.	3	.2
LEMON JUICE:			
Fresh (USDA)	1 T. (.5 oz.)	4	1.2
Plastic container, *ReaLemon*	1 T. (.5 oz.)	3	.8
*Frozen (Minute Maid) unsweetened	1 fl. oz.	7	2.2
***LEMON-LIMEADE DRINK,** mix:			
Regular:			
(Minute Maid)	6 fl. oz.	80	20.0
Country Time	6 fl. oz.	65	16.2
Dietetic, *Crystal Light*	6 fl. oz.	3	.1
LEMON PEEL, CANDIED (USDA)	1 oz.	90	22.9
LEMON & PEPPER SEASONING:			
(French's)	1 tsp.	6	1.0
(McCormick)	1 tsp.	7	.8
LENTIL:			
Whole:			
Dry:			
(USDA)	½ lb.	771	136.3
(USDA)	1 cup (6.7 oz.)	649	114.8
(Sinsheimer)	1 oz.	95	17.0
Cooked (USDA) drained	½ cup (3.6 oz.)	107	19.5
Split (USDA) dry	½ lb.	782	140.2

(USDA): United States Department of Agriculture
(HEW/FAO):   Health, Education and Welfare/Food and Agriculture
            Organization
* Prepared as Package Directs

Food and Description	Measure or Quantity	Calories	Carbo-hydrates (grams)
LETTUCE (USDA):			
Bibb, untrimmed	1 lb.	47	8.4
Bibb, untrimmed	7.8-oz. head (4″ dia.)	23	4.1
Boston, untrimmed	1 lb.	47	8.4
Boston, untrimmed	7.8-oz. head (4″ dia.)	23	4.1
Butterhead varieties (See Bibb & Boston)			
Cos (See Romaine)			
Dark green (See Romaine)			
Grand Rapids	1 lb. (weighed untrimmed)	52	10.2
Great Lakes	1 lb. (weighed untrimmed)	56	12.5
Great Lakes, trimmed	1-lb. head (4¾″ dia.)	59	13.2
Iceberg:			
Untrimmed	1 lb.	56	12.5
Trimmed	1-lb. head (4¾″ dia.)	59	13.2
Leaves	1 cup (2.3 oz.)	9	1.9
Chopped	1 cup (2 oz.)	8	1.7
Chunks	1 cup (2.6 oz.)	10	2.1
Looseleaf varieties (See Salad Bowl)			
New York	1 lb. (weighed untrimmed)	56	12.5
New York	1-lb. head (4¾″ dia.)	59	13.2
Romaine:			
Untrimmed	1 lb.	52	10.2
Trimmed, shredded & broken into pieces	½ cup	4	.8
Salad Bowl	1 lb. (weighed untrimmed)	52	10.2
Salad Bowl	2 large leaves (1.8 oz.)	9	1.8
Simpson	1 lb. (weighed untrimmed)	52	10.2
Simpson	2 large leaves (1.8 oz.)	9	1.8
White Paris (See Romaine)			

Food and Description	Measure or Quantity	Calories	Carbo-hydrates (grams)
LIFE, cereal (Quaker) regular or cinnamon	⅔ cup (1 oz.)	105	19.7
LIL' ANGELS (Hostess)	1-oz. piece	78	14.2
LIME, fresh (USDA) peeled fruit	2″ dia. lime (1.8 oz.)	15	4.9
*LIMEADE, frozen (Minute Maid)	6 fl. oz.	75	20.1
LIME JUICE, *ReaLime*	1 T.	2	.5
LINGCOD, raw (USDA):			
Whole	1 lb. (weighed whole)	130	0.
Meat only	34 oz.	95	0.
LINGUINI WITH CLAM SAUCE, frozen (Stouffer's)	10½-oz. pkg.	285	36.0
LIQUEUR (See individual kinds)			
LITCHI NUT (USDA):			
Fresh:			
Whole	4 oz. (weighed in shell with seeds)	44	11.2
Flesh only	4 oz.	73	18.6
Dried:			
Whole	4 oz. (weighed in shell with seeds)	145	36.9
Flesh	2 oz.	157	40.1
LIVER:			
Beef:			
(USDA):			
Raw	1 lb.	635	24.0
Fried	4 oz.	260	6.0

(USDA): United States Department of Agriculture
(HEW/FAO):   Health, Education and Welfare/Food and Agriculture
                    Organization
* Prepared as Package Directs

Food and Description	Measure or Quantity	Calories	Carbo-hydrates (grams)
(Swift) packaged, True-Tender, sliced, cooked	⅕ of 1-lb. pkg.	141	3.1
Calf (USDA):			
Raw	1 lb.	635	18.6
Fried	4 oz.	296	4.5
Chicken:			
Raw	1 lb.	585	13.2
Simmered	4 oz.	187	3.5
Goose, raw (USDA)	1 lb.	826	24.5
Hog (USDA):			
Raw	1 lb.	594	11.8
Fried	4 oz.	273	2.8
Lamb (USDA):			
Raw	1 lb.	617	13
LONGAN (USDA):			
Fresh:			
Whole	1 lb. (weighed with shell & seeds)	147	38.0
Flesh only	4 oz.	69	17.9
Dried:			
Whole	1 lb. (weighed with shell & seeds)	467	120.8
Flesh only	4 oz.	324	83.9
LONG ISLAND TEA COCKTAIL (Mr. Boston) 12½% alcohol	3 fl. oz.	94	9.0
LOQUAT, fresh, flesh only (USDA)	2 oz.	27	7.0
LUCKY CHARMS, cereal (General Mills)	1 cup (1 oz.)	110	24.0
LUNCHEON MEAT (See also individual listings such as **BOLOGNA, HAM,** etc.):			
All meat (Oscar Mayer)	1-oz. slice	98	.4
Banquet loaf (Eckrich)	¾-oz. slice	50	1.0

Food and Description	Measure or Quantity	Calories	Carbo-hydrates (grams)
Bar-B-Que Loaf:			
(Eckrich)	1-oz. slice	35	1.0
(Hormel)	1 slice	45	.5
(Oscar Mayer) 90% fat free	1-oz. slice	49	1.4
Beef, jellied (Hormel) loaf	1 slice	45	0.
Gourmet loaf (Eckrich):			
Regular	1-oz. slice	35	2.0
Smorgas Pac	¾-oz. slice	25	2.0
Ham & cheese (See **HAM & CHEESE)**			
Ham roll sausage (Oscar Mayer)	1-oz. slice	43	.6
Honey loaf:			
(Eckrich):			
Regular	1-oz. slice	40	3.0
Smorgas Pac	¾-oz. slice	30	2.0
Smorgas Pac	1-oz. slice	35	3.0
(Hormel)	1 slice	45	.5
(Oscar Mayer) 95% fat free	1-oz. slice	37	1.1
Iowa Brand (Hormel)	1 slice	45	0.
Liver cheese (Oscar Mayer)	1.3-oz. slice	114	.6
Liver loaf (Hormel)	1 slice	80	6.5
Luxury loaf (Oscar Mayer)	1-oz. slice	39	1.5
Macaroni-cheese loaf (Eckrich)	1-oz. slice	70	3.0
Meat loaf (USDA)	1-oz. serving	57	.9
New England Brand sliced sausage:			
(Eckrich)	1-oz. slice	35	1.0
(Hormel)	1 slice	50	0.
(Oscar Mayer) 92% fat free	.8-oz. slice	34	.5
Old fashioned loaf:			
(Eckrich):			
Regular	1-oz. slice	70	3.0
Smorgas Pac	¾-oz. slice	50	2.0
(Oscar Mayer)	1-oz. slice	65	2.3
Olive loaf:			
(Eckrich)	1-oz. slice	80	2.0

(USDA): United States Department of Agriculture
(HEW/FAO):   Health, Education and Welfare/Food and Agriculture
                     Organization
* Prepared as Package Directs

Food and Description	Measure or Quantity	Calories	Carbo-hydrates (grams)
(Hormel)	1 slice	55	1.5
(Oscar Mayer)	1-oz. slice	65	2.8
Peppered loaf:			
(Eckrich)	1-oz. slice	40	1.0
(Oscar Mayer) 93% fat free	1-oz. slice	42	1.3
Pickle loaf:			
(Eckrich):			
Regular	1-oz. slice	80	2.0
Smorgas Pac	¾-oz. slice	50	1.0
(Hormel)	1 slice	60	1.5
Pickle & pimiento loaf (Oscar Mayer)	1-oz. slice	65	3.0
Picnic loaf (Oscar Mayer)	1-oz. slice	64	1.6
Spiced (Hormel)	1 slice	75	.5
LUNG, raw (USDA):			
Beef	1 lb.	435	0.
Calf	1 lb.	481	0.
Lamb	1 lb.	467	0.

Food and Description	Measure or Quantity	Calories	Carbo-hydrates (grams)

M

MACADAMIA NUT (Royal Hawaiian) | 1 oz. | 197 | 4.5

MACARONI & CHEESE:
Frozen:
  (Banquet):

Buffet Supper	2-lb. pkg.	1344	148.0
Casserole	8-oz. pkg.	344	36.0
Cookin' Bag	5-oz. pkg.	227	25.0
(Green Giant) *Boil 'N Bag*	9-oz. entree	290	36.0
(Morton):			
Casserole	8-oz. casserole	270	36.0
Dinner	11-oz. dinner	320	54.0
Family Meal	2-lb. pkg.	1040	136.0
(Stouffer's)	6-oz. serving	260	24.0
(Swanson):			
Regular	12-oz. entree	440	43.0
TV Brand	12¼-oz. dinner	380	48.0
(Van de Kamp's)	5-oz. serving	150	23.0
Mix:			
(Golden Grain) deluxe	¼ of 7¼-oz. pkg.	202	38.1
*(Lipton)	¼ of pkg.	210	25.0
*(Prince)	¾ cup	268	34.6

MACARONI & CHEESE PIE,
frozen (Swanson) | 7-oz. pie | 210 | 25.0

MACARONI SALAD, canned
(Nalley's) | 4-oz. serving | 206 | 15.9

MACE (French's) | 1 tsp. | 10 | .8

(USDA): United States Department of Agriculture
(HEW/FAO): Health, Education and Welfare/Food and Agriculture Organization
* Prepared as Package Directs

Food and Description	Measure or Quantity	Calories	Carbo-hydrates (grams)
MACKEREL:			
Atlantic:			
Raw:			
Whole	1 lb. (weighed whole)	468	0.
Meat only	4 oz.	217	0.
Broiled with butter	4 oz.	268	0.
Canned, solids & liq.		208	0.
Pacific:			
Raw:			
Dressed	1 lb. (weighed with bones & skin)	519	0.
Meat only	4 oz.	180	0.
Canned, solids & liq.	4 oz.	204	0.
Salted	4 oz.	346	0.
Smoked	4 oz.	248	0.
MADEIRA WINE (Leacock) 19% alcohol	3 fl. oz.	120	6.3
MALT, dry (USDA)	1 oz.	104	21.9
MALTED MILK MIX (Carnation);			
Chocolate	3 heaping tsps. (.7 oz.)	85	18.0
Natural	3 heaping tsps. (.7 oz.)	88	15.8
MALT LIQUOR, *Champale,* 6¼% alcohol	12 fl. oz.	179	
MALT-O-MEAL cereal:			
Regular	1 T. (.3 oz.)	33	7.3
Chocolate flavored	1 T. (.3 oz.)	33	7.0
MAMEY or MAMMEE APPLE, fresh (USDA)	1 lb. (weighed with skin & seeds)	143	35.2

Food and Description	Measure or Quantity	Calories	Carbo-hydrates (grams)
MANDARIN ORANGE (See **TANGERINE**)			
MANGO, fresh (USDA):			
Whole	1 lb. (weighed with seeds & skin)	201	51.1
Flesh only, diced or sliced	½ cup	54	13.8
MANHATTAN COCKTAIL (Mr. Boston) 20% alcohol	3 fl. oz.	123	6.3
MAPLE SYRUP (See **SYRUP,** Maple)			
MARGARINE, salted or unsalted:			
Regular:			
(USDA)	1 lb.	3266	1.8
(USDA)	1 cup (8 oz.)	1633	.9
(Autumn) soft or stick	1 T.	80	Tr.
(Blue Bonnet) soft or stick	1 T. (.5 oz.)	100	0.
(Chiffon):			
Soft	1 T.	90	0.
Stick	1 T.	100	0.
(Fleischmann's) soft or stick	1 T. (.5 oz.)	100	0.
(Golden Mist)	1 T.	100	0.
(Holiday)	1 T. (.5 oz.)	102	0.
(Imperial) soft or stick	1 T. (.5 oz.)		
Whipped:			
(Blue Bonnet)	1 T. (9 grams)	70	0.
(Chiffon)	1 T.	70	0.
(Fleischmann's) soft	1 T.	70	0.
(Imperial)	1 T. (9 grams)	50	Tr.
(Parkay) cup	1 T.	67	Tr.

(USDA): United States Department of Agriculture
(HEW/FAO):   Health, Education and Welfare/Food and Agriculture
            Organization
* Prepared as Package Directs

Food and Description	Measure or Quantity	Calories	Carbo-hydrates (grams)
MARGARITA COCKTAIL,			
(Mr. Boston) 12½% alcohol:			
Regular	3 fl. oz.	105	10.8
Strawberry	3 fl. oz.	138	18.9
MARINADE MIX:			
Chicken (Adolph's)	1-oz. packet	64	14.4
Meat:			
(Adolph's)	.8-oz. pkg.	38	8.5
(Durkee)	1-oz. pkg.	47	9.0
(French's)	1-oz. pkg.	80	16.0
(Kikkoman)	1-oz. pkg.	64	12.5
MARJORAM (French's)	1 tsp. (1.2 grams)	4	.8
MARMALADE:			
Sweetened:			
(USDA)	1 T. (.7 oz.)	51	14.0
(Keiller)	1 T.	60	15.0
(Smucker's)	1 T. (.7 oz.)	53	13.5
Dietetic:			
(Dia-Mel; Louis Sherry)	1 T. (.6 oz.)	6	0.
(Featherweight)	1 T.	16	4.0
(S&W) *Nutradiet*, red label	1 T.	12	3.0
MARSHMALLOW FLUFF	1 heaping tsp.	59	14.4
MARSHMALLOW KRISPIES,			
cereal (Kellogg's)	1¼ cups (1.3 oz.)	140	33.0
MARTINI COCKTAIL (Mr.			
Boston) 20% alcohol:			
Gin, extra dry	3 fl. oz.	99	0.
Vodka	3 fl. oz.	102	.9
MASA HARINA (Quaker)	⅓ cup (1.3 oz.)	237	27.4
MASA TRIGO (Quaker)	⅓ cup (1.3 oz.)	149	24.7

Food and Description	Measure or Quantity	Calories	Carbo-hydrates (grams)
MATZO:			
(Goodman's):			
Diet-10s	1 sq.	109	23.0
Unsalted	1 matzo (1 oz.)	109	23.0
(Horowitz-Margareten)			
unsalted	1 matzo	135	28.2
(Manischewitz):			
Regular	1.1-oz. matzo	114	28.1
Egg	1.2-oz. matzo	133	26.6
Thin tea	1-oz. matzo	114	24.8
Whole wheat	1.2-oz. matzo	124	24.2
MATZO MEAL (Manischewitz)	1 cup (4.1 oz.)	438	96.2
MAYONNAISE:			
Real, *Hellmann's* (Best Foods)	1 T. (.5 oz.)	103	.1
Imitation or dietetic:			
(Dia-Mel)	1 T. (.5 oz.)	106	0.
Diet Delight) *Mayo-Lite*	1 T. (.5 oz.)	24	0.
(Featherweight) *Soyamaise*	1 T.	100	0.
(Tillie Lewis) *Tasti Diet,*			
Maylonaise	1 T.	25	1.0
(Weight Watchers)	1 T.	40	1.0
MAYPO, cereal:			
30-second	¼ cup (.8 oz.)	89	16.4
Vermont style	¼ cup (1.1 oz.)	121	22.0
McDONALD'S:			
Big Mac	1 hamburger	563	40.6
Cheeseburger	1 cheeseburger	307	29.8
Chicken McNuggets	1 serving	314	15.4
Chicken McNuggets Sauce:			
Barbecue	1.1-oz. serving	60	13.7
Honey	.5-oz. serving	50	12.4
Hot mustard	1.1-oz. serving	63	10.5
Sweet & sour	1.1-oz. serving	64	15.0

(USDA): United States Department of Agriculture
(HEW/FAO): Health, Education and Welfare/Food and Agriculture Organization
* Prepared as Package Directs

Food and Description	Measure or Quantity	Calories	Carbo-hydrates (grams)
Cookies:			
Chocolate chip	1 package	342	44.8
McDonaldland	1 package	308	48.7
Egg McMuffin	1 serving	327	31.0
Egg, scrambled	1 serving	180	2.5
English muffin, with butter	1 muffin	186	29.5
Filet-O-Fish	1 sandwich	432	37.4
Grapefruit juice	6 fl. oz.	80	17.9
Hamburger	1 hamburger	255	29.5
Hot cakes with butter & syrup	1 serving	500	93.9
MEAT LOAF DINNER, frozen:			
(Banquet):			
Buffet Supper	30-oz. pkg.	1510	60.0
Cookin' Bag	5-oz. pkg.	251	10.0
Dinner:			
American Favorites	11-oz. dinner	437	30.0
Extra Helping	19-oz. dinner	984	80.0
(Morton):			
Regular	11-oz. dinner	340	28.0
Family Meal, & tomato			
sauce	1-lb. pkg.	800	68.0
(Swanson) *TV Brand:*			
Dinner	10¾-oz. dinner	490	48.0
Entree, with tomato sauce			
& whipped potatoes	9-oz. entree	340	28.0
MEAL LOAF SEASONING MIX:			
(Contadina)	3¾-oz. pkg.	360	72.4
(French's)	1.5-oz. pkg.	160	40.0
MEAT, POTTED:			
(Hormel)	1 T.	30	0.
(Libby's)	1-oz. serving	55	0.
MEAT TENDERIZER:			
Regular (Adolph's;			
McCormick)	1 tsp.	2	.5
Seasoned (McCormick)	1 tsp.	5	.8

Food and Description	Measure or Quantity	Calories	Carbo-hydrates (grams)
MELBA TOAST, salted (Old London):			
Garlic, onion or white rounds	1 piece	10	1.8
Pumpernickel, rye, wheat or white	1 piece	17	3.4
Sesame, flat	1 piece	18	3.0
MELON BALL, in syrup, frozen (USDA)	½ cup (4.1 oz.)	72	18.2
MENHADEN, Atlantic, canned (USDA) solids & liq.	4 oz.	195	0.
MERLOT WINE (Louis M. Martini) 12½% alcohol	3 fl. oz.	60	.2
MEXICAN DINNER, frozen: (Banquet):			
Regular	12-oz. dinner	483	62.0
Combination	12-oz. dinner	518	72.0
Extra Helping	20-oz. dinner	721	86.9
(Morton)	11-oz. dinner	300	45.0
(Swanson):			
3-course	18-oz. dinner	630	67.0
TV Brand	16-oz. dinner	590	66.0
(Van de Kamp's)	11-oz. dinner	421	43.0
MILK BREAK BARS (Pillsbury):			
Chocolate	1 bar	230	22.0
Chocolate mint	1 bar	230	21.0
Natural	1 bar	230	21.0
Peanut butter	1 bar	220	21.0
MILK, CONDENSED, sweetened, canned: (USDA)	1 T. (.7 oz.)	61	10.4

(USDA): United States Department of Agriculture
(HEW/FAO):   Health, Education and Welfare/Food and Agriculture
                    Organization
* Prepared as Package Directs

Food and Description	Measure or Quantity	Calories	Carbo-hydrates (grams)
(Carnation)	1 fl. oz.	123	20.8
(Milnot) *Dairy Sweet*	1 fl. oz. (1.3 oz.)	119	19.3
MILK, DRY:			
Whole (USDA) packed cup	1 cup (5.1 oz.)	728	55.4
*Nonfat, instant:			
(USDA)	8 fl. oz.	82	10.8
(Alba):			
Regular	8 fl. oz.	81	11.6
Chocolate flavor	8 fl. oz.	80	12.9
(Carnation)	8 fl. oz.	80	12.0
(Pet)	1 cup	80	12.0
(Sanalac)	1 cup	80	11.0
MINT, LEAVES, raw, trimmed			
(HEW/FAO)	½ oz.	4	.8
MOLASSES:			
Barbados (USDA)	1 T. (.7 oz.)	51	13.3
Blackstrap (USDA)	1 T. (.7 oz.)	40	10.4
Dark (Brer Rabbit)	1 T. (.7 oz.)	33	10.6
Light (USDA)	1 T. (.7 oz.)	48	12.4
Medium (USDA)	1 T.	44	11.4
Unsulphured (Grandma's)	1 T.	60	15.0
MORTADELLA, sausage			
(USDA)	1 oz.	89	.2
MOST, cereal (Kellogg's)	½ cup (1 oz.)	100	22.0
MOUSSE, canned, dietetic			
(Featherweight) chocolate	½ cup (4 oz.)	100	22.0
MUFFIN:			
Blueberry:			
Home recipe (USDA)	1.4-oz. muffin	112	16.8
(Hostess)	1¾-oz. muffin	127	21.9
(Morton):			
Regular	1.6-oz. muffin	120	23.0
Rounds	1.5-oz. muffin	110	21.0
(Pepperidge Farm)	1.9-oz. muffin	180	27.0

Food and Description	Measure or Quantity	Calories	Carbo-hydrates (grams)
Bran:			
Home recipe (USDA)	1.4-oz. muffin	104	17.2
(Arnold) *Bran'nola*	2.3-oz. muffin	160	30.0
(Pepperidge Farm)	1 muffin	180	28.0
Corn:			
Home recipe (USDA) prepared with whole-ground cornmeal	1.4-oz. muffin	115	17.0
(Morton)	1.7-oz. muffin	130	17.0
(Pepperidge Farm)	1.9-oz. muffin	180	27.0
(Thomas')	2-oz. muffin	184	25.8
English:			
(Arnold) extra crisp	2.3-oz. muffin	150	30.0
(Pepperidge Farm):			
Plain or wheat	2-oz. muffin	130	25.0
Cinnamon apple or sourdough	2-oz. muffin	140	27.0
Cinnamon raisin	2-oz. muffin	150	28.0
Roman Meal	2.3-oz. muffin	150	29.8
(Thomas's):			
Regular or frozen	2-oz. muffin	133	25.7
Honey wheat	2-oz. muffin	135	27.0
Raisin	2.2-oz. muffin	153	30.4
(Wonder)	2-oz. muffin	133	26.1
Orange-cranberry (Pepperidge Farm)	2.1-oz. muffin	190	30.0
Plain (USDA) home recipe	1.4-oz. muffin	118	16.9
Raisin:			
(Arnold)	2½-oz. muffin	170	35.0
(Wonder)	2-oz. muffin	150	27.8
Sourdough (Wonder)	2-oz. muffin	131	25.6
MUFFIN MIX:			
*Apple (Betty Crocker) spiced	1 muffin	120	18.0
Blueberry:			
*(Betty Crocker) wild	1 muffin	120	18.0
(Duncan Hines)	1/12 of pkg.	99	17.0

(USDA): United States Department of Agriculture
(HEW/FAO):   Health, Education and Welfare/Food and Agriculture
               Organization
* Prepared as Package Directs

Food and Description	Measure or Quantity	Calories	Carbo-hydrates (grams)
Bran:			
(Duncan Hines)	¹⁄₁₂ of pkg.	97	16.3
(Elam's) natural	1 T. (.25 oz.)	23	5.3
*Cherry (Betty Crocker)	¹⁄₁₂ of pkg.	120	18.0
Corn:			
*(Betty Crocker)	1 muffin	160	25.0
*(Dromedary)	1 muffin	130	20.0
*(Flako)	1 muffin	140	23.0
MULLIGAN STEW, canned, *Dinty Moore, Short Orders,* (Hormel)	7½-oz. can	230	14.0
MUSCATEL WINE (Gallo) 14% alcohol	3 fl. oz.	86	7.9
MUSHROOM:			
Raw (USDA):			
Whole	½ lb. (weighed untrimmed)	62	9.7
Trimmed, sliced	½ cup (1.2 oz.)	10	1.5
Canned (Green Giant) solids & liq., whole or sliced:			
Regular	2-oz. serving	14	2.0
B in B	1½-oz. serving	18	2.3
In butter sauce	1¾-oz. serving	26	3.5
Frozen (Green Giant) in butter sauce	½ cup	70	5.0
MUSHROOM, CHINESE, dried (HEW/FAO):			
Dry	1 oz.	81	18.9
Soaked, drained	1 oz.	12	2.4
MUSKELLUNGE, raw (USDA):			
Whole	1 lb. (weighed whole)	242	0.
Meat only	4 oz.	234	0.
MUSKMELON (See **CANTALOUPE, CASABA or HONEYDEW**)			

Food and Description	Measure or Quantity	Calories	Carbo-hydrates (grams)
MUSKRAT, roasted (*SDA)	4 oz.	174	0.
MUSSEL, (USDA):			
Atlantia & Pacific, raw:			
In Shell	1 lb. (weighed in shell)	153	7.2
Meat only	4 oz.	108	3.7
Pacific, canned, drained	4 oz.	129	1.7
MUSTARD:			
Powder (French's)	1 tsp. (1.5 grams)	9	.3
Prepared:			
Brown (French's; Gulden's)	1 tsp.	5	.3
Dijon, *Grey Poupon*	1 tsp. (.2 oz.)	6	Tr.
Horseradish (French's)	1 tsp. (.2 oz.)	5	.3
Medford (French's)	1 tsp.	5	.3
Onion (French's)	1 tsp.	8	1.6
Unsalted (Featherweight)	1 tsp.	5	.3
Yellow (Gulden's)	1 tsp.	5	.4
MUSTARD GREENS:			
Raw (USDA) whole	1 lb. (weighed untrimmed)	98	17.8
Boiled (USDA) drained	1 cup (7.8 oz.)	51	8.8
Canned (Sunshine) chopped, solids & liq.	½ cup (4.1 oz.)	22	3.2
Frozen, chopped:			
(Birds Eye)	⅓ of 10-oz. pkg.	25	3.2
(McKenzie)	⅓ of 10-oz. pkg.	20	3.0
(Southland)	⅕ of 16-oz. pkg.	20	3.0
MUSTARD SPINACH (USDA):			
Raw	1 lb.	100	17.7
Boiled, drained, no added salt	4-oz. serving	18	3.2

(USDA): United States Department of Agriculture
(HEW/FAO):   Health, Education and Welfare/Food and Agriculture
                        Organization
* Prepared as Package Directs

Food and Description	Measure or Quantity	Calories	Carbo-hydrates (grams)

N

NATURAL CEREAL:

Heartland	¼ cup (1 oz.)	138	17.9
(Quaker):			
Hot, whole wheat	⅓ cup (1 oz.)	106	21.8
100% natural	¼ cup (1 oz.)	138	17.4
100% natural, with apple & cinnamon	¼ cup (1 oz.)	135	18.0
100% natural with raisins & dates	¼ cup (1 oz.)	134	18.0

NATURE SNACKS (Sun-Maid):

Carob Crunch	1 oz.	143	16.8
Carob Peanut	1¼ oz.	190	18.0
Carob Raisin or Yogurt Raisin	1¼ oz.	160	25.0
Nuts Galore	1 oz.	170	5.0
Raisin Crunch or Rocky Road	1 oz.	126	19.1
Sesame Nut Crunch	1 oz.	154	14.6
Tahitian Treat or Yogurt Crunch	1 oz.	123	19.4
Yogurt Peanut	1¼ oz.	200	18.0

NECTARINE, fresh (USDA):

Whole	1 lb. (weighed with pits)	267	71.4
Flesh only	4 oz.	73	19.4

NEW ZEALAND SPINACH (USDA):

Raw	1 lb.	86	14.1
Boiled, drained	4 oz.	15	2.4

NOODLE. Plain noodle products are essentially the same in caloric value and carbohydrate content on the same weight basis. The longer they are

Food and Description	Measure or Quantity	Calories	Carbo-hydrates (grams)
cooked, the more water is absorbed and this affects the nutritive values. (USDA):			
Dry	1 oz.	110	20.4
Dry, 1½″ strips	1 cup (2.6 oz.)	283	52.6
Cooked	1 oz.	35	6.6
NOODLES & BEEF:			
Canned (Hormel) *Short Orders*	7½-oz. can	230	16.0
Frozen (Banquet) *Buffet Supper*	2-lb. pkg.	754	83.6
NOODLES & CHICKEN:			
Canned (Hormel) *Dinty Moore, Short Orders*	7½-oz. can	210	15.0
Frozen (Swanson) *TV Brand*	10½-oz. dinner	270	37.0
NOODLE, CHOW MEIN (La Choy)	½ cup (1 oz.)	150	17.0
NOODLE MIX:			
*(Betty Crocker):			
Fettucini Alfredo	¼ of pkg.	220	23.0
Parisienne	¼ of pkg.	160	26.0
Romanoff	¼ of pkg.	230	23.0
Stroganoff	¼ of pkg.	240	26.0
Noodle Roni, parmesano	⅕ of 6-oz. pkg.	130	22.5
*(Lipton) *Egg Noodles & Sauce:*			
Beef, butter or chicken	¼ of pkg.	190	26.0
Butter and herb	¼ of pkg.	180	23.0
Cheese	¼ of pkg.	200	24.0
NOODLE, RICE (La Choy)	1 oz.	130	21.0
NOODLE ROMANOFF, frozen (Stouffer's)	⅓ of 12-oz. pkg.	170	16.0

(USDA): United States Department of Agriculture
(HEW/FAO):   Health, Education and Welfare/Food and Agriculture
                      Organization
* Prepared as Package Directs

Food and Description	Measure or Quantity	Calories	Carbo-hydrates (grams)
NUT, MIXED:			
Dry roasted:			
(Flavor House) salted	1 oz.	172	5.4
(Planters)	1 oz.	160	7.0
Oil roasted (Planters) with or without peanuts	1 oz.	180	6.0
NUTMEG (French's)	1 tsp. (1.9 grams)	11	.9
NUTRI-GRAIN, cereal (Kellogg's):			
Corn	½ cup (1 oz.)	110	24.0
Wheat	⅔ cup (1 oz.)	110	24.0
Wheat & Raisin	⅔ cup (1.4 oz.)	140	33.0
NUTRIMATO (Mott's)	6 fl. oz.	70	17.0

0

Food and Description	Measure or Quantity	Calories	Carbo- hydrates (grams)
OAT FLAKES, cereal (Post)	⅔ cup (1 oz.)	107	20.6
OATMEAL:			
Dry:			
Regular:			
(USDA)	½ cup (1.2 oz.)	140	44.5
(Elam's):			
Scotch style or stone ground	1 oz.	108	18.2
Steel cut, whole grain	¼ cup (1.6 oz.)	174	30.4
(H-O) old fashioned	1 T. (.14 oz.)	15	2.6
(Quaker) old fashioned	⅓ cup (1 oz.)	109	18.5
(3-Minute Brand)	⅓ cup (1 oz.)	110	18.1
Instant:			
(Harvest Brand):			
Regular	1 oz.	108	17.3
Apple & cinnamon	1¼ oz.	136	25.7
Cinnamon & spice	1⅝ oz.	183	35.5
Maple & brown sugar	1.5 oz.	171	25.6
Peaches & cream	⅓ cup (1¼ oz.)	140	25.6
(H-O):			
Regular, boxed	1 T.	15	2.6
Regular, packets	1-oz. packet	105	17.9
With bran & spice	1½-oz. packet	157	29.0
Country apple & brown sugar	1.1-oz. packet	121	22.7
With maple & brown sugar flavor	1½-oz. packet	160	31.8
Sweet & mellow	1.4-oz. packet	149	28.7
(Quaker):			
Regular	1-oz. packet	105	18.1
Apple & cinnamon	1¼-oz. packet	134	26.0

(USDA): United States Department of Agriculture
(HEW/FAO):   Health, Education and Welfare/Food and Agriculture Organization
* Prepared as Package Directs

Food and Description	Measure or Quantity	Calories	Carbo-hydrates (grams)
Bran & raisin	1.5-oz. packet	153	29.2
Cinnamon & spice	1⅝-oz. packet	176	34.8
Honey & graham	1¼-oz. packet	136	26.6
Maple & brown sugar	1.5-oz. packet	163	31.9
Raisins & spice	1½-oz. packet	159	31.4
(3-Minute Brand)	1½-oz. packet	162	25.9
Quick:			
(Harvest Brand)	⅓ cup (1 oz.)	110	18.1
(H-O)	½ cup (1.2 oz.)	129	22.2
(Quaker)	⅓ cup (1 oz.)	109	18.5
(Ralston Purina)	⅓ cup (1 oz.)	110	18.0
(3-Minute Brand)	⅓ cup	110	18.1
Cooked, regular (USDA)	1 cup (8.5 oz.)	132	23.3
OCTOPUS, raw (USDA) meat only	4 oz.	83	0.
OIL, SALAD OR COOKING:			
(USDA) all kinds, including olive	1 T. (.5 oz.)	124	0.
(USDA) all kinds, including olive	½ cup (3.9 oz.)	972	0.
Crisco, Fleischmann's; Mazola	1 T. (.5 oz.)	126	0.
(Golden Thistle)	1 T. (.5 oz.)	130	0.
Mrs. Tucker's, corn or soybean	1 T.	130	0.
(Planters) peanut or popcorn	1 T.	130	0.
Sunlite; Wesson	1 T.	120	0.
OKRA:			
Raw (USDA) whole	1 lb. (weighed untrimmed)	140	29.6
Boiled (USDA) drained:			
Whole	½ cup (3.1 oz.)	26	5.3
Pods	8 pods (3 oz.)	25	5.1
Slices	½ cup (2.8 oz.)	23	4.8
Frozen:			
(Birds Eye)			
Whole, baby	⅓ of 10-oz. pkg.	36	6.7
Cut	⅓ of 10-oz. pkg.	30	5.7
(McKenzie):			
Cut	3.3 oz.	25	6.0
Whole	3.3 oz.	30	7.0

Food and Description	Measure or Quantity	Calories	Carbo- hydrates (grams)
(Seabrook Farms) cut	⅓ of 10-oz. pkg.	32	6.1
(Southland):			
Cut	⅕ of 16-oz. pkg.	25	5.0
Whole	⅕ of 16-oz. pkg.	35	7.0
OLD FASHIONED COCKTAIL			
(Hiram Walker) 62 proof	3 fl. oz.	165	3.0
OLIVE:			
Green style (USDA):			
With pits, drained	1 oz.	77	2.0
Pitted, drained	1 oz.	96	2.5
Green (USDA)	1 oz.	33	.4
Ripe, by variety (USDA):			
Ascalano, any size, pitted & drained	1 oz.	37	.7
Manzanilla, any size	1 oz.	37	.7
Mission	3 small or 2 large	18	.3
Mission, slices	½ cup (2.2 oz.)	26	6.1
Ripe, by size (Lindsay):			
Colassal	1 olive	13	.3
Extra large	1 olive	5	.1
Giant	1 olive	8	.2
Jumbo	1 olive	10	.2
Large	1 olive	5	.1
Mammoth	1 olive	6	.1
Medium	1 olive	4	.1
Select	1 olive	3	.1
Super colossal	1 olive	16	.3
Super supreme	1 olive	18	.3
ONION (See also **ONION, GREEN** and **ONION, WELCH**):			
Raw (USDA):			
Whole	1 lb. (weighed untrimmed)	157	35.9

(USDA): United States Department of Agriculture
(HEW/FAO):   Health, Education and Welfare/Food and Agriculture
Organization
* Prepared as Package Directs

Food and Description	Measure or Quantity	Calories	Carbo-hydrates (grams)
Whole	3.9-oz. onion (2½" dia.)	38	8.7
Chopped	½ cup (3 oz.)	33	7.5
Chopped	1 T. (.4 oz.)	4	1.0
Grated	1 T. (.5 oz.)	5	1.2
Slices	½ cup (2 oz.)	21	4.9
Boiled, drained (USDA):			
Whole	½ cup (3.7 oz.)	30	6.8
Whole, pearl onions	½ cup (3.2 oz.)	27	6.0
Halves or pieces	½ cup (3.2 oz.)	26	5.8
Canned, *O & C* (Durkee):			
Boiled	1-oz. serving	8	2.0
In cream sauce	1-oz. serving	143	17.0
Dehydrated:			
Flakes:			
(USDA)	1 tsp. (1.3 grams)	5	1.1
(Gilroy)	1 tsp.	5	1.2
Powder (Gilroy)	1 tsp.	9	2.0
Frozen:			
(Birds Eye):			
Chopped	1 oz.	8	2.0
Small, whole	¼ of 16-oz. pkg.	44	9.6
Small, with cream sauce	⅓ of 9-oz. pkg.	118	11.2
(Green Giant) small, in cheese sauce	½ cup	90	9.0
(McKenzie) chopped	1 oz.	8	2.0
(Mrs. Paul's) rings, breaded & fried	½ of 5-oz. pkg.	167	22.2
(Southland) chopped	⅕ of 10-oz. pkg.	20	5.0
ONION BOUILLON:			
(Herb-Ox):			
Cube	1 cube	10	1.3
Packet	1 packet	14	2.1
MBT	1 packet	16	2.0
ONION, GREEN, raw (USDA):			
Whole	1 lb. (weighed untrimmed)	157	35.7
Bulb & entire top	1 oz.	10	2.3
Bulb without green top	3 small onions (.9 oz.)	11	2.6

Food and Description	Measure or Quantity	Calories	Carbo-hydrates (grams)
Slices, bulb & white portion of top	½ cup (1.8 oz.)	22	5.2
Tops only	1 oz.	8	1.6
ONION SALAD SEASONING (French's) instant	1 T.	15	3.0
ONION SALT (French's)	1 tsp.	6	1.0
ONION SOUP (See **SOUP**, Onion)			
ONION, WELCH, raw (USDA):			
Whole	1 lb. (weighed untrimmed)	100	19.2
Trimmed	4 oz.	39	7.4
OPOSSUM (USDA) roasted, meat only	4 oz.	251	0.
ORANGE, fresh (USDA):			
California Navel:			
Whole	1 lb. (weighed with rind & seeds)	157	39.3
Whole	6.3-oz. orange (2⅘" dia.)	62	15.5
Sections	1 cup (8.5 oz.)	123	30.6
California Valencia:			
Whole	1 lb. (weighed with rind & seeds)	174	42.2
Fruit, including peel	6.3-oz. orange (2⅝" dia.)	72	27.9
Sections	1 cup (8.6 oz.)	123	29.9
Florida, all varieties:			
Whole	1 lb. (weighed with rind & seeds)	158	40.3

(USDA): United States Department of Agriculture
(HEW/FAO):   Health, Education and Welfare/Food and Agriculture
              Organization
* Prepared as Package Directs

Food and Description	Measure or Quantity	Calories	Carbo-hydrates (grams)
Whole	7.4-oz. orange (3″ dia.)	73	18.6
Sections	1 cup (8.5 oz.)	113	28.9
ORANGE-APRICOT JUICE COCKTAIL, *Musselman's*	8 fl. oz.	100	23.0
ORANGE DRINK:			
Canned:			
Capri Sun, natural	6¾-fl.-oz. can	103	26.1
(Hi-C)	6 fl. oz.	92	23.0
(Lincoln)	6 fl. oz.	100	24.0
*Mix:			
Regular (Hi-C)	6 fl. oz.	91	17.0
Dietetic, *Crystal Light*	6 fl. oz. (6.3 oz.)	4	.4
ORANGE EXTRACT (Virginia Dare) 79% alcohol	1 tsp.	22	0.
ORANGE-GRAPEFRUIT JUICE:			
Canned:			
(Del Monte):			
Sweetened	6 fl. oz.	91	21.1
Unsweetened	6 fl. oz.	79	18.3
(Libby's) unsweetened	6 fl. oz.	80	19.0
*Frozen (Minute Maid) unsweetened	6 fl. oz.	76	19.1
ORANGE JUICE:			
Fresh (USDA):			
California Navel	½ cup (4.4 oz.)	60	14.0
California Valencia	½ cup (4.4 oz.)	58	13.0
Florida, early or midseason	½ cup (4.4 oz.)	50	11.4
Florida Temple	½ cup (4.4 oz.)	67	16.0
Florida Valencia	½ cup (4.4 oz.)	56	13.0
Canned, unsweetened:			
(USDA)	½ cup (4.4 oz.)	60	13.9
(Del Monte)	6 fl. oz. (6.5 oz.)	80	19.0
(Sunkist)	½ cup (4.4 oz.)	60	14.0
(Texsun)	6 fl. oz.	83	20.0

Food and Description	Measure or Quantity	Calories	Carbo-hydrates (grams)
Canned, sweetened:			
(USDA)	6 fl. oz.	66	15.4
(Del Monte)	6 fl. oz.	76	17.4
Chilled (Minute Maid)	6 fl. oz.	83	19.7
*Dehydrated crystals (USDA)	½ cup (4.4 oz.)	57	13.4
*Frozen:			
(USDA)	½ cup (4.4 oz.)	56	13.3
(Birds Eye) *Orange Plus*	6 fl. oz.	99	24.0
Bright & Early, imitation	6 fl. oz.	90	21.6
(Minute Maid)	6 fl. oz.	86	20.5
(Snow Crop)	6 fl. oz.	86	20.5
(Sunkist)	6 fl. oz.	92	21.7
ORANGE, MANDARIN (See **TANGERINE**)			
ORANGE PEEL, CANDIED			
(USDA)	1 oz.	90	22.9
ORANGE-PINEAPPLE DRINK, canned (Lincoln)	6 fl. oz.	128	
ORANGE-PINEAPPLE JUICE, canned (Texsun)	8 fl. oz.	89	21.0
OREGANO (French's)	1 tsp.	6	1.0
OVALTINE:			
Chocolate	¾ oz.	78	17.9
Malt	¾ oz.	88	17.6
OVEN FRY (General Foods):			
Crispy crumb for pork	4.2-oz. envelope	484	78.0
Crispy crumb for chicken	4.2-oz. envelope	460	82.4
Homestyle flour recipe	3.2-oz. envelope	304	64.8

(USDA): United States Department of Agriculture
(HEW/FAO):   Health, Education and Welfare/Food and Agriculture
                        Organization
* Prepared as Package Directs

Food and Description	Measure or Quantity	Calories	Carbo-hydrates (grams)
OYSTER:			
Raw (USDA):			
Eastern, meat only	19–31 small or 13–19 med.	158	8.2
Pacific & Western, meat only	6–9 small or 4–6 med. (8.5 oz.)	218	15.4
Canned (Bumble Bee) shelled, whole, solids & liq.	1 cup (8.5 oz.)	218	15.4
Fried (USDA) dipped in milk, egg & breadcrumbs	4 oz.	271	21.1
OYSTER STEW (USDA):			
Home recipe:			
1 part oysters to 1 part milk by volume	1 cup (8.5 oz., 6–8 oysters)	245	14.2
1 part oysters to 2 parts milk by volume	1 cup (8.5 oz.)	233	10.8
1 part oysters to 3 parts milk by volume	1 cup (8.5 oz.)	206	11.3
Frozen:			
Prepared with equal volume milk	1 cup (8.5 oz.)	201	14.2
Prepared with equal volume water	1 cup (8.5 oz.)	122	8.2

Food and Description	Measure or Quantity	Calories	Carbo-hydrates (grams)

P

Food and Description	Measure or Quantity	Calories	Carbo-hydrates (grams)
PAC-MAN CEREAL			
(General Mills)	1 cup (1 oz.)	110	25.0
*PANCAKE BATTER			
FROZEN (Aunt Jemima):			
Plain	4″ pancake	70	14.1
Blueberry or buttermilk	4″ pancake	68	13.8
Buttermilk	4″ pancake	68	14.2
PANCAKE DINNER OR			
ENTREE, frozen			
(Swanson):			
& blueberries, in sauce,			
TV Brand	7-oz. entree	400	70.0
& sausage	6-oz. entree	440	48.0
*PANCAKE & WAFFLE MIX:			
Plain:			
(Aunt Jemima):			
Original	4″ pancake	73	8.7
Complete	4″ pancake	80	15.7
(Log Cabin):			
Regular	4″ pancake	60	8.7
Complete	4″ pancake	58	11.2
(Pillsbury) *Hungry Jack:*			
Complete:			
Bulk	4″ pancake	63	13.0
Packets	4″ pancake	70	10.0
Extra Lights	4″ pancake	70	10.0
Golden Blend:			
Regular	4″ pancake	67	8.7
Complete	4″ pancake	80	14.3

(USDA): United States Department of Agriculture
(HEW/FAO):   Health, Education and Welfare/Food and Agriculture
                Organization
* Prepared as Package Directs

Food and Description	Measure or Quantity	Calories	Carbo-hydrates (grams)
Panshakes	4″ pancake	83	14.3
Blueberry (Pillsbury)			
Hungry Jack	4″ pancake	107	13.3
Buckwheat (Aunt Jemima)	4″ pancake	67	8.3
Buttermilk:			
(Aunt Jemima):			
Regular	4″ pancake	100	13.3
Complete	4″ pancake	80	15.3
(Betty Crocker):			
Regular	4″ pancake	93	13.0
Complete	4″ pancake	70	13.7
(Pillsbury) *Hungry Jack:*			
Regular	4″ pancake	80	9.7
Complete	4″ pancake	63	13.0
Whole wheat (Aunt Jemima)	4″ pancake	83	10.7
Dietetic:			
(Dia-Mel)	3″ pancake	33	7.0
(Featherweight) low sodium	4″ pancake	43	8.0
(Tillie Lewis) *Tasti Diet*	4″ pancake	47	8.7

PANCAKE & WAFFLE SYRUP (See **SYRUP,** Pancake & Waffle)

PASSION FRUIT JUICE, fresh (HEW/FAO)	4 oz.	50	11.5
PASTINA, DRY (USDA):			
Carrot	1 oz.	105	21.5
Egg	1 oz.	109	20.4
Spinach	1 oz.	104	21.2
PASTOSO (Petri) 12% alcohol	3 fl. oz.	71	1.2
PASTRAMI, packaged:			
(Eckrich) sliced	1-oz. slice	47	1.3
(Vienna)	2 oz.	86	0.
PANCREAS, raw (USDA):			
Beef, lean only	4 oz.	160	0.
Calf	4 oz.	183	0.
Hog or hog sweetbread	4 oz.	274	0.

Food and Description	Measure or Quantity	Calories	Carbo-hydrates (grams)
PAPAW, fresh (USDA):			
Whole	1 lb. (weighed with rind & seeds)	289	57.2
Flesh only	4 oz.	96	19.1
PAPAYA, fresh (USDA):			
Whole	1 lb. (weighed with skin & seeds)	119	30.4
Cubed	1 cup (6.4 oz.)	71	18.2
PAPAYA JUICE, canned (HEW/FAO)	4 oz.	77	19.6
PAPRIKA, domestic (French's)	1 tsp.	7	1.1
PARSLEY, fresh (USDA):			
Whole	½ lb.	100	19.3
Chopped	1 T. (4 grams)	2	.3
PARSLEY FLAKES, dehydrated (French's)	1 tsp. (1.1 grams)	4	.6
PARSNIP (USDA):			
Raw, whole	1 lb. (weighed unprepared)	293	67.5
Boiled, drained, cut in pieces	½ cup (3.7 oz.)	70	15.8
PASSION FRUIT, fresh (USDA):			
Whole	1 lb. (weighed with shell)	212	50.0
Pulp & seeds	4 oz.	102	24.0
PASSION FRUIT JUICE, fresh (HEW/FAO)	4 oz.	50	11.5

(USDA): United States Department of Agriculture
(HEW/FAO):   Health, Education and Welfare/Food and Agriculture
Organization
* Prepared as Package Directs

Food and Description	Measure or Quantity	Calories	Carbo-hydrates (grams)
PASTINA, DRY (USDA):			
Carrot	1 oz.	105	21.5
Egg	1 oz.	109	20.4
Spinach	1 oz.	104	21.2
PASTOSO (Petri) 12% alcohol	3 fl. oz.	71	1.2
PASTRAMI, packaged:			
(Eckrich) sliced	1 oz. slice	47	1.3
(Vienna)	1 oz.	86	0.
PASTRY SHEET, PUFF, frozen			
(Pepperidge Farm)	1 sheet (4.3 oz.)	510	45.0
PASTRY SHELL, frozen			
(Pepperidge Farm)	1 shell (1.7 oz.)	210	17.0
PÂTÉ:			
De foie gras (USDA)	1 T. (.5 oz.)	69	.7
Liver:			
(Hormel)	1 T.	35	.3
(Sell's)	½ of 4.8-oz. can	223	2.7
PDQ:			
Chocolate	1 T. (.6 oz.)	66	15.1
Egg Nog	2 heaping T. (1 oz.)	113	27.5
Strawberry	1 T. (.5 oz.)	60	15.0
PEA, green:			
Raw (USDA):			
In pod	1 lb. (weighed in pod)	145	24.8
Shelled	1 lb.	381	65.3
Shelled	½ cup (2.4 oz.)	58	9.9
Boiled (USDA) drained			
Canned, regular pack:			
(USDA):			
Alaska, early or June:			
Solids & liq.	½ cup (4.4 oz.)	82	15.5
Solids only	½ cup (3 oz.)	76	14.4

Food and Description	Measure or Quantity	Calories	Carbo-hydrates (grams)
Sweet:			
Solids & liq.	½ cup (4.4 oz.)	71	12.9
Solids only	½ cup (3 oz.)	69	12.9
Drained liquid	4 oz.	25	4.9
(Del Monte) seasoned or sweet, regular size solids & liq.	½ cup	60	11.0
(Green Giant) solids & liq.:			
Early with onions, sweet or sweet with onions	¼ of 17-oz. can	60	10.0
Sweet, mimi	¼ of 17-oz. can	64	10.9
(Le Sueur) early June or sweet mini, solids & liq.	¼ of 17-oz. can	60	11.0
(Libby's) sweet, solids & liq.	½ cup (4.2 oz.)	66	11.6
(USDA):			
Alaska, early or June:			
Solids & liq.	4 oz.	62	11.1
Solids only	4 oz.	88	16.2
Sweet:			
Solids & liq.	4 oz.	53	9.5
Solids only	4 oz.	82	14.7
(Del Monte) No Salt Added, sweet, solids & liq.	½ cup (4.3 oz.)	60	11.0
(Diet Delight) solids & liq.	½ cup (4.3 oz.)	50	8.0
(Featherweight) sweet, solids & liq.	½ cup (4 oz.)	70	12.0
(S&W) *Nutradiet,* green label, solids & liq.	½ cup	40	8.0
Frozen:			
(Birds Eye):			
Regular	⅓ of 10-oz. pkg.	78	13.3
In butter sauce	⅓ of 10-oz. pkg.	85	12.6
In cream sauce	⅓ of 8-oz. pkg.	84	14.3
Tiny, tender, deluxe	⅓ of 10-oz. pkg.	64	10.7
(Green Giant):			
In cream sauce	½ cup	100	12.0

(USDA): United States Department of Agriculture
(HEW/FAO):   Health, Education and Welfare/Food and Agriculture
Organization
* Prepared as Package Directs

Food and Description	Measure or Quantity	Calories	Carbohydrates (grams)
Early June or sweet, polybag	½ cup	60	10.0
Early & sweet in butter sauce	½ cup	90	14.0
Sweet, *Harvest Fresh*	½ cup	80	14.0
(McKenzie):			
Regular	3.3 oz.	80	13.0
Tiny	3.3 oz.	60	11.0
PEA & CARROT:			
Canned, regular pack, solids & liq.:			
(Del Monte)	½ cup (4 oz.)	50	10.0
(Libby's)	½ cup (4.2 oz.)	56	10.3
Canned, dietetic pack, solids & liq.:			
(Diet Delight)	½ cup (4.3 oz.)	40	6.0
(S&W) *Nutradiet*, green label	½ cup	35	7.0
Frozen:			
(Birds Eye)	⅓ of 10-oz. pkg.	61	11.2
(McKenzie)	3.3-oz. serving	60	11.0
PEA, CROWDER, frozen:			
(Birds Eye)	⅕ of 16-oz. pkg.	130	22.6
(McKenzie)	3-oz. serving	130	23.0
(Southland)	⅓ of 16-oz. pkg.	120	21.0
PEA, MATURE SEED, dry (USDA):			
Whole	1 lb.	1542	272.5
Whole	1 cup	680	120.6
Split	1 lb.	1579	284.4
Split	1 cup (7.2 oz.)	706	127.3
Cooked, split, drained solids	½ cup (3.4 oz.)	112	20.2
PEA & ONION, frozen (Birds Eye)	⅓ of 10-oz. pkg.	67	117
PEA POD:			
Raw (USDA) edible podded or Chinese	1 lb. (weighed untrimmed)	228	51.7

Food and Description	Measure or Quantity	Calories	Carbo- hydrates (grams)
Boiled (USDA) drained	4 oz.	49	10.8
Frozen (La Choy)	6-oz. pkg.	70	12.0
PEACH:			
Fresh (USDA):			
Whole, without skin	1 lb. (weighed unpeeled)	150	38.3
Whole	4-oz. peach (2" dia.)	38	9.6
Diced	½ cup (4.7 oz.)	51	12.9
Sliced	½ cup (3 oz.)	31	8.2
Canned, regular pack, solids & liq.:			
(USDA):			
Extra heavy syrup	4 oz.	110	28.5
Heavy syrup	2 med. halves & 2 T. syrup (4.1 oz.)	91	23.5
Juice pack	4 oz.	51	13.2
Light syrup	4 oz.	66	17.1
(Del Monte):			
Cling:			
Halves or slices	½ cup (4 oz.)	80	22.0
Spices	3½ oz.	80	20.0
Freestone	½ cup (4 oz.)	90	23.0
(Libby's) heavy syrup:			
Halves	½ cup (4.5 oz.)	105	25.4
Slices	½ cup (4.5 oz.)	102	24.7
Canned, dietetic pack, solids & liq.:			
(Del Monte) Lite:			
Cling	½ cup (4 oz.)	50	13.0
Freestone	½ cup (4 oz.)	60	13.0
(Diet Delight) Cling:			
Juice pack	½ cup (4.4 oz.)	50	14.0
Water pack	½ cup (4.3 oz.)	30	2.0

(USDA): United States Department of Agriculture
(HEW/FAO):   Health, Education and Welfare/Food and Agriculture
            Organization
* Prepared as Package Directs

Food and Description	Measure or Quantity	Calories	Carbo-hydrates (grams)
(Featherweight):			
Cling or Freestone, juice pack	½ cup	50	12.0
Cling, water pack	½ cup	30	8.0
(S&W) *Nutradiet,* Cling:			
Juice pack	½ cup	60	14.0
Water pack	½ cup	30	8.0
Dehydrated (USDA):			
Uncooked	1 oz.	96	24.9
Cooked, with added sugar, solids & liq.	½ cup (5.4 oz.)	184	47.6
Dried (USDA):			
Uncooked	½ cup	231	60.1
Cooked:			
Unsweetened	½ cup	111	28.9
Sweetened	½ cup (5.4 oz.)	181	46.8
Frozen (Birds Eye) quick thaw	5-oz. serving	141	34.1
PEACH BUTTER (Smucker's)	1 T. (.7 oz.)	45	16.0
PEACH DRINK, canned (Hi-C):			
Canned	6 fl. oz.	90	23.0
*Mix	6 fl. oz.	72	18.0
PEACH LIQUEUR (DeKupyer)	1 fl. oz.	82	8.3
PEACH NECTAR, canned (Libby's)	6 fl. oz.	90	23.0
PEACH PRESERVE OR JAM:			
Sweetened (Smucker's)	1 T. (.7 oz.)	53	13.5
Dietetic (Dia-Mel)	1 T.	6	0.
PEANUT:			
Raw (USDA):			
In shell	1 lb. (weighed in shell)	1868	61.6
With skins	1 oz.	160	5.3
Without skins	1 oz.	161	5.0
Roasted:			
(USDA):			
Whole	1 lb. (weighed in shell)	1769	62.6

Food and Description	Measure or Quantity	Calories	Carbo-hydrates (grams)
Chopped	½ cup	404	13.0
Halves	½ cup	421	13.5
(Fisher):			
In shell, salted	1 oz.	105	3.7
Shelled:			
Dry roasted, salted or unsalted	1 oz.	163	5.0
Oil roasted, salted	1 oz.	166	5.3
(Frito-Lay's):			
In shell, salted	1 oz, shelled	163	5.7
Shelled	1 oz.	172	6.2
(Planters):			
Dry roasted	1 oz. (jar)	170	5.4
Oil roasted	¾-oz. bag	133	3.7
Spanish roasted:			
(Frito-Lay's)	1 oz.	168	6.6
(Planter's):			
Dry roasted	1 oz. (jar)	175	3.4
Oil roasted	1 oz. (can)	182	3.4

PEANUT BUTTER:
Regular:

(Elam's) natural, with defatted wheatgerm	1 T. (.6 oz.)	109	2.1
(Jif) creamy	1 T. (.6 oz.)	93	2.7
(Peter Pan):			
Crunchy	1 T. (.6 oz.)	101	3.0
Smooth	1 T. (.6 oz.)	94	3.1
(Planter's)	1 T. (.6 oz.)	95	3.0
(Skippy):			
Creamy or super chunk	1 T.	108	3.0
Creamy, old fashioned	1 T.	107	2.8
Dietetic:			
(Featherweight) low sodium	1 T. (.5 oz.)	90	2.0
(Peter Pan) low sodium	1 T.	106	2.3
(S&W) *Nutradiet,* low sodium	1 T.	93	2.0

(USDA): United States Department of Agriculture
(HEW/FAO):   Health, Education and Welfare/Food and Agriculture
                       Organization
* Prepared as Package Directs

Food and Description	Measure or Quantity	Calories	Carbo-hydrates (grams)
PEANUT BUTTER BAKING CHIPS (Reese's)	3 T. (1 oz.)	151	12.8
PEAR:			
Fresh (USDA):			
Whole	1 lb. (weighed with stems & core)	252	63.2
Whole	6.4-oz. pear (3″ × 2½″ dia.)	101	25.4
Quartered	1 cup (6.8 oz.)	117	29.4
Slices	½ cup (6.8 oz.)	50	12.5
Canned, regular pack, solids & liq.:			
(USDA):			
Extra heavy syrup	4 oz.	104	26.8
Heavy syrup	½ cup	87	22.3
Juice pack	4 oz.	52	13.4
Light syrup	4 oz.	69	17.7
(Del Monte) Bartlett, halves or slices	½ cup (4. oz.)	80	22.0
(Libby's) halves, heavy syrup	½ cup (4.5 oz.)	102	25.1
Canned, dietetic pack, solids & liq.:			
(Del Monte) Lite, Bartlett halves or slices	½ cup (4 oz.)	50	14.0
(Diet Delight):			
Juice pack	½ cup	60	16.0
Water pack	½ cup	35	9.0
(Featherweight) Bartlett, halves:			
Juice pack	½ cup	60	15.0
Water pack	½ cup	40	10.0
(Libby's) water pack	½ cup	60	15.0
(S&W) *Nutradiet,* halves, quarters or slices, white or blue label	½ cup	35	10.0
Dried (Sun-Maid)	½ cup (3.5 oz.)	260	70.0
PEAR, CANDIED (USDA)	1 oz.	86	21.5
PEAR NECTAR, canned:			
(Del Monte)	6 fl. oz. (6.6 oz.)	122	11.5
(Libby's)	6 fl. oz.	100	25.0

Food and Description	Measure or Quantity	Calories	Carbo-hydrates (grams)
PEAR-PASSION FRUIT			
NECTAR, canned (Libby's)	6 fl. oz.	60	14.0
PEBBLES, cereal:			
Cocoa	⅞ cup (1 oz.)	117	24.4
Fruity	⅞ cup (1 oz.)	116	24.5
PECAN:			
In shell (USDA)	1 lb. (weighed in shell)	1652	35.1
Shelled (USDA):			
Whole	1 lb. (weighed in shell)	3116	66.2
Chopped	½ cup (1.8 oz.)	357	7.6
Chopped	1 T. (7 grams)	48	1.0
Halves	12–14 halves (.5 oz.)	96	2.0
Halves	½ cup (1.9 oz.)	371	7.9
Oil dipped (Fisher) salted	¼ cup	410	8.9
Roasted, dry:			
(Fisher) salted	¼ cup (1.1 oz.)	220	4.5
(Flavor House)	1 oz.	195	4.1
(Planters)	1 oz.	206	3.5
PECTIN, FRUIT:			
Certo	6-oz. pkg.	19	4.8
Sure-Jell:			
Regular	1¾-oz. pkg.	170	42.6
Light	1¾-oz. pkg.	160	40.0
PEPPER:			
Black (French's)	1 tsp. (2.3 grams)	9	1.5
Seasoned (French's)	1 tsp.	8	1.0
PEPPER, CHILI:			
Raw, green (USDA) without seeds	4 oz.	42	10.3

(USDA): United States Department of Agriculture
(HEW/FAO):   Health, Education and Welfare/Food and Agriculture Organization
* Prepared as Package Directs

Food and Description	Measure or Quantity	Calories	Carbo-hydrates (grams)
Canned:			
(Del Monte):			
Green, whole	½ cup (4 oz.)	20	5.0
Jalapeno or chili, whole	½ cup (4 oz.)	30	6.0
Yellow, whole	½ cup (3.9 oz.)	30	4.0
Old El Paso, green, chopped or whole	1 oz.	7	1.4
(Ortega):			
Green, diced, strips or whole	1 oz.	6	1.1
Jalapeno, diced or whole	1 oz.	9	1.7
PEPPERMINT EXTRACT			
(Durkee) imitation	1 tsp.	15	DNA
PEPPERONI:			
(Eckrich)	1-oz. serving	135	1.0
(Hormel):			
Regular, chub, Rosa or Rosa Grande	1 oz.	140	0.
Packaged, sliced	1 slice	40	0.
PEPPER & ONION, frozen			
(Southland):			
Diced	2-oz. serving	15	3.0
Red & green	2-oz. serving	20	4.0
PEPPER STEAK, frozen			
(Stouffer's)	10½-oz. pkg.	350	35.0
PEPPER, STUFFED:			
Home recipe (USDA) with beef & crumbs	2¾" × 2½" pepper with 1⅛ cups stuffing	314	31.1
Frozen:			
(Green Giant) green, baked	½ of pkg.	200	15.0
(Stouffer's) green with beef in tomato sauce	7¾-oz. serving	225	18.0
(Weight Watchers) with veal stuffing, one-compartment meal	11¾-oz. meal	240	22.0

Food and Description	Measure or Quantity	Calories	Carbo-hydrates (grams)
PEPPER, SWEET:			
Raw (USDA):			
Green:			
Whole	1 lb. (weighed untrimmed)	82	17.9
Without stem & seeds	1 med. pepper (2.6 oz.)	13	2.9
Chopped	½ cup (2.6 oz.)	16	3.6
Slices	½ cup (1.4 oz.)	9	2.0
Red:			
Whole	1 lb. (weighed untrimmed)	112	25.8
Without stem & seeds	1 med. pepper (2.2 oz.)	19	2.4
Boiled, green, without salt, drained	1 med. pepper (2.6 oz.)	13	2.8
Frozen:			
(McKenzie)	1-oz. serving	6	1.0
(Southland):			
Green	2-oz. serving	10	3.0
Red & green	2-oz. serving	15	3.0
PERCH, OCEAN:			
Raw Atlantic, (USDA):			
Whole	1 lb. (weighed whole)	124	0.
Meat only	4 oz.	108	0.
Pacific, raw, whole	1 lb. (weighed whole)	116	0.
Frozen:			
(Banquet)	8¾-oz. dinner	434	49.8
(Mrs. Paul's) fillet, breaded & fried	2-oz. piece	145	10.5
(Van de Kamp's):			
Regular batter, dipped, french fried	2-oz. piece	145	10.0
Today's Catch	4 oz.	110	0.

(USDA): United States Department of Agriculture
(HEW/FAO): Health, Education and Welfare/Food and Agriculture
Organization
* Prepared as Package Directs

Food and Description	Measure or Quantity	Calories	Carbo-hydrates (grams)
PERNOD (Julius Wile)	1 fl. oz.	79	1.1
PERSIMMON (USDA):			
Japanese or Kaki, fresh:			
With seeds	4.4-oz. piece	79	20.1
Seedless	4.4-oz. piece	81	20.7
Native, fresh, flesh only	4-oz. serving	144	38.0
PHEASANT, raw (USDA) meat only	4-oz. serving	184	0.
PICKLE:			
Cucumber, fresh or bread & butter			
(USDA)	3 slices (.7 oz.)	15	3.8
(Fannings)	1.2-oz. serving	17	3.9
(Featherweight) low sodium	1-oz. pickle	12	3.0
(Nalley's) chip	1-oz. serving	27	6.5
Dill:			
(USDA)	4.8-oz. pickle	15	3.0
(Claussen) halves	2 oz.	7	1.3
(Featherweight) low sodium, whole kosher	1-oz. serving	4	1.0
(Smucker's):			
Candied sticks	4″ piece (.8 oz.)	45	11.0
Hamburger, sliced	1 slice (.13 oz.)	Tr.	0.
Polish, whole	3½″ pickle (1.8 oz.)	8	1.0
Spears	3½″ spear (1.4 oz.)	6	1.0
Hamburger (Nalley's) chips	1-oz. serving	3	.6
Kosher dill:			
(Claussen) halves or whole	2-oz. serving	7	1.3
(Featherweight) low sodium	1-oz. serving	4	1.0
(Smucker's):			
Baby	2¾-oz. long pickle	4	.5
Slices	1 slice (.1 oz.)	Tr.	0.
Whole	2½″ long pickle (.5 oz.)	8	1.0
Sour (USDA) cucumber	1 oz.	3	.6
Sweet:			
(Nalley's) *Nubbins*	1-oz. serving	28	7.9

Food and Description	Measure or Quantity	Calories	Carbohydrates (grams)
(Smucker's):			
Candied mix	1 piece (.3 oz.)	14	3.3
Gherkins	2″ long pickle (9 grams)	15	3.5
Slices	1 slice (.2 oz.)	11	2.3
Whole	2½″ long pickle	18	4.0
Sweet & sour (Claussen) slices	1 slice	3	.8

PIE:

Regular, non-frozen:			
Apple:			
Home recipe (USDA), two crust	⅙ of 9″ pie	404	60.2
(Hostess)	4½-oz. pie	409	51.1
Banana, home recipe (USDA), cream or custard	⅙ of 9″ pie	336	46.7
Berry (Hostess)	4½-oz. pie	404	51.1
Blackberry, home recipe (USDA) two crust	⅙ of 9″ pie	384	54.4
Blueberry:			
Home recipe (USDA), two-crust	⅙ of 9″ pie	382	55.1
(Hostess)	4½-oz. pie	394	49.9
Boston cream (USDA), home recipe	¹⁄₁₂ of 8″ pie	208	34.4
Butterscotch (USDA), home recipe, 1-crust	⅙ of 9″ pie	406	58.2
Cherry:			
Home recipe (USDA), 2-crust	⅙ of 9″ pie	412	60.7
(Hostess)	4½-oz. pie	429	56.2
Chocolate chiffon (USDA) home recipe, made with vegetable shortening	⅙ of 9″ pie	459	61.2
Chocolate meringue (USDA), home recipe, made with vegetable shortening	⅙ of 9″ pie	353	46.9

(USDA): United States Department of Agriculture
(HEW/FAO): Health, Education and Welfare/Food and Agriculture Organization
* Prepared as Package Directs

Food and Description	Measure or Quantity	Calories	Carbo- hydrates (grams)
Coconut custard (USDA), home recipe	⅙ of 9″ pie	357	37.8
Lemon (Hostess)	4½-oz. pie	415	52.4
Mince, home recipe, (USDA) 2-crust	⅙ of 9″ pie	428	65.1
Peach (Hostess)	4½-oz. pie	409	52.4
Pecan:			
Home recipe (USDA) 1-crust, made with lard or vegetable shortening	⅙ of 9″ pie	577	70.8
Pineapple, custard, home recipe (USDA) made with lard or vegetable shortening	⅙ of 9″ pie (5.4 oz.)	400	60.2
Pineapple, home recipe (USDA) 1 crust, made with lard or vegetable shortening	⅙ of 9″ pie	344	48.8
Pumpkin, home recipe (USDA) 2-crust, made with lard or vegetable shortening	⅙ of 9″ pie (5.4 oz.)	321	37.2
Raisin, home recipe (USDA) 2-crust, made with lard or vegetable shortening	⅙ of 9″ pie (5.6 oz.)	427	67.9
Rhubarb, home recipe (USDA) 2-crust, made with lard or vegetable shortening	⅙ of 9″ pie (5.6 oz.)	400	60.4
Strawberry, home recipe (USDA) made with lard or vegetable shortening	⅙ of 9″ pie (5.6 oz.)	313	48.8
Frozen:			
Apple:			
(Banquet):			
Regular	8-oz. pie	578	88.0
Family size	⅕ of 20-oz. pie	253	37.0

Food and Description	Measure or Quantity	Calories	Carbo-hydrates (grams)
(Morton):			
Regular	⅙ of 24-oz. pie	290	41.0
Great Little Desserts:			
Regular	8-oz. pie	590	88.0
Dutch	7¾-oz. pie	600	94.0
(Sara Lee):			
Regular	⅙ of 31-oz. pie	376	43.2
Dutch	⅙ of 30-oz. pie	354	50.6
Banana cream:			
(Banquet)	⅙ of 14-oz. pie	177	21.0
(Morton):			
Regular	⅙ of 14-oz. pie	160	19.0
Great Little Desserts	3½-oz. pie	250	27.0
Blackberry (Banquet)	⅙ of 20-oz. pie	268	40.0
Blueberry:			
(Banquet)	⅙ of 20-oz. pie	266	40.0
(Morton):			
Great Little Desserts	8-oz. pie	580	86.0
Regular	⅙ of 24-oz. pie	280	39.0
(Sara Lee)	⅙ of 31-oz. pie	449	44.8
Cherry:			
(Banquet):			
Regular	8-oz. pie	575	87.0
Family size	⅙ of 24-oz. pie	252	36.0
(Morton):			
Regular	⅙ of 24-oz. pie	300	423.0
Great Little Desserts	8-oz. pie	590	87.0
(Sara Lee)	⅙ of 31-oz. pie	397	48.0
Chocolate (Morton)	⅙ of 14-oz. pie	180	20.0
Chocolate cream:			
(Banquet)	⅙ of 14-oz. pie	185	24.0
(Morton) *Great Little Desserts*	3½-oz. pie	270	29.0
Coconut cream:			
(Banquet)	⅙ of 14-oz. pie	187	22.0
(Morton) *Great Little Desserts*	3½-oz. pie	270	25.0

(USDA): United States Department of Agriculture
(HEW/FAO):   Health, Education and Welfare/Food and Agriculture
            Organization
* Prepared as Package Directs

Food and Description	Measure or Quantity	Calories	Carbo-hydrates (grams)
Coconut custard (Morton)			
Great Little Desserts	6½-oz. pie	370	53.0
Lemon (Morton)	⅙ of 14-oz. pie	160	18.0
Lemon cream:			
(Banquet)	⅙ of 14-oz. pie	173	23.0
(Morton) *Great Little*			
Desserts	3½-oz. pie	250	27.0
Mince:			
(Banquet)	⅙ of 20-oz. pie	258	38.0
(Morton)	⅙ of 24-oz. pie	310	46.0
Peach:			
(Banquet):			
Regular	8-oz. pie	553	82.0
Family size	⅙ of 20-oz. pie	244	35.0
(Morton):			
Regular	⅙ of 24-oz. pie	280	39.0
Great Little Desserts	8-oz. pie	590	91.0
(Sara Lee)	⅙ of 31-oz. pie	458	56.2
Pumpkin:			
(Banquet)	⅙ of 20-oz. pie	197	29.0
(Morton) regular	⅙ of 24-oz. pie	230	36.0
(Sara Lee)	⅛ of 45-oz. pie	354	49.4
Strawberry cream (Banquet)	⅙ of 14-oz. pie	168	22.0
PIECRUST:			
Home recipe (USDA), 9″ pie, baked, made with vegetable shortening	1 crust	900	78.8
Frozen (Banquet) 9″ shell:			
Regular	1 crust (5 oz.)	614	61.9
Deep Dish	1 crust (6 oz.)	751	78.8
Refrigerated (Pillsbury)	2 crusts	1920	184
*PIECRUST MIX:			
(Betty Crocker):			
Regular	¹⁄₁₆ of pkg.	120	10.0
Stick	⅛ of stick	120	10.0
(Flako)	⅙ of 9″ pie shell	245	25.2
(Pillsbury) mix or stick	⅙ of 2-crust pie	270	25.0

Food and Description	Measure or Quantity	Calories	Carbo- hydrates (grams)
PIE FILLING (See also **PUDDING OR PIE FILLING**):			
Apple (Comstock)	⅙ of 21-oz. can	110	24.0
Apple rings or slices (See **APPLE,** canned)			
Apricot (Comstock)	⅙ of 21-oz. can	110	24.0
Banana cream (Comstock)	⅙ of 21-oz. can	110	22.0
Blueberry (Comstock)	⅙ of 21-oz. can	120	26.0
Cherry (Comstock)	⅙ of 21-oz. can	120	26.0
Chocolate (Comstock)	⅙ of 21-oz. can	140	27.0
Coconut cream (Comstock)	⅙ of 21-oz. can	120	24.0
Coconut custard (USDA) home recipe, made with egg yolk & milk	5 oz. (inc. crust)	288	41.3
Lemon (Comstock)	⅙ of 21-oz. can	160	33.0
Mincemeat (Comstock)	⅙ of 21-oz. can	170	36.0
Peach (Comstock)	⅙ of 21-oz. can	130	27.0
Pineapple (Comstock)	⅙ of 21-oz. can	110	25.0
Pumpkin: (See also **PUMPKIN,** canned)			
(Libby's)	1 cup	210	58.0
(Comstock)	⅙ of 27-oz. can	170	38.0
Raisin (Comstock)	⅙ of 21-oz. can	140	30.0
Strawberry (Comstock)	⅙ of 21-oz. can	130	28.0
*PIE MIX (Betty Crocker) Boston cream	⅛ of pie	260	48.0
PIEROGIES, frozen (Mrs. Paul's) potato & cheese	1 pierogi (1.7 oz.)	93	14.7
PIGEON, (SEe **SQUAB**)			
PIGEON PEA (USDA):			
Raw, immature seeds in pods	1 lb.	207	37.7
Dry seeds	1 lb.	1551	288.9

(USDA): United States Department of Agriculture
(HEW/FAO): Health, Education and Welfare/Food and Agriculture Organization
* Prepared as Package Directs

Food and Description	Measure or Quantity	Calories	Carbo-hydrates (grams)
PIGNOLLA (See **PINE NUT**)			
PIGS FEET, pickled (USDA):			
Blue:			
Whole	1 lb. (weighed whole)	180	0.
Meat only	4 oz.	102	0.
Northern:			
Whole	1 lb. (weighed whole)	104	0.
Meat only	4 oz.	100	0.
Walleye:			
Whole	1 lb. (weighed whole)	140	0.
Meat only	4 oz.	105	0.
PIMIENTO, canned:			
(Dromedary) drained	1-oz. serving	10	2.0
(Ortega) drained	¼ cup	6	1.3
(Sunshine) diced or sliced, solids & liq.	1 T.	4	.9
PIÑA COLADA (Mr. Boston)			
12½% alcohol	3 fl. oz.	240	34.2
PINEAPPLE:			
Fresh (USDA):			
Whole	1 lb. (weighed untrimmed)	123	32.3
Diced	½ cup (2.8 oz.)	41	10.7
Sliced	¾″ × 3½″ slice (3. oz.)	44	11.5
Canned, regular pack, solids & liq.:			
(USDA):			
Heavy syrup:			
Crushed	½ cup (5.6 oz.)	97	25.4
Slices	1 large slice & 2 T. syrup (4.3 oz.)	90	23.7
Tidbits	½ cup (4.6 oz.)	95	25.0

Food and Description	Measure or Quantity	Calories	Carbo-hydrates (grams)
Juice pack	4 oz.	66	17.1
Light syrup	5 oz.	76	17.5
(Del Monte):			
Juice pack:			
Chunks, slice or tidbits	½ cup (4 oz.)	70	18.0
Spears	2 spears		
	(3.1 oz.)	50	14.0
Syrup pack	½ cup (4 oz.)	90	23.0
(Dole)			
Juice pack, chunk, crushed or sliced	½ cup (4 oz.)	70	17.5
Heavy syrup, chunk, crushed or sliced	½ cup	95	24.8
Canned, unsweetened or dietetic, solids & liq.:			
(Diet Delight) juice pack	½ cup (4.4 oz.)	70	18.0
(Featherweight):			
Juice pack	½ cup	70	18.0
Water pack	½ cup	60	15.0
(Libby's) Lite	½ cup (4.4 oz.)	60	16.0
(S&W) *Nutradiet*, blue label	1 slice	30	7.5
PINEAPPLE, CANDIED			
(USDA)	1-oz. serving	90	22.7
PINEAPPLE FLAVORING			
(Durkee) imitation	1 tsp.	6	DNA
PINEAPPLE & GRAPEFRUIT JUICE DRINK, canned:			
(Del Monte) regular or pink	6 fl. oz.	90	24.0
(Dole) pink	6 fl. oz.	101	25.4
(Texsun)	6 fl. oz.	91	22.0
PINEAPPLE JUICE:			
Canned:			
(Del Monte) unsweetened	6 fl. oz.		
	(6.6 oz.)	100	25.0

(USDA): United States Department of Agriculture
(HEW/FAO):   Health, Education and Welfare/Food and Agriculture Organization
* Prepared as Package Directs

Food and Description	Measure or Quantity	Calories	Carbo-hydrates (grams)
(Dole) unsweetened	6 fl. oz.	103	25.4
(Texsun) unsweetened	6 fl. oz.	97	24.0
*Frozen (Minute Maid)	6 fl. zo.	92	22.7
PINEAPPLE-ORANGE DRINK, canned (Hi-C)	6 fl. oz.	94	23.0
PINEAPPLE-ORANGE JUICE:			
Canned (Del Monte)	6 fl. oz. (6.6 oz.)	90	24.0
*Frozen (Minute Maid)	6 fl. oz.	94	23.0
PINEAPPLE PRESERVE OR JAM, sweetened (Smucker's)	1 T. (.7 oz.)	53	13.5
PINE NUT (USDA):			
Pignolias, shelled	4 oz.	626	13.2
Pinon, whole	4 oz. (weighed in shell)	418	13.5
Pinon, shelled	4 oz.	720	23.2
PINOT CHARDONNAY WINE (Paul Masson) 12% alcohol	3 fl. oz.	71	2.4
PISTACHIO NUT:			
Raw (USDA):			
In shell	4 oz. (weighed in shell)	337	10.8
Shelled	½ cup (2.2 oz.)	368	11.8
Shelled	1 T. (8 grams)	46	1.5
Roasted:			
(Fisher) Salted:			
In shell	1 oz.	84	2.7
Shelled	1 oz.	174	5.4
(Flavor House) dry roasted	1 oz.	168	5.4
(Frito-Lay's)	1 oz.	175	4.8
(Planters) dry roasted	1 oz.	170	6.0
PITANGA, Fresh (USDA)			
Whole	1 lb. (weighed whole)	187	45.9
Flesh only	4 oz.	58	14.2

Food and Description	Measure or Quantity	Calories	Carbo-hydrates (grams)
PIZZA PIE:			
Regular, non-frozen:			
Home recipe (USDA) with cheese topping	⅛ of 14″ pie	177	21.2
(Pizza Hut):			
Cheese	½ of 10″ pie	436	53.2
Pepperoni	½ of 10″ pie	459	54.4
Frozen:			
Canadian style bacon (Celeste):			
Small	8-oz. pie	483	50.5
Large	¼ of 19-oz. pie	288	30.0
Cheese:			
(Celeste):			
Small	7-oz. pie	472	57.1
Large	¼ of 19-oz. pie	309	31.6
(Stouffer's) French Bread	½ of 10⅜-oz. pkg.	330	43.0
(Weight Watchers)	6-oz. pie	350	37.0
Combination:			
(Celeste) Chicago style	¼ of 24-oz. pie	360	36.2
(La Pizzeria)	½ of 13½-oz. pie	420	43.0
(Van de Kamp's)	¼ of 23½-oz. pie	310	24.0
(Weight Watchers) deluxe	7¼-oz. pie	340	38.0
Deluxe:			
(Celeste):			
Small	½ of 9-oz. pie	281	31.3
Large	¼ of 23½-oz. pie	368	37.4
(Stouffer's) French Bread	½ of 12⅜-oz. pkg.	400	46.0
Hamburger (Stouffer's) French Bread	½ of 12¼-oz. pkg.	400	39.0
Mexican style (Van de Kamp's)	½ of 11-oz. pkg.	420	27.0

(USDA): United States Department of Agriculture
(HEW/FAO):   Health, Education and Welfare/Food and Agriculture
            Organization
* Prepared as Package Directs

Food and Description	Measure or Quantity	Calories	Carbo-hydrates (grams)
Mushroom (Stouffer's)			
French Bread	½ of 12-oz. pkg.	340	43.0
Pepperoni:			
(Celeste):			
Regular:			
Small	7¼-oz. pie	568	54.1
Large	¼ of 20-oz. pie	347	34.8
Chicago style	¼ of 24-oz. pie	374	36.7
(Stouffer's) French Bread	½ of		
	11¼-oz. pkg.	410	44.0
(Van de Kamp's)	¼ of 22-oz. pie	370	38.0
Sausage:			
(Celeste):			
Regular:			
Small	½ of 8-oz. pie	262	29.8
Large	¼ of 22-oz. pie	359	34.7
Chicago style	¼ of 24-oz. pie	382	36.6
(Stouffer's) French Bread	½ of 12-oz. pkg.	420	44.0
(Weight Watchers) veal	6¾-oz. pie	350	35.1
Sausage & mushroom:			
(Celeste):			
Small	9-oz. pie	555	56.8
Large	¼ of 24-oz. pie	365	34.1
(Stouffer's) French Bread	½ of		
	12½-oz. pkg.	395	40.0
Sicilian style (Celeste)			
deluxe	¼ of 26-oz. pie	408	45.4
Suprema (Celeste):			
Regular:			
Small	10-oz. pie	590	52.2
Large	¼ of 24-oz. pie	354	31.3
Without meat:			
Small	8-oz. pie	434	49.1
Large	⅓ of 20-oz. pie	272	30.8
Vegetable (Weight Watchers)	7¼-oz. pie	350	39.0
*Mix (Ragu) *Pizza Quick*	¼ of pie	300	37.0
PIZZA SAUCE:			
(Contadina):			
Regular or with cheese	½ cup (4.2 oz.)	80	10.0
With pepperoni	½ cup (4.2 oz.)	90	10.0

Food and Description	Measure or Quantity	Calories	Carbo-hydrates (grams)
(Ragu) *Pizza Quick:*			
Regular	3 T. (1.7 oz.)	35	6.0
Chunky	3 T. (1.9 oz.)	45	6.0
PIZZA SEASONING SPICE			
(French's)	1 tsp. (.1 oz.)	5	1.0
PLANTAIN, raw (USDA):			
Whole	1 lb. (weighed with skin)	389	101.9
Flesh only	4 oz.	135	35.4
PLUM:			
Fresh (USDA):			
Damson:			
Whole	1 lb. (weighed with pits)	272	73.5
Flesh only	4 oz.	75	20.2
Japanese & hybrid:			
Whole	1 lb. (weighed with pits)	205	52.5
	2.1-oz. plum (2″ dia.)	27	6.9
Diced	½ cup (2.9 oz.)	39	10.1
Halves	½ cup (3.1 oz.)	42	10.8
Slices	½ cup (3 oz.)	40	10.3
Prune type:			
Whole	1 lb. (weighed with pits)	320	84.0
Halves	½ cup (2.8 oz.)	60	52.8
Canned, purple, regular pack solids & liq.:			
(USDA):			
Extra heavy syrup	4 oz.	116	30.3
Heavy syrup, with pits	½ cup (4.5 oz.)	106	27.6
Heavy syrup, without pits	½ cup (4.2 oz.)	100	25.9
Light syrup	4 oz.	71	18.8
(Stokely-Van Camp)	½ cup	120	30.0

(USDA): United States Department of Agriculture
(HEW/FAO):   Health, Education and Welfare/Food and Agriculture
                        Organization
* Prepared as Package Directs

Food and Description	Measure or Quantity	Calories	Carbo-hydrates (grams)
Canned, unsweetened or low calorie, solids & liq.: (Diet Delight) purple:			
Juice pack	½ cup (4.4 oz.)	70	19.0
Water pack	½ cup (4.4 oz.)	50	13.0
(Featherweight) purple:			
Juice pack	½ cup	80	18.0
Water pack	½ cup	40	9.0
(S&W) *Nutradiet,* purple, juice pack	½ cup	80	20.0
PLUM JELLY:			
Sweetened (Smucker's)	1 T. (.7 oz.)	53	13.5
Dietetic or low calorie (Featherweight)	1 T.	16	4.0
PLUM PRESERVE or JAM, sweetened (Smucker's)	1 T. (.7 oz.)	53	13.5
PLUM PUDDING (Richardson & Robbins)	2″ wedge (3.6 oz.)	270	61.0
POLISH STYLE SAUSAGE (See **SAUSAGE**)			
POLYNESIAN-STYLE DINNER, frozen (Swanson) *TV Brand*	12-oz. dinner	350	46.0
POMEGRANATE, raw (USDA):			
Whole	1 lb. (weighed whole)	160	41.7
Pulp only	4 oz.	71	18.6
PONDEROSA RESTAURANT:			
A-1 Sauce	1 tsp.	4	1.0
Beef, chopped patty only (See Also Bun):			
Regular	3½ oz.	209	0.
Big	4.8-oz.	295	0.

Food and Description	Measure or Quantity	Calories	Carbo-hydrates (grams)
Double Deluxe	5.9 oz.	362	0.
Junior (*Square Shooter*)	1.6 oz.	98	0.
Steakhouse Deluxe	2.96 oz.	181	0.
Beverages:			
Coca-Cola	8 fl. oz.	96	24.0
Coffee	6 fl. oz.	2	.5
Dr. Pepper	8 fl. oz.	96	24.8
Lemon	8 fl. oz.	110	28.5
Milk:			
Regular	8 fl. oz.	159	12.0
Chocolate	8 fl. oz.	208	25.9
Orange drink	8 fl. oz.	110	30.0
Root beer	8 fl. oz.	104	25.6
Sprite	8 fl. oz.	95	24.0
Tab	8 fl. oz.	1	.1
Bun:			
Regular	2.4-oz. bun	190	35.0
Hot dog	1 bun	108	18.9
Junior	1.4-oz. bun	118	21.0
Steakhouse deluxe	2.4-oz. bun	190	35.0
Chicken strips:			
Adult portion	2¾ oz.	282	15.8
Children's portion	1.4 oz.	141	7.9
Cocktail sauce	1½ oz.	57	.2
Filet Mignon	3.8 oz. (edible portion)	152	.2
Filet of sole, fish only (See also Bun)	3-oz. piece	125	4.4
Fish, baked	4.9-oz. serving	268	11.6
Gelatin dessert	½ cup	97	23.5
Gravy, au jus	1 oz.	3	Tr.
Ham & cheese:			
Bun (See Bun)			
Cheese, Swiss	2 slices (.8 oz.)	76	.5
Ham	2½ oz.	184	1.4
Hot dog, child's, meat only (See also Bun)	1.6-oz. hot dog	140	2.0

(USDA): United States Department of Agriculture
(HEW/FAO): Health, Education and Welfare/Food and Agriculture
                Organization
* Prepared as Package Directs

Food and Description	Measure or Quantity	Calories	Carbo-hydrates (grams)
Margarine:			
Pat	1 pat	36	Tr.
On potato, as served	½ oz.	100	.1
Mustard sauce, sweet & sour	1 oz.	50	9.5
New York strip steak	6.1 oz. (edible portion)	362	0.
Onion, chopped	1 T. (.4 oz.)	4	.9
Pickle, dill	3 slices (.7 oz.)	2	.2
Potato:			
Baked	7.2-oz. potato	145	32.8
French fries	3-oz. serving	230	30.2
Prime ribs:			
Regular	4.2 oz. (edible portion)	286	0.
Imperial	8.4 oz. (edible portion)	572	0.
King	6 oz. (edible portion)	409	0.
Pudding:			
Butterscotch	4½ oz.	200	27.4
Chocolate	4½ oz.	213	27.1
Vanilla	4½ oz.	195	27.5
Ribeye	3.2 oz. (edible portion)	197	0.
Ribeye & Shrimp:			
Ribeye	3.2 oz.	197	0.
Shrimp	2.2 oz.	139	0.
Roll, kaiser	2.2-oz. roll	184	33.0
Salad bar:			
Bean sprouts	1 oz.	13	1.5
Beets	1 oz.	5	.9
Broccoli	1 oz.	9	1.7
Cabbage, red	1 oz.	9	2.0
Carrots	1 oz.	12	2.8
Cauliflower	1 oz.	8	1.5
Celery	1 oz.	4	1.1
Chickpeas (Garbanzos)	1 oz.	102	17.3
Cucumber	1 oz.	4	.7
Mushrooms	1 oz.	8	1.2
Onion, white	1 oz.	11	2.6
Pepper, green	1 oz.	6	1.4

Food and Description	Measure or Quantity	Calories	Carbo-hydrates (grams)
Radish	1 oz.	5	1.0
Tomato	1 oz.	6	1.3
Salad dressing:			
Blue cheese	1 oz.	129	2.1
Italian, creamy	1 oz.	138	2.8
Low calorie	1 oz.	14	.8
Oil & vinegar	1 oz.	124	.9
Sweet'n Tart	1 oz.	129	9.2
Thousand Island	1 oz.	117	6.7
Shrimp dinner	7 pieces (3½ oz.)	220	9.8
Sirloin:			
Regular	3.3 oz. (edible portion)	197	0.
Super	6½ oz. (edible portion)	383	0.
Tips	4 oz. (edible portion)	192	0.
Steak sauce	1 oz.	23	4.0
Tartar sauce	1.5 oz.	285	4.5
T-Bone	4.3 oz. (edible portion)	240	0.
Tomato (See also Salad Bar):			
Slices	2 slices (.9 oz.)	5	1.2
Whole, small	3.5 oz.	22	4.7
Topping, whipped	¼ oz.	19	1.2
Worcestershire sauce	1 tsp.	4	.9
POPCORN:			
*Plain, popped fresh:			
(Jiffy Pop)	½ of 5-oz. pkg.	244	29.8
(Pillsbury) Microwave Popcorn:			
Regular	1 cup	70	6.5
Butter flavor	1 cup	65	6.0
(Super Pop):			
Dry popped	1 oz.	100	20.0
Oil popped	1 oz.	220	20.0

(USDA): United States Department of Agriculture
(HEW/FAO):   Health, Education and Welfare/Food and Agriculture
                          Organization
* Prepared as Package Directs

Food and Description	Measure or Quantity	Calories	Carbo-hydrates (grams)
Packaged:			
Plain (Bachman)	1 oz.	160	13.0
Caramel-coated:			
(Bachman)	1-oz. serving	110	25.0
(Old London) without peanuts	1¾-oz. serving	195	43.6
Cheese flavored (Bachman)	1-oz. serving	180	14.0
Cracker Jack	¾-oz. serving	90	16.7
POPOVER:			
Home recipe (USDA)	1 average popover (2 oz.)	128	14.7
*Mix (Flako)	1 popover	170	25.0
POPPY SEED (French's)	1 tsp.	13	.8
POPSICLE, twin	3-fl-oz. pop	70	17.0
PORGY, raw (USDA):			
Whole	1 lb. (weighed whole)	208	0.
Meat only	4 oz.	127	0.
PORK, medium-fat:			
Fresh (USDA):			
Boston butt:			
Raw:	1 lb. (weighed with bone & skin)	1220	0.
Roasted, lean & fat	4 oz.	400	0.
Roasted, lean only	4 oz.	277	0.
Chop:			
Broiled, lean & fat	1 chop (4 oz., weighed with bone)	295	0.
Broiled, lean & fat	1 chop (4 oz., weighed with bone)	332	0.
Broiled, lean & fat	1 chop (3 oz., weighed without bone)	230	0.
Fat, separable cooked	1 oz.	219	0.

Food and Description	Measure or Quantity	Calories	Carbo-hydrates (grams)
Ham (see also **HAM**):			
Raw	1 lb. (weighed with bone & skin)	1188	0.
Roasted, lean & fat	4 oz.	424	0.
Roasted, lean only	4 oz.	246	0.
Loin:			
Raw	1 lb. (weighed with bone)	1065	0.
Roasted, lean & fat	4 oz.	411	0.
Roasted, lean only	4 oz.	288	0.
Picnic:			
Raw	1 lb. (weighed with bone & skin)	1083	0.
Simmered, lean & fat	4 oz.	424	0.
Simmered, lean only	4 oz.	240	0.
Spareribs:			
Raw, with bone	1 lb. (weighed with bone)	976	0.
Braised, lean & fat	4 oz.	499	0.
Cured, light commercial cure:			
Bacon (see **BACON**)			
Bacon butt (USDA):			
Raw	1 lb. (weighed with bone & skin)	1227	0.
Roasted, lean & fat	4 oz.	374	0.
Roasted, lean only	4 oz.	276	0.

PORK & BEANS (See **BEAN, BAKED**)

PORK, CANNED, chopped luncheon meat (USDA):

Regular	1 oz.	83	.4
Chopped	1 cup (4.8 oz.)	400	1.8
Diced	1 cup	415	1.8

(USDA): United States Department of Agriculture
(HEW/FAO):   Health, Education and Welfare/Food and Agriculture
             Organization
* Prepared as Package Directs

Food and Description	Measure or Quantity	Calories	Carbo-hydrates (grams)
PORK DINNER, frozen (Swanson) *TV Brand*	11¼-oz. dinner	270	20.0
PORK, PACKAGED (Eckrich)	1-oz. serving	45	1.0
PORK RINDS, *Baken-Ets*	1-oz. serving	150	1.0
PORK STEAK, BREADED, FROZEN (Hormel)	3-oz. serving	220	11.0
PORK, SWEET & SOUR, frozen (La Choy)	½ of 15-oz. pkg.	229	45.2
PORT WINE:			
(Gallo) 16% alcohol	3 fl. oz.	94	7.8
(Louis M. Martini) 19½% alcohol	3 fl. oz.	165	2.0
***POSTUM**, instant, regular or coffee flavored	6 fl. oz.	11	2.6
POTATO:			
Cooked (USDA)			
Au gratin, with cheese	½ cup (4.3 oz.)	177	16.6
Baked, peeled	2½" dia. potato (3.5 oz.)	92	20.9
Boiled, peeled before boiling, no salt	4.3-oz. potato	79	17.7
French-fried in deep fat, no salt	10 pieces (2 oz.)	156	20.5
Hash-browned, home recipe, after holding overnight	½ cup (3.4 oz.)	223	28.4
Mashed, milk & butter added	½ cup (3.5 oz.)	92	12.1
Canned, solids & liq.:			
(Del Monte) sliced or whole	½ cup (4 oz.)	45	10.0
(Sunshine) whole	½ cup (4.4 oz.)	51	10.5
Frozen:			
(Birds Eye):			
Cottage fries	2.8-oz. serving	119	17.3
Crinkle cuts:			
Regular	3-oz. serving	115	18.4
Deep Gold	3-oz. serving	138	25.5

Food and Description	Measure or Quantity	Calories	Carbo-hydrates (grams)
Farm style wedge	3-oz. serving	109	17.9
French fries:			
Regular	3-oz. serving	113	16.8
Deep Gold	3-oz. serving	161	24.4
Hash browns:			
Regular	4-oz. serving	74	16.5
Shredded	¼ of 12-oz. pkg.	61	13.1
Shoestring	3-oz. serving	126	17.8
Steak fries	3-oz. serving	109	17.9
Tasti Fries	2½-oz. serving	136	16.5
Tasti Puffs	¼ of 10-oz. pkg.	192	19.4
Tiny Taters	⅕ of 16.oz. pkg.	204	22.0
Triangles	1½-oz. serving	73	5.9
Whole, peeled	3.2-oz. serving	59	12.8
(Green Giant):			
Sliced, in butter sauce	½ cup	80	14.0
& sweet peas in bacon cream sauce	½ cup	110	15.0
(McKenzie) whole, white, boiled	3.2-oz. serving	60	13.0
(Stouffer's):			
Au gratin	⅓ of 11½-oz. pkg.	135	13.0
Scalloped	⅓ of 12-oz. pkg.	125	14.0
POTATO & BACON, canned (Hormel) *Short Orders,* au gratin	7½ oz. can	240	20.0
POTATO & BEEF, canned, *Dinty Moore* (Hormel) *Short Orders*	7½-oz. can	250	25.0
POTATO CHIP:			
(Bachman):			
Regular	1 oz.	160	14.0
BBQ or sour cream & onion	1 oz.	150	14.0

(USDA): United States Department of Agriculture
(HEW/FAO):   Health, Education and Welfare/Food and Agriculture
                    Organization
* Prepared as Package Directs

Food and Description	Measure or Quantity	Calories	Carbo- hydrates (grams)
(Featherweight) unsalted	1 oz.	160	14.0
(Frtio-Lay's) natural	1 oz.	157	15.1
Lay's:			
BBQ or sour cream & onion flavor	1 oz.	160	14.0
Regular	1 oz.	150	14.0
Pringle's:			
Regular or *Cheez-Ums*	1 oz.	167	10.5
Light	1 oz.	148	16.5
Rippled	1 oz.	168	13.4
POTATO & HAM, canned (Hormel) *Short Orders,* scalloped	7½-oz. can	250	19.0
*POTATO MIX:			
Au gratin:			
(Betty Crocker)	½ cup	150	21.0
(French's) *Big Tate*, tangy	½ cup	150	25.0
(Libby's) *Potato Classics*	¾ cup	130	22.0
Creamed (Betty Crocker)	½ cup	160	20.0
Hash browns (Betty Crocker) with onion	½ cup	150	23.0
Hickory smoke cheese (Betty Crocker)	½ cup	150	21.0
Julienne (Betty Crocker) with mild cheese sauce	½ cup	130	17.0
Mashed:			
(American Beauty)	½ cup	120	17.0
(Betty Crocker) *Buds*	½ cup	130	15.0
(French's):			
Big Tate	½ cup	140	16.0
Idaho	½ cup	120	16.0
(Pillsbury) *Hungry Jack*, flakes	½ cup	140	17.0
Scalloped:			
(Betty Crocker)	½ cup	140	19.0
(French's) *Big Tate*	½ cup	160	25.0
(Libby's) *Potato Classics*	¾ cup	130	24.0
Sour cream & chive:			
(Betty Crocker)	½ cup	150	19.0
(French's)	½ cup	170	24.0

Food and Description	Measure or Quantity	Calories	Carbo-hydrates (grams)
*POTATO PANCAKE MIX			
(French's) *Big Tate*	3″ pancake	43	5.7
POTATO SALAD:			
Home recipe (USDA):			
With cooked salad dressing seasonings	4 oz.	112	18.5
With mayonnaise & French dressing, hard-cooked eggs, seasonings	4 oz.	164	15.2
Canned (Nally's):			
Regular	4-oz. serving	139	17.0
German style	4-oz. serving	143	18.2
POTATO STICKS (Durkee)			
O & C	1½-oz. serving	231	22.0
POTATO, STUFFED, BAKED, frozen (Green Giant):			
With cheese flavored topping	½ of 10-oz. pkg.	200	33.0
With sour cream & chives	½ of 10-oz. pkg.	230	31.0
POTATO TOPPERS (Libby's)	1 T.	30	4.0
POUND CAKE (See **CAKE,** Pound)			
PRESERVE OR JAM (See individual flavors)			
PRETZEL:			
(Bachman) regular or butter	1 oz.	110	21.0
(Estee) unsalted	1 piece (1.3 grams)	5	1.0
(Featherweight) unsalted	1 piece (.1 oz.)	7	1.3
(Nabisco) *Mister Salty:*			
Regular	1 piece (.2 oz.)	20	4.0

(USDA): United States Department of Agriculture
(HEW/FAO):   Health, Education and Welfare/Food and Agriculture
                        Organization
* Prepared as Package Directs

Food and Description	Measure or Quantity	Calories	Carbo-hydrates (grams)
Dutch	1 piece (.5 oz.)	55	11.0
Little Shapes	1 piece (.2 oz.)	6	1.2
Sticks	1 piece (.1 oz.)	1	.2
(Pepperidge Farm):			
Nuggets	1¼-oz. serving	148	26.3
Sticks, thin	1¼-oz. serving	145	26.3
Twist, tiny	1-oz. serving	116	21.6
(Rokeach):			
Baldies, unsalted,			
Dutch style	1-oz. serving	110	20.0
Party cannister	1-oz. serving	110	23.0
PRICKLY PEAR, fresh			
(USDA):			
Whole	1 lb. (weighed with rind & seeds)	84	21.8
Flesh only	4 oz.	48	12.4
PRODUCT 19, cereal (Kellogg's)	1 cup (1 oz.)	110	24.0
PROSCIUTTO (Hormel) boneless	1 oz.	90	0.
PRUNE:			
Canned:			
(Featherweight) stewed, water pack	½ cup	130	35.0
(Sunsweet) stewed	½ cup (4.6 oz.)	120	32.0
Dried:			
(Del Monte):			
Moist Pak	2 oz.	120	30.0
Uncooked:			
With pits	2 oz.	120	31.0
Pitted	2 oz.	140	35.0
(Sunsweet):			
Whole	2 oz.	120	31.0
Pitted	2 oz.	140	36.0
PRUNE JUICE:			
(Del Monte)	6 fl. oz. (6.7 oz.)	120	33.0

Food and Description	Measure or Quantity	Calories	Carbo-hydrates (grams)
(Mott's) regular (Sunsweet):	6 fl. oz.	140	34.0
Regular	6 fl. oz.	140	33.0
Home style with pulp	6 fl. oz.	130	32.0
PRUNE NECTAR, canned (Mott's)	6 fl. oz.	100	25.0
PRUNE WHIP (USDA) home recipe	1 cup (4.8 oz.)	211	49.8
PUDDING OR PIE FILLING:			
Home recipe (USDA):			
Rice, made with raisins	½ cup (4.7 oz.)	1983	35.2
Tapioca:			
Apple	½ cup (4.4 oz.)	146	36.8
Cream	½ cup (2.9 oz.)	110	14.0
Canned, regular pack:			
Banana:			
(Del Monte) *Pudding Cup*	5-oz. container	181	30.1
(Hunt's) *Snack Pack*	5-oz. container	180	24.0
Butterscotch:			
(Del Monte) *Pudding Cup*	5-oz. container	184	30.8
(Hunt's) *Snack Pack*	5-oz. container	170	27.0
Chocolate:			
(Del Monte) *Pudding Cup:*			
Regular	5-oz. container	201	32.9
Fudge	5-oz. container	193	30.9
(Hunt's) *Snack Pack*	5-oz. container	180	28.0
Rice:			
(Betty Crocker)	4¼-oz. container	150	25.0
(Comstock; Menner's)	½ of 7½-oz. can	120	23.0
Tapioca:			
(Betty Crocker)	4¼-oz. container	150	22.0
(Del Monte) *Pudding Cup*	5-oz. container	172	30.1
(Hunt's) *Snack Pack*	5-oz. container	140	23.0
Vanilla (Del Monte)	5-oz. container	1188	32.1

(USDA): United States Department of Agriculture
(HEW/FAO): Health, Education and Welfare/Food and Agriculture
            Organization
* Prepared as Package Directs

Food and Description	Measure or Quantity	Calories	Carbohydrates (grams)
Canned, dietetic pack (Sego) all flavors	4-oz. serving	125	
Chilled, *Swiss Miss:*			
Butterscotch, chocolate malt or vanilla	4-oz. container	150	24.0
Chocolate or double rich	4-oz. container	160	24.0
Chocolate malt	4-oz. container	150	22.0
Chocolate sundae	4-oz. container	170	26.0
Rice	4-oz. container	150	24.0
Tapioca	4-oz. container	130	22.0
Vanilla sundae	4-oz. container	170	25.0
Frozen (Rich's):			
Banana	3-oz. container	142	19.3
Butterscotch or vanilla	4½-oz. container	199	27.4
Chocolate	4½-oz. container	214	27.1
*Mix, sweetened, regular & instant:			
Banana:			
(Jell-O) cream:			
Regular	½ cup	161	26.7
Instant	½ cup	174	30.0
(Royal) regular	½ cup	160	27.0
Butter pecan (Jell-O) instant	½ cup	175	29.1
Butterscotch:			
(Jell-O):			
Regular	½ cup	172	29.7
Instant	½ cup	175	30.0
(My-T-Fine) regular	½ cup	143	28.0
(Royal) regular	½ cup	160	27.0
Chocolate:			
(Jell-O):			
Plain:			
Regular	½ cup	174	28.8
Instant	½ cup	181	30.6
Fudge:			
Regular	½ cup	169	27.8
Instant	½ cup	182	30.9
Milk:			
Regular	½ cup	171	28.2
Instant	½ cup	184	34.0
(My-T-Fine) regular	½ cup	169	

Food and Description	Measure or Quantity	Calories	Carbohydrates (grams)
Coconut:			
(Jell-O) cream:			
Regular	½ cup	176	24.4
Instant	½ cup	182	26.1
(Royal) instant	½ cup	170	30.0
Custard:			
Jell-O Americana	½ cup	164	23.2
(Royal) Regular	½ cup	150	22.0
Flan (Royal) regular	½ cup	150	22.0
Lemon:			
(Jell-O):			
Regular	½ cup	181	38.8
Instant	½ cup	179	31.1
(My-T-Fine) regular	½ cup	164	30.0
Lime (Royal) Key Lime, regular	½ cup	160	30.0
Pineapple (Jell-O) cream, instant	½ cup	176	30.4
Pistachio (Jell-O) instant	½ cup	174	28.4
Raspberry (Salada) *Danish Dessert*	½ cup	130	32.0
Rice, *Jell-O Americana*	½ cup	176	29.9
Strawberry (Salada) *Danish Dessert*	½ cup	130	32.0
Tapioca:			
Jell-O Americana:			
Chocolate	½ cup	173	27.8
Vanilla	½ cup	162	27.4
(My-T-Fine) vanilla	½ cup	130	
Vanilla:			
(Jell-O):			
Plain, instant	½ cup	179	31.0
French, regular	½ cup	172	29.7
(Royal)	½ cup	180	29.0
*Mix, dietetic:			
Butterscotch:			
(Dia-Mel)	½ cup	50	9.0

(USDA): United States Department of Agriculture
(HEW/FAO):   Health, Education and Welfare/Food and Agriculture Organization
* Prepared as Package Directs

Food and Description	Measure or Quantity	Calories	Carbo-hydrates (grams)
(D-Zerta)	½ cup	68	12.0
(Estee)	½ cup	70	13.0
(Featherweight) artifically sweetened	½ cup	60	9.0
Chocolate:			
(Dia-Mel)	½ cup	50	9.0
(D-Zerta)	½ cup (4.6 oz.)	68	11.5
(Estee)	½ cup	70	11.5
(Featherweight)	½ cup	60	9.0
(Louis Sherry)	½ cup (4.2 oz.)	50	9.0
Lemon:			
(Dia-Mel)	½ cup (4.2 oz.)	14	4.0
(Estee)	½ cup	70	12.0
Vanilla:			
(Dia-Mel)	½ cup (4.2 oz.)	50	9.0
(D-Zerta)	½ cup	71	12.7
(Estee)	½ cup	70	13.0
(Featherweight) artificially sweetened	½ cup	60	9.0
PUFFED RICE:			
(Malt-O-Meal)	1 cup (.5 oz.)	50	12.0
(Quaker)	1 cup	55	12.7
PUFFED WHEAT:			
(Malt-O-Meal)	1 cup (.5 oz.)	50	11.0
(Quaker)	1 cup (.5 oz.)	54	10.8
PUMPKIN:			
Fresh (USDA):			
Whole	1 lb. (weighed with rind & seeds)	83	20.6
Flesh only	4 oz.	29	7.4
Canned:			
(Del Monte)	½ cup (4.3 oz.)	35	9.0
(Festal)	½ cup	45	9.5
(Libby's) solids pack	½ of 16-oz. can	40	10.0
(Stokely-Van Camp)	½ cup (4.3 oz.)	45	9.5
PUMPKIN SEED, dry (USDA):			
Whole	4 oz. (weighed in hull)	464	12.6
Hulled	4 oz.	627	17.0

Food and Description	Measure or Quantity	Calories	Carbo-hydrates (grams)

Q

QUAIL, raw (USDA) meat & skin	4 oz.	195	0.
QUIK (Nestlé):			
Chocolate	1 tsp. (.4 oz.)	45	9.5
Strawberry	1 tsp. (.4 oz.)	45	11.0
QUISP, cereal	1⅙ cup (1 oz.)	121	23.1

(USDA): United States Department of Agriculture
(HEW/FAO):   Health, Education and Welfare/Food and Agriculture
              Organization
* Prepared as Package Directs

Food and Description	Measure or Quantity	Calories	Carbo-hydrates (grams)

R

RABBIT (USDA)
Domesticated:

Raw, ready-to-cook	1 lb. (weighed with bones)	581	0.
Stewed, flesh only	4 oz.	245	0.
Wild, ready-to-cook	1 lb. (weighed with bones)	490	0.

RACCOON (USDA):
Common, raw:

Without tops	½ lb. (weighed untrimmed)	34	7.4
Trimmed, whole	4 small radishes (1.4 oz.)	7	1.4
Trimmed sliced	½ cup (2 oz.)	10	2.1
Oriental, raw, without tops	½ lb. (weighed unpared)	34	7.4
Oriental, raw, trimmed & pared	4 oz.	22	4.8

RAISIN:
Dried:
  (USDA):

Whole, pressed down	½ cup (2.9 oz.)	237	63.5
Chopped	½ cup (2.9 oz.)	234	62.7
Ground	½ cup (4.7 oz.)	387	103.7
(Del Monte):			
Golden	3 oz.	260	68.0
Thompson	3 oz.	250	68.0
(Sun-Maid) seedless, natural			
Thompson	1 oz.	96	23.0
Cooked, (USDA) added sugar solids & liq.	½ cup (4.3 oz.)	260	68.8

RAISINS, RICE & RYE, cereal

(Kellogg's)	¾ cup (1.3 oz.)	140	31.0

Food and Description	Measure or Quantity	Calories	Carbo-hydrates (grams)
RALSTON, cereal, regular or instant	¼ cup (1 oz.)	90	20.0
RASPBERRY:			
Black (USDA):			
Fresh:			
Whole	1 lb. (weighed with caps & stems)	160	34.6
Without caps & stems	½ cup (2.4 oz.)	49	10.5
Canned, water pack unsweetened, solids & liq.	4 oz.	58	12.1
Red:			
Fresh (USDA):			
Whole	1 lb. (weighed with caps & stems)	126	29.9
Without caps & stems	½ cup (2.5 oz.)	41	9.8
Canned, water pack, unsweetened or low calorie, solids & liq. (USDA)	4 oz.	40	10.0
Frozen (Birds Eye) quick thaw:			
Regular	5-oz. serving	155	37.0
In lite syrup	5-oz. serving	110	25.7
RASPBERRY PRESERVE OR JAM:			
Sweetened (Smucker's)	1 T. (.7 oz.)	53	13.5
Dietetic:			
(Dia-Mel; Louis Sherry)	1 T. (.6 oz.)	6	0.
(Featherweight) red	1 T.	16	4.0
(S&W) *Nutradiet*, red label	1 T.	12	3.0
RATATOUILLE, frozen (Stouffer's)	5-oz. serving	60	9.0

(USDA): United States Department of Agriculture
(HEW/FAO): Health, Education and Welfare/Food and Agriculture Organization
* Prepared as Package Directs

Food and Description	Measure or Quantity	Calories	Carbo-hydrates (grams)
RAVIOLI:			
Canned, regular pack (Franco-American):			
Beef:			
In meat sauce	7½-oz. can	230	36.0
RavioliOs	7½-oz. serving	210	34.0
Cheese, in tomato sauce,			
RavioliOs	7½-oz. can	260	39.0
Canned, dietetic:			
(Dia-Mel) beef	8-oz. can	260	35.0
(Featherweight) beef	8-oz. serving	260	35.0
RED & GRAY SNAPPER, raw (USDA):			
Whole	1 lb. (weighed whole)	219	0.
Meat only	4 oz.	105	0.
RELISH:			
Hamburger (Nalley's)	1 T. (.6 oz.)	17	4.1
Hot dog (Nalley's)	1 T. (.7 oz.)	24	4.8
Sour (USDA)	1 T. (.5 oz.)	3	.4
Sweet (Smucker's)	1 T. (.6 oz.)	23	4.8
RENNET MIX (Junket):			
*Powder, any flavor:			
Made with skim milk	½ cup	90	15.0
Made with whole milk	½ cup	120	15.0
Tablet	1 tablet	1	0.
RHINE WINE:			
(Great Western) 12% alcohol	3 fl. oz.	73	2.9
(Taylor) 12½% alcohol	3 fl. oz.	75	.3
RHUBARB (USDA)			
Cooked, sweetened, solids & liq.	½ cup (4.2 oz.)	169	43.2
Fresh:			
Partly trimmed	1 lb. (weighed with part leaves, ends & trimmings)	54	12.6
Trimmed	4 oz.	18	4.2
Diced	½ cup (2.2 oz.)	10	2.3

Food and Description	Measure or Quantity	Calories	Carbo-hydrates (grams)
*RICE:			
Brown (Uncle Ben's) parboiled, with added butter & salt	⅔ cup	152	26.4
White:			
(USDA) instant or pre-cooked	⅔ cup (3.3 oz.)	101	22.5
(Minute Rice) instant, no added butter	⅔ cup (4.3 oz.)	120	27.4
(River)	½ cup	100	22.0
(Success) long grain	½ cup	110	23.0
White & wild (Carolina)	½ cup	90	20.0
RICE BRAN (USDA)	1 oz.	78	14.4
RICE, FRIED (See also **RICE MIX**):			
*Canned (La Choy)	⅓ of 11-oz. can	190	40.0
Frozen:			
(Birds Eye)	3.7-oz. serving	104	22.8
(Green Giant) *Boil 'N Bag*	10-oz. entree	300	49.0
(La Choy) & pork	8-oz. serving	280	52.0
RICE, FRIED, SEASONING MIX:			
*(Durkee)	1 cup	213	46.5
(Kikkoman)	1-oz. pkg.	91	15.6
RICE KRINKLES, cereal			
(Post) frosted	⅞ cup (1 oz.)	109	25.9
RICE KRISPIES, cereal			
(Kellogg's):			
Regular	1 cup (1 oz.)	110	25.0
Frosted	¾ cup (1 oz.)	110	25.0

(USDA): United States Department of Agriculture
(HEW/FAO): Health, Education and Welfare/Food and Agriculture Organization
* Prepared as Package Directs

Food and Description	Measure or Quantity	Calories	Carbo-hydrates (grams)
RICE MIX:			
Beef:			
*(Carolina) *Bake-It-Easy*	¼ of pkg.	110	23.0
*(Minute Rice) rib roast	½ cup (4.1 oz.)	149	25.1
Rice-A-Roni	⅙ of 8-oz. pkg.	129	26.0
*Brown & Wild (Uncle Bens') with butter	½ cup	150	24.7
Chicken:			
*(Carolina) *Bake-It-Easy*	¼ of pkg.	110	23.0
*(Minute Rice) drumstick	½ cup (3.8 oz.)	153	25.4
Rice-A-Roni	⅕ of 8-oz. pkg.	160	33.2
*Fried (Minute Rice)	½ cup (3.4 oz.)	156	25.2
*Long grain & wild (Minute Rice)	½ cup (4.1 oz.)	148	25.0
(Uncle Ben's):			
Without butter	½ cup	97	20.6
With butter	½ cup	112	20.6
*Oriental (Carolina) *Bake-It-Easy*	¼ of pkg.	120	23.0
Spanish:			
*(Carolina) *Bake-It-Easy*	¼ of pkg.	110	23.0
*(Minute Rice)	½ cup (5.2 oz.)	150	25.6
Rice-A-Roni	⅙ of 7½-oz. pkg.	124	25.9
RICE, SPANISH:			
Home recipe (USDA)	4 oz.	99	18.8
Canned:			
Regular pack (Comstock; Menner's)	½ of 7½-oz. can	140	27.0
Dietetic (Featherweight) low sodium	7½-oz. serving	140	30.0
Frozen (Birds Eye)	3.7-oz. serving	122	26.1
RICE & VEGETABLE, frozen:			
(Birds Eye):			
French style	3.7-oz. serving	117	25.0
Peas with mushrooms	2⅓-oz. serving	109	23.1
(Green Giant) *Rice Originals:*			
& broccoli in cheese flavored sauce	½ cup	140	19.0
& herb butter sauce	½ cup	150	21.0

Food and Description	Measure or Quantity	Calories	Carbo-hydrates (grams)
Italian blend	½ cup	160	21.0
Long grain & white	½ cup	110	23.0
Medley	½ cup	120	20.0
Pilaf	½ cup	120	23.0
RICE WINE (HEW/FAO):			
Chinese, 20.7% alcohol	1 fl. oz.	38	1.1
Japanese, 10.6% alcohol	1 fl. oz.	72	13.1
ROCK & RYE (Mr. Boston) 27% alcohol	1 fl. oz.	74	7.2
ROE (USDA):			
Raw:			
Carp, cod haddock, herring, pike or shad	4 oz.	147	1.7
Salmon, sturgeon or turbont	4 oz.	235	1.6
Baked or broiled, cod & shad	4 oz.	143	2.2
Canned, cod, haddock or herring, solids & liq.	4 oz.	134	.3
ROLL OR BUN:			
Commercial type, non-frozen:			
Biscuit (Wonder)	1¼-oz. piece	99	17.0
Brown & serve:			
(Pepperidge Farm):			
Club	1.3-oz. piece	100	20.0
French	3.3-oz. piece	260	48.0
French	5-oz. piece	380	72.0
Hearth	.7-oz. piece	80	29.0
(Roman Meal)	1-oz. piece	78	12.6
(Wonder):			
Buttermilk	1-oz. piece	84	13.1
French	1-oz. piece	87	13.6
Gem style	1-oz. piece	72	13.1

(USDA): United States Department of Agriculture
(HEW/FAO):   Health, Education and Welfare/Food and Agriculture Organization
* Prepared as Package Directs

Food and Description	Measure or Quantity	Calories	Carbo-hydrates (grams)
Half & Half	1-oz. piece	81	12.8
Home bake	1-oz. piece	73	12.8
Crescent (Pepperidge Farm) butter	1-oz. piece	110	14.0
Croissant (Pepperidge Farm):			
Almond or Walnut	2-oz. piece	210	21.0
Butter	2-oz. piece	200	19.0
Chocolate	2.4-oz. piece	260	25.0
Cinnamon	2-oz. piece	200	23.0
Honey sesame	2-oz. piece	200	22.0
Raisin	2-oz. piece	200	24.0
Dinner:			
Home Pride	1-oz. piece	85	14.2
(Pepperidge Farm)	.7-oz. piece	60	10.0
(Wonder)	1¼-oz. piece	99	17.0
Dinner party rounds (Arnold)	.7-oz. piece	55	10.0
Finger (Pepperidge Farm) sesame or poppy seed	.6-oz. piece	60	9.0
Frankfurter:			
(Arnold) Hot Dog	1.3-oz. piece	110	20.0
(Pepperidge Farm)	1¾-oz. piece	110	18.0
(Wonder)	2-oz. piece	157	28.4
French:			
(Arnold) *Francisco:*			
Regular	2-oz. roll	160	31.0
Sourdough	1.1-oz. piece	90	16.0
(Pepperidge Farm):			
Small	1.3-oz. piece	110	20.0
Large	3-oz. piece	240	44.0
Golden Twist (Pepperidge Farm)	1-oz. piece	120	20.0
Hamburger:			
(Arnold)	1.4-oz. piece	110	21.0
(Pepperidge Farm)	1.5-oz. piece	130	23.0
Roman Meal	1.8-oz. piece	193	36.1
(Wondera)	2-oz. piece	157	28.4
Hard (USDA)	1.8-oz. piece	156	29.8
Hoggie (Wonder)	6-oz. piece	465	81.8
Honey (Hostess) glazed	3¾-oz. piece	422	52.2
Kaiser (Wonder)	6-oz. piece	465	81.8

Food and Description	Measure or Quantity	Calories	Carbo-hydrates (grams)
Old fashioned (Pepperidge Farm)	.6-oz. piece	60	23.0
Pan (Wonder)	1¼-oz. piece	99	17.0
Parkerhouse (Pepperidge Farm)	.6-oz. piece	60	9.0
Party (Pepperidge Farm)	.4-oz. piece	45	22.0
Sandwich:			
(Arnold):			
Franciso	2-oz. piece	160	30.0
Soft, plain or with poppy seed	1.3-oz. piece	110	18.0
Soft with sesame seeds	1.3-oz. piece	110	19.0
(Pepperidge Farm):			
Regular, with or without seeds	1.6-oz. piece	130	22.0
Onion with poppy seeds	1.9-oz. piece	150	27.0
Soft (Pepperidge Farm)	1¼-oz. piece	110	18.0
Sourdough french (Pepperidge Farm)	1.3-oz. piece	100	19.0
Frozen:			
Apple crunch (Sara Lee)	1-oz. piece	102	13.5
Caramel pecan (Sara Lee)	1.3-oz. piece	161	17.4
Caramel sticky (Sara Lee)	1-oz. piece	116	15.2
Cinnamon (Sara Lee)	.9-oz. piece	100	13.9
Croissant (Sara Lee)	.9-oz. piece	109	11.2
Crumb (Sara Lee):			
Blueberry	1¾-oz. piece	169	26.8
French	1¾-oz. piece	188	29.9
Danish (Sara Lee):			
Apple	1.3-oz. piece	120	17.4
Apple country	1.8-oz. piece	156	22.9
Cheese	1.3-oz. piece	130	13.9
Cheese country	1.5-oz. piece	146	13.5
Cherry	1.3-oz. piece	125	16.4
Cinnamon raisin	1.3-oz. piece	147	17.3
Pecan	1.3-oz. piece	148	18.3

(USDA): United States Department of Agriculture
(HEW/FAO):   Health, Education and Welfare/Food and Agriculture Organization
* Prepared as Package Directs

Food and Description	Measure or Quantity	Calories	Carbo-hydrates (grams)
Honey (Morton):			
Regular	2.3-oz. piece	230	31.0
Mini	1.3-oz. piece	133	18.0
*ROLL OR BUN DOUGH:			
Frozen (Rich's):			
Cinnamon	2¼-oz. piece	173	32.8
Danish, round	1 piece	202	24.0
Frankfurter	1 piece	136	24.9
Hamburger, regular	1 piece	134	25.0
Onion, deluxe	1 piece	204	38.3
Parkerhouse	1 piece	82	13.4
Refrigerated (Pillsbury):			
Apple danish, *Pipin' Hot*	1 piece	250	33.0
Butterflake	1 piece	110	16.0
Caramel danish, with nuts	1 piece	155	19.5
Cinnamon:			
Regular *Pipin'Hot*	1 piece	220	27.0
With icing:			
Regular, *Pipin' Hot*	1 piece	115	17.0
Hungry Jack	1 piece	145	18.5
& raisin	1 piece	145	19.5
Crescent	1 piece	100	11.0
Parkerhouse	1 piece	75	13.5
White, bakery style	1 piece	100	20.0
*ROLL MIX, HOT (Pillsbury)	1 piece	100	17.0
ROMAN MEAL CEREAL:			
2- or 5-minute	⅓ cup (1 oz.)	103	20.0
5-minute with oats	⅓ cup (1 oz.)	105	15.5
ROSEMARY LEAVES			
(French's)	1 tsp	5	.8
ROSE WINE:			
(Great Western) 12% alcohol	3 fl. oz.	80	2.4
(Paul Masson):			
Regular, 11.8% alcohol	3 fl. oz.	76	4.2
Light, 7.1% alcohol	3 fl. oz.	49	3.9

Food and Description	Measure or Quantity	Calories	Carbohydrates (grams)
RUTABAGA:			
Raw (USDA):			
Without tops	1 lb. (weighed with skin)	177	42.4
Diced	½ cup (2.5 oz.)	32	7.7
Boiled (USDA) drained, diced	½ cup (3 oz.)	30	7.1
Canned (Sunshine) solids & liq.	½ cup (4.2 oz.)	32	6.9
Frozen (Southland)	⅕ of 20-oz. pkg.	50	13.0
RYE, whole grain (USDA)	1 oz.	95	20.8

RYE FLOUR (See **FLOUR**)

RYE WHISKEY (See **DISTILLED LIQUOR**)

(USDA): United States Department of Agriculture
(HEW/FAO):   Health, Education and Welfare/Food and Agriculture
                        Organization
* Prepared as Package Directs

Food and Description	Measure or Quantity	Calories	Carbo-hydrates (grams)
	S		
SABLEFISH, raw (USDA):			
Whole	1 lb. (weighed whole)	362	0.
Meat only	4 oz.	215	0.
SAFFLOWER SEED (USDA) in hull	1 oz.	89	1.8
SAGE (French's)	1 tsp.	4	.6
SAKE WINE (HEW/FAO) 19.8% alcohol	1 fl. oz.	39	1.4
SALAD CRUNCHIES (Libby's)	1 T.	35	4.0
SALAD DRESSING:			
Regular:			
Bacon (Seven Seas) creamy	1 T.	60	1.0
Bleu blue cheese:			
(USDA)	1 T. (.5 oz.)	76	1.1
(Bernstein) Danish	1 T.	60	.6
(Wish-Bone) chunky	1 T.	70	Tr.
Boiled (USDA) home recipe	1 T. (.6 oz.)	26	2.4
Caesar:			
(Pfeiffer)	1 T.	70	.5
(Seven Seas) *Viva*	1 T.	60	1.0
Capri (Seven Seas)	1 T.	70	3.0
Cheddar & bacon (Wish-Bone)	1 T. (.5 oz.)	70	1.0
Cucumber (Wish-Bone) creamy	1 T.	80	2.0
French:			
Home recipe (USDA)	1 T.	101	.6
(Bernstein's) creamy	1 T. (.5 oz.)	56	2.1
(Seven Seas) creamy	1 T.	60	2.0
(Wish-Bone):			
Deluxe	1 T.	50	2.0

Food and Description	Measure or Quantity	Calories	Carbohydrates (grams)
Garlic or herbal	1 T.	60	2.0
Spice	1 T.	60	3.0
Garlic (Wish-Bone) creamy	1 T.	80	2.0
Green Goddess:			
(Seven Seas)	1 T.	60	0.
(Wish-Bone)	1 T.	70	1.0
Herb & spice (Seven Seas)	1 T.	60	1.0
Italian:			
(Bernstein's)	1 T.	50	.8
(Pfeiffer) chef	1 T.	60	.5
(Seven Seas) VIVA!	1 T.	70	1.0
(Wish-Bone):			
Regular or robusto	1 T.	80	1.0
Creamy	1 T.	80	2.0
Herbal	1 T.	70	1.0
Red wine vinegar & oil			
(Seven Seas)	1 T.	60	1.0
Roquefort:			
(USDA)	1 T. (.5 oz.)	76	1.1
(Bernstein's)	1 T.	65	.8
(Marie's)	1 T.	105	1.1
Russian:			
(USDA)	1 T.	74	1.6
(Pfeiffer)	1 T.	65	2.0
(Wish-Bone)	1 T.	50	7.0
Spin Blend (Hellman's)	1 T. (.6 oz.)	57	2.6
Thousand Island:			
(USDA)	1 T.	80	2.5
(Pfeiffer)	1 T.	65	2.0
(Wish-Bone):			
Regular	1 T.	60	2.0
Southern recipe:			
Plain	1 T.	70	3.0
Bacon	1 T.	60	2.0
Vinaigrette (Bernstein's)			
French	1 T.	49	.2

(USDA): United States Department of Agriculture
(HEW/FAO):   Health, Education and Welfare/Food and Agriculture
                        Organization
* Prepared as Package Directs

Food and Description	Measure or Quantity	Calories	Carbo-hydrates (grams)
Dietetic or low calorie:			
Bleu or blue cheese:			
(Dia-Mel)	1 T. (.5 oz.)	2	Tr.
(Featherweight) imitation	1 T.	4	1.0
(Tillie Lewis) *Tasti-Diet*	1 T.	12	Tr.
(Walden Farms) chunky	1 T.	27	1.7
(Wish-Bone) chunky	1 T.	40	3.0
Caesar:			
(Estee) garlic	1 T. (.5 oz.)	4	1.0
(Featherweight) creamy	1 T.	14	2.0
Cucumber:			
(Dia-Mel) creamy	1 T. (.5 oz.)	2	Tr.
(Featherweight)	1 T.	12	0.
(Wish-Bone) creamy	1 T.	40	1.0
Cucumber & onion			
(Featherweight) creamy	1 T.	4	1.0
French:			
(Dia-Mel)	1 T. (.5 oz.)	1	0.
(Featherweight):			
Low calorie	1 T.	6	1.0
Low sodium	1 T.	60	0.
(Tillie Lewis) *Tatsi Diet*	1 T.	6	Tr.
(Walden Farms)	1 T.	33	2.6
(Wish-Bone):			
Regular	1 T.	30	2.0
Sweet & spicy	1 T.	30	4.0
Garlic (Dia-Mel)	1 T. (.5 oz.)	1	0.
Herb garden (Estee)	1 T.	4	1.0
Herb & spice			
(Featherweight)	1 T.	6	1.0
Italian:			
(Dia-Mel) regular or creamy	1 T. (.5 oz.)	1	0.
(Estee) spicy	1 T.	4	1.0
(Featherweight)	1 T.	4	1.0
(Tillie Lewis) *Tasti Diet*	1 T.	2.	0.
(Walden Farm):			
Regular or low sodium	1 T.	9	1.5
No sugar added	1 T.	6	Tr.
(Weight Watchers)	1 T.	50	2.0
(Wish-Bone) regular or creamy	1 T.	30	1.0

Food and Description	Measure or Quantity	Calories	Carbo-hydrates (grams)
Onion & chive (Wish-Bone)	1 T.	40	3.0
Onion & cucumber (Estee)	1 T. (.5 oz.)	6	2.0
Red wine/vinegar:			
(Dia-Mel)	1 T.	1	0.
(Featherweight)	1 T.	6	1.0
Russian:			
(Featherweight) creamy	1 T.	6	1.0
(Tillie Lewis) *Tasti Diet*	1 T.	6	Tr.
(Weight Watchers)	1 T.	50	2.0
(Wish-Bone)	1 T. (.5 oz.)	25	5.0
Tahiti (Dia-Mel)	1 T.	2	Tr.
Thousand Island:			
(Dia-Mel)	1 T.	2	Tr.
(Walden Farms)	1 T.	24	3.1
(Weight Watchers)	1 T.	50	2.0
(Wish-Bone)	1 T.	25	3.0
2-Calorie Low Sodium			
(Featherweight)	1 T.	2	0.
Whipped:			
(Dia-Mel)	1 T.	24	Tr.
(Tillie Lewis) *Tasti Diet*	1 T.	18	1.0
Yogurt-buttermilk (Dia-Mel)	1 T.	2	Tr.
SALAD DRESSING MIX:			
*Regular (Good Seasons):			
Blue cheese	1 T. (.6 oz.)	84	.3
Buttermilk, farm style	1 T. (.6 oz.)	58	1.2
Classic herb	1 T.	83	.3
Farm style	1 T.	53	.7
French, old fashioned	1 T.	83	.5
Garlic, cheese	1 T.	85	.5
Garlic & herb	1 T.	84	.7
Italian:			
Regular, cheese or zesty	1 T. (.6 oz.)	84	.6
Mild	1 T. (.6 oz.)	86	1.2
Tomato & herb	1 T. (.6 oz.)	85	1.0

(USDA): United States Department of Agriculture
(HEW/FAO):   Health, Education and Welfare/Food and Agriculture
                    Organization
* Prepared as Package Directs

Food and Description	Measure or Quantity	Calories	Carbo-hydrates (grams)
Dietetic:			
*Blue cheese			
(Weight Watchers)	1 T.	10	1.0
*French (Weight Watchers)	1 T.	4	1.0
Garlic (Dia-Mel) (creamy)	½-oz. pkg.	21	1.0
*Italian:			
(Good Seasons):			
Regular	1 T.	8	1.8
Lite	1 T.	27	.8
(Weight Watchers):			
Regular	1 T.	2	0.
Creamy	1 T.	4	1.0
*Russian (Weight Watchers)	1 T.	4	1.0
*Thousand Island			
(Weight Watchers)	1 T.	12	1.0
SALAD LIFT SPICE (French's)	1 tsp. (4 grams)	6	1.0
SALAD SEASONING (Durkee):			
Regular	1 tsp.	4	.7
Cheese	1 tsp.	10	.4
SALAD SUPREME			
(McCormick)	1 tsp. (.1 oz.)	11	.5
SALAMI:			
(USDA):			
Dry	1 oz.	128	.3
Cooked	1 oz.	88	.4
(Eckrich):			
For beer or cooked	1 oz.	70	1.0
Cotto:			
Beef	.7-oz. slice	50	1.0
Meat	1-oz. slice	70	1.0
Hard	1 oz.	130	1.0
(Hormel):			
Beef	1 slice	25	0.
Cotto:			
Chib	1 oz.	100	0.
Sliced	1 slice	60	5.
Genoa:			
Packaged, sliced	1 slice	35	0.

Food and Description	Measure or Quantity	Calories	Carbo- hydrates (grams)
Whole:			
Regular or Gran Value	1 oz.	110	0.
Di Lusso	1 oz.	100	0.
Hard:			
Packaged, sliced	1 slice	40	0.
Whole:			
Regular	1 oz.	110	0.
National Brand	1 oz.	120	0.
Party slice	1 oz.	90	0.
Piccolo, stick	1 oz.	120	0.
(Oscar Mayer):			
For beer:			
Regular	.8-oz. slice	54	.4
Beef	.8-oz. slice	76	.2
Cotto:			
Regular	.8-oz. slice	52	.4
Regular	1-oz. slice	63	.5
Beef	.5-oz. slice	34	.4
Beef	.8-oz. slice	52	.6
SALISBURY STEAK, frozen:			
(Banquet):			
Buffet Supper	2-lb. pkg.	1410	30.0
Cookin' Bag	5-oz. pkg.	251	5.0
Dinner:			
American Favorites	11-oz. dinner	395	24.0
Extra Helping	19-oz. dinner	1024	71.0
(Green Giant):			
Baked with gravy	½ of entree	280	11.0
Boil 'n bag, with creole sauce	9-oz. entree	410	11.0
Twin pouch, with mashed potatoes	11-oz. entree	450	27.0
(Morton):			
Regular:			
Dinner	11-oz. dinner	290	25.0
Entree	5-oz. pkg.	150	7.0
Country Table	15-oz. dinner	500	62.0

(USDA): United States Department of Agriculture
(HEW/FAO): Health, Education and Welfare/Food and Agriculture
Organization
* Prepared as Package Directs

Food and Description	Measure or Quantity	Calories	Carbo-hydrates (grams)
King Size:			
Dinner	19-oz. dinner	780	65.0
Entree	10.3-oz. dinner	500	36.0
(Stouffer's):			
Regular, with onion gravy	12-oz. pkg.	500	10.0
Lean Cuisine, with Italian			
style sauce & vegetables	9½-oz. pkg.	270	14.0
(Swanson):			
Regular, with gravy	10-oz. entree	410	14.0
Hungry Man:			
Dinner	17-oz. dinner	780	63.0
Entree	12½-oz. entree	640	34.0
3-Course	16-oz. dinner	500	50.0
TV Brand:			
Regular	11½-oz. dinner	430	43.0
With crinkle cut potatoes	5½-oz. entree	350	30.0
SALMON:			
Atlantic (USDA):			
Raw:			
Whole	1 lb. (weighed whole)	640	0.
Meat only	4 oz.	246	0.
Canned, solids & liq., including bones	4 oz.	230	9.
Chinook or King (USDA)			
Raw:			
Steak	1 lb. (weighed whole)	886	0.
Meat only	4 oz.	252	0.
Canned, solids & liq., including bones	4 oz.	238	0.
Chum, canned (USDA), solids & liq., including bones	4 oz.	158	0.
Coho, canned (USDA) solids & liq., including bones	4 oz.	174	0.
Keta, canned (Bumble Bee) solids & liq., including bones	½ cup (3.9 oz.)	153	0.
Pink or Humpback (USDA):			
Raw:			
Steak	1 lb. (weighed whole)	475	0.
Meat only	4 oz.	135	0.

Food and Description	Measure or Quantity	Calories	Carbo- hydrates (grams)
Canned, solids & liq.:			
(USDA) including bones	4 oz.	135	0.
(Bumble Bee) including bones	½ cup (4 oz.)	155	0.
(Del Monte)	7¾-oz. can	277	0.
Sockeye or Red or Blueback, canned, solids & liq.:			
(USDA)	4 oz.	194	0.
(Bumble Bee) including bones	½ cup (4 oz.)	155	0.
(Del Monte)	½ of 7¾-oz. can	165	0.
Unspecified kind of salmon			
(USDA) baked or broiled	4.2 oz. steak (approx. 4″ × 3″ × ½″)	218	0.
SALMON, SMOKED (USDA)	4 oz.	200	0.
SALT:			
Regular:			
Butter-flavored (French's) imitation	1 tsp. (3.6 grams)	8	0.
Garlic (Lawry's)	1 tsp. (4 grams)	5	1.0
Hickory smoke (French's)	1 tsp. (4 grams)	2	Tr.
Onion (Lawry's)	1 tsp.	4	.9
Seasoned (Lawry's)	1 tsp.	1	.1
Table:			
(USDA)	1 tsp.	0	0.
(Morton) iodized	1 tsp. (7 grams)	0	0.
Lite Salt (Morton) iodized	1 tsp. (6 grams)	0	0.
Substitute:			
(Adolph's):			
Regular	1 tsp. (6 grams)	1	Tr.
Packet	8-gram packet	<1	Tr.
Seasoned	1 tsp.	6	1.1
(Dia-Mel) *Salt-It*	½ tsp.	0	0.
(Estee)	½ tsp.	0	0.

(USDA): United States Department of Agriculture
(HEW/FAO):   Health, Education and Welfare/Food and Agriculture
                        Organization
* Prepared as Package Directs

Food and Description	Measure or Quantity	Calories	Carbo-hydrates (grams)
(Morton):			
Regular	1 tsp. (6 grams)	Tr.	Tr.
Seasoned	1 tsp. (6 grams)	3	.5
SALT PORK, raw (USDA):			
With skin	1 lb. (weighed with skin)	3410	0.
Without skin	1 oz.	222	0.
SALT 'N SPICE SEASONING (McCormick)	1 tsp. (.1 oz.)	3	.5
SANDWICH SPREAD:			
(USDA)	1 T. (.5 oz.)	57	2.4
(USDA)	½ cup (4.3 oz.)	466	19.5
(Hellmann's)	1 T. (.5 oz.)	65	2.2
(Oscar Mayer)	1-oz. serving	68	3.2
SANGRIA (Taylor) 11.6% alcohol	3 fl. oz.	99	10.8
SARDINE:			
Raw (HEW/FAO):			
Whole	1 lb. (weighed whole)	321	0.
Meat only	4 oz.	146	0.
Canned:			
Atlantic:			
(USDA) in oil: Solids & liq.	3¾-oz. can	330	.6
(Drained solids, with skin & bones	3¾-oz. can	187	DNA
(Del Monte) in tomato sauce, solids & liq.	7½-oz. can	330	4.0
Imported (Underwood):			
In mustard sauce	3¾-oz. can	230	Tr.
In tomato sauce	3¾-oz. can	230	1.0
Norwegian:			
King Oscar Brand:			
In mustard sauce, solids & liq.	3¾-oz. can	240	2.0
In oil, drained	3-oz. can	260	1.0

Food and Description	Measure or Quantity	Calories	Carbo-hydrates (grams)
In tomato sauce, solids & liq.	3¾-oz. can	240	2.0
(Underwood)	3¾-oz. can	380	Tr.
Pacific (USDA) in brine or mustard, solids & liq.	4 oz.	222	1.9
SAUCE:			
Regular:			
A-1	1 T. (.6 oz.)	12	3.1
Barbecue:			
(USDA)	1 cup (8.8 oz.)	228	20.0
Chris & Pitt's	1 T.	15	4.0
(French's) regular or smoky	1 T. (.6 oz.)	25	5.0
(Gold's)	1 T.	16	3.9
Open Pit (General Foods):			
Original	1 T.	24	5.1
Original with minced onion	1 T.	25	5.7
Hot & spicy	1 T.	24	5.4
Smoke flavor	1 T.	24	5.5
Burrito (Del Monte)	¼ cup (2 oz.)	20	4.0
Chili (See **CHILI SAUCE**)			
Cocktail (See also Seafood):			
(Gold's)	1 oz.	31	7.5
(Pfeiffer)	1-oz. serving	50	6.0
Escoffier Sauce Diable	1 T.	20	4.3
Escoffier Sauce Robert	1 T. (.6 oz.)	20	5.1
Famous Sauce	1 T.	69	2.2
Hot, *Frank's*	1 tsp.	1	0.
Italian (See also **SPAGHETTI SAUCE** or **TOMATO SAUCE**):			
(Contadina)	4-fl.-oz. serving (4.4 oz.)	71	10.5
(Ragu) red cooking	3½-oz. serving	45	6.0
Salsa Mexicana (Contadina)	4 fl. oz. (4.4 oz.)	38	6.8

(USDA): United States Department of Agriculture
(HEW/FAO): Health, Education and Welfare/Food and Agriculture Organization
* Prepared as Package Directs

Food and Description	Measure or Quantity	Calories	Carbo- hydrates (grams)
Salsa Picante (Del Monte):			
Regular	¼ cup (2 oz.)	20	4.0
Hot & chunky	¼ cup	15	3.0
Salsa Roja (Del Monte)	¼ cup (2 oz.)	20	4.0
Seafood cocktail			
(Del Monte)	1 T. (.6 oz.)	21	4.9
Soy:			
(USDA)	1 oz.	19	2.7
(Gold's)	1 T.	10	1.0
(Kikkoman):			
Regular	1 T. (.6 oz.)	12	.9
Light	1 T.	9	.7
(La Choy)	1 T. (.5 oz.)	8	.9
Spare rib (Gold's)	1 T.	51	11.7
Steak (Dawn Fresh) with			
mushrooms	1 oz. serving	9	1.7
Steak Supreme	1 T. (.6 oz.)	20	5.1
Sweet & sour:			
(Contadina)	4 fl. oz. (4.4 oz.)	150	29.6
(La Choy)	1-oz. serving	51	12.6
Tabasco	¼ tsp.	Tr.	Tr.
Taco:			
Old El paso, hot or mild	1-oz. serving	10	2.3
(Ortega)	1 T. (.6 oz.)	22	5.1
Tartar:			
(USDA)	1 T. (.5 oz.)	74	.6
(Hellmann's)	1 T. (.5 oz.)	73	.2
(Nalley's)	1 T.	89	.3
Teriyaki (Kikkoman)	1 T. (.6 oz.)	16	3.1
V-8	1-oz. serving	25	6.0
White (USDA) home recipe:			
Thin	¼ cup (2.2 oz.)	74	4.5
medium	¼ cup (2.5 oz.)	103	5.6
Thick	¼ cup (2.2 oz.)	122	6.8
Worcestershire:			
(French's) regular or smoky	1 T. (.6 oz.)	10	2.0
(Gold's)	1 T.	42	3.3
(Lea & Pearins)	1 T. (.6 oz.)	12	3.0
Deitetic:			
Barbecue (Estee)	1 T. (.6 oz.)	16	4.0

Food and Description	Measure or Quantity	Calories	Carbo-hydrates (grams)
Cocktail (Estee)	1 T. (.5 oz.)	10	3.0
Tartar (USDA)	1 T. (.5 oz.)	31	.9
SAUCE MIX:			
Regular:			
A la King (Durkee)	1.1 oz. pkg.	133	14.0
*Cheese:			
(Durkee)	½ cup	168	9.5
(French's)	½ cup	160	14.0
Hollandaise:			
(Durkee)	1-oz. pkg.	173	11.0
*(French's)	1 T.	15	.7
*Sour cream:			
(Durkee)	⅔ cup	214	15.0
(French's)	2½ T.	60	5.0
*Stroganoff (French's)	⅓ cup	110	11.0
Sweet & sour:			
*(Durkee)	½ cup	115	22.5
*(French's)	½ cup	55	14.0
(Kikkoman)	2⅛-oz. pkg.	228	51.0
Teriyaki:			
*(French's)	1 T.	17	3.5
(Kikkoman)	1.5-oz. pkg.	125	22.3
*White (Durkee)	½ cup	119	20.5
*Dietetic (Weight Watchers)			
lemon butter	1 T.	8	1.0
SAUERKRAUT, canned:			
(USDA):			
Solids & liq.	½ cup (4.1 oz.)	21	4.7
Drained solids	½ cup (2.5 oz.)	15	3.1
(Claussen) drained	½ cup (2.7 oz.)	16	2.8
(Del Monte) solids & liq.	½ cup (4 oz.)	25	6.0
(Silver Floss) solids & liq.:			
Regular, can	½ cup (4 oz.)	30	5.0
Regular, jar	½ cup (4 oz.)	25	5.0
Bavarian Kraut	½ cup	35	8.0

(USDA): United States Department of Agriculture
(HEW/FAO):   Health, Education and Welfare/Food and Agriculture
                     Organization
* Prepared as Package Directs

Food and Description	Measure or Quantity	Calories	Carbo-hydrates (grams)
Krispy Kraut	½ cup	25	5.0
Polybag	½ cup	20	4.0
SAUERKRAUT JUICE, canned			
(USDA) 2% salt	½ cup (4.3 oz.)	12	2.8
SAUSAGE:			
*Brown & serve:			
(USDA)	1 oz.	120	.8
(Hormel)	1 sausage	70	0.
Country style (USDA) smashed	1 oz.	98	0.
Patty (Hormel) hot or mild	1 patty	150	0.
Polish-style:			
(Eckrich) meat:			
Regular	1 oz.	95	1.0
Skinless	1-oz. link	90	1.0
Skinless	1-oz. link	180	2.0
(Hormel):			
Regular	1 sausage	85	0.
Kielbasa, skinless	½ a link	180	1.0
Kolbase	3 oz.	220	1.0
(Vinna) beef	3 oz.	240	1.3
Pork:			
*(USDA)	1 oz.	135	Tr.
(Eckrich):			
Links	1-oz. link	110	.5
Patty	2-oz. patty	240	1.0
Roll, hot	2-oz. serving	240	1.0
*(Hormel):			
Little Sizzlers	1 link	51	0.
Midget links	1 link	71	0.
Smoked	1 oz.	96	.3
(Jimmy Dean)	2-oz. serving	227	Tr.
*(Oscar Mayer):			
Little Friers	1 link	82	.2
Patty, Southern Brand	1 oz.	81	0.
Roll (Eckrich) minced	1-oz. slice	80	1.0
Smoked:			
(Eckrich):			
Beef:			
Regular	2 oz.	190	1.0
Smok-Y-Links	.8-oz. link	70	1.0

Food and Description	Measure or Quantity	Calories	Carbo-hydrates (grams)
Cheese	2 oz.	180	2.0
Ham, Smok-Y-Links	.8-oz. link	75	1.0
Maple flavored, Smok-Y-Links	.8-oz.	75	1.0
Meat:			
Regular	2 oz.	190	1.0
Hot	2.7-oz. link	240	3.0
Skinless:			
Regular	2-oz. link	180	2.0
Smok-Y-Links	.8-oz. link	75	1.0
(Hormel) Smokies:			
Regular	1 link	80	.5
Cheese	1 link	84	.5
(Oscar Mayer):			
Beef	1½-oz. link	132	.9
Cheese	1½-oz. link	142	.4
Meat	2-oz. link	359	1.5
Thuringer (See **THURINGER**)			
*Turkey (Louis Rich) links or tube	1-oz. serving	45	Tr.
Vienna, canned:			
(USDA)	1 link (5-oz. can)	38	Tr.
(Hormel) drained:			
Regular	1 link	50	.3
Chicken	1 link	45	.3
(Libby's):			
In barbecue sauce	2½-oz. serving	180	2.0
In beef broth	1 link	46	.3
SAUTERNE:			
(Great Western)	3 fl. oz.	79	4.5
(Taylor)	3 fl. oz.	81	4.8
SAVORY (French's)	1 tsp.	5	1.0

SCALLION (See **ONION, GREEN**)

(USDA): United States Department of Agriculture
(HEW/FAO): Health, Education and Welfare/Food and Agriculture
Organization
* Prepared as Package Directs

Food and Description	Measure or Quantity	Calories	Carbo-hydrates (grams)
SCALLOP:			
Raw (USDA) muscle only	4-oz. serving	92	3.7
Steamed (USDA)	4-oz. serving	127	DNA
Frozen:			
(Mrs. Paul's) breaded & fried	3½-oz. serving	210	23.0
(Stouffer's) *Lean Cuisine*, oriental, & vegetable with rice	11-oz. pkg.	230	32.0
SCALLOPS & SHRIMP MARINER frozen (Stouffer's) with rice	10¼-oz. pkg.	400	40.0
SCHNAPPS:			
Apple (Mr. Boston) 27% alcohol	1 fl. oz.	76	8.0
Cinnamon (Mr. Boston) 27% alcohol	1 fl. oz.	76	8.0
Peppermint:			
(De Kuyper)	1 fl. oz.	79	7.5
(Mr. Boston)	1 fl. oz.	115	8.0
Spearmint (Mr. Boston)	1 fl. oz.	76	8.0
Strawberry (Mr. Boston)	1 fl. oz.	66	7.0
SCREWDRIVER COCKTAIL (Mr. Boston) 12½% alcohol	3 fl. oz.	111	12.0
SEA BASS, raw (USDA) meat only	4 oz.	109	0.
SEASON-ALL SEASONING (McCormick)	1 tsp.	4	.6
SEAFOOD PLATTER, frozen (Mrs. Paul's) breaded & fried, combination	9-oz. serving	510	49.0
SEAFOOD SEASONING (French's)	1 tsp. (.2 oz.)	2	Tr.
SEAWEED, dried (HEW/FAO):			
Agar	1 oz.	88	23.7
Lavar	1 oz.	67	12.6

Food and Description	Measure or Quantity	Calories	Carbo-hydrates (grams)
SEGO DIET FOOD, canned:			
Milk chocolate, very chocolate, very chocolate fudge, very chocolate malt, very chocolate marshmallow, very coconut or very dutch chocolate	10-fl.-oz. can	25	39.0
Very banana, very butter-scotch, very cherry vanilla, very French vanilla, very strawberry, very vanilla	10-fl.-oz. can	225	34.0
SESAME NUT MIX, canned (Planters) oil roasted	1 oz.	160	8.0
SESAME SEEDS, dry (USDA):			
Whole	1 oz.	160	6.1
Hulled	1 oz.	165	5.0
SHAD (USDA):			
Raw:			
Whole	1 lb. (weighed whole)	370	0.
Meat only	4 oz.	193	0.
Cooked, home recipe:			
Baked with butter or marga-rine & bacon slices	4 oz.	228	0.
Creole	4 oz.	172	1.8
Canned, solids & liq.	4 oz.	172	0.
SHAD, GIZZARD, raw (USDA):			
Whole	1 lb. (weighed whole)	229	0.
Meat only	4 oz.	227	0.
SHREDDED WHEAT:			
(Nabisco):			
Regular size	¾-oz. biscuit	90	19.0
Spoon Size	⅔ cup (1 oz.)	110	23.0
(Quaker)	1 biscuit (.6 oz.)	52	11.0

(USDA): United States Department of Agriculture
(HEW/FAO):   Health, Education and Welfare/Food and Agriculture
                        Organization
* Prepared as Package Directs

Food and Description	Measure or Quantity	Calories	Carbo-hydrates (grams)
SHRIMP:			
Raw (USDA):			
Whole	1 lb. (weighed in shell)	285	4.7
Meat only	4 oz.	103	1.7
Canned (Bumble Bee) solids & liq.	4½-oz. can	90	.9
Frozen (Mrs. Paul's) fried	3-oz. serving	190	15.0
SHRIMP DINNER, frozen:			
(Stouffer's) Newburg	6½-oz. serving	300	4.0
(Van de Kamp's)	10-oz. dinner	370	40.0
SHRIMP PASTE, canned (USDA)	1 oz.	51	.4
SKATE, raw (USDA) meat only	4 oz.	111	0.
SLENDER (Carnation):			
Bar:			
Chocolate or chocolate chip	1 bar	135	13.0
Chocolate peanut butter or vanilla	1 bar	135	12.0
Dry	1 packet	110	21.0
Liquid	10-fl.-oz. can	220	34.0
SLOPPY HOT DOG SEASONING MIX (French's)	1½-oz. pkg.	160	28.0
SLOPPY JOE:			
Canned:			
(Hormel) *Short Orders*	7½-oz. can	340	15.0
(Libby's):			
Beef	⅓ cup (2.5 oz.)	110	7.0
Pork	⅓ cup	120	6.0
Frozen (Banquet) *Cookin' Bag*	5-oz. pkg.	210	12.0
SLOPPY JOE SEASONING MIX:			
*(Durkee)			
Regular	1¼ cup	128	32.0
Pizza flavor	1¼ cup	746	26.0

Food and Description	Measure or Quantity	Calories	Carbo-hydrates (grams)
(French's)	1.5-oz. pkg.	128	32.0
(McCormick)	1.3-oz. pkg.	103	23.4
SMELT, Atlantic, jack & bar (USDA): Raw:			
Whole	1 lb. (weighed whole)	244	0.
Meat only	4 oz.	111	0.
Canned, solids & liq.	4 oz.	227	0.
SMURF BERRY CRUNCH, cereal (Post)	1 cup (1 oz.)	116	25.4
SMOKED SAUSAGE (See **SAUSAGE**)			
SNACK (See **CRACKER, POPCORN, POTATO CHIP,** etc.)			
SNACK BAR (Pepperidge Farm):			
Apple nut	1.7-oz. piece	170	33.0
Apricot raspberry or blueberry	1.7-oz. piece	170	36.0
Brownie nut or date nut	1½-oz. piece	190	30.0
Chocolate chip or coconut macaroon	1½-oz. piece	210	28.0
Raisin spice	1½-oz. piece	180	31.0
SNAIL, raw (USDA):			
Unspecified kind	4 oz.	102	2.3
Giant African	4 oz.	83	5.0
SNAPPER (See **RED SNAPPER**)			
SNO BALL (Hostess)	1½-oz. piece	148	27.3

(USDA): United States Department of Agriculture
(HEW/FAO):   Health, Education and Welfare/Food and Agriculture
              Organization
* Prepared as Package Directs

Food and Description	Measure or Quantity	Calories	Carbo-hydrates (grams)
SOAVE WINE (Antinori) 12% alcohol	3 fl. oz.	84	6.3
SOFT DRINK:			
Sweetened:			
Birch beer (Canada Dry)	6 fl. oz.	82	21.0
Bitter lemon:			
(Canada Dry)	6 fl. oz. (6.5 oz.)	75	19.5
(Schweppes)	6 fl. oz. (6.5 oz.)	84	20.8
Bubble Up	6 fl. oz.	73	18.4
Cactus Cooler (Canada Dry)	6 fl. oz. (6.5 oz.)	90	21.8
Cherry:			
(Canada Dry) wild	6 fl. oz. (6.5 oz.)	98	24.0
(Shasta) black	6 fl. oz.	79	21.5
Chocolate (Yoo-Hoo)	6 fl. oz.	93	18.0
Club	Any quantity	0	0.
Cola:			
Coca-Cola:			
Regular	6 fl. oz.	72	19.0
Caffeine-free	6 fl. oz.	76	20.0
Jamaica (Canada Dry)	6 fl. oz. (6.5 oz.)	82	20.2
Pepsi-Cola, regular or *Pepsi Free*	6 fl. oz.	79	19.8
RC 100, caffeine free	6 fl. oz.	78	19.5
(Royal Crown)	6 fl. oz.	78	19.5
(Shasta):			
Regular	6 fl. oz.	72	19.5
Cherry	6 fl. oz.	68	18.5
Collins mix (Canada Dry)	6 fl. oz. (6.5 oz.)	60	15.0
Cream:			
(Canada Dry) vanilla	6 fl. oz. (6.6 oz.)	97	24.0
(Schweppes) red	6 fl. oz.	86	21.3
(Shasta)	6 fl. oz.	75	20.5
Dr. Pepper	6 fl. oz. (6.5 oz.)	75	19.4

Food and Description	Measure or Quantity	Calories	Carbo-hydrates (grams)
Fruit punch:			
(Nehi)	6 fl. oz.	91	22.8
(Shasta)	6 fl. oz.	84	23.0
Ginger ale:			
(Canada Dry):			
Regular	6 fl. oz.	68	15.8
Golden	6 fl. oz.	75	18.0
(Fanta)	6 fl. oz.	63	16.0
(Nehi)	6 fl. oz.	69	16.6
(Schweppes)	6 fl. oz.	66	16.3
(Shasta)	6 fl. oz.	59	16.0
Ginger beer (Schweppes)	6 fl. oz.	72	16.8
Grape:			
(Canada Dry) concord	6 fl. oz.		
	(6.6 oz.)	97	24.0
(Fanta)	6 fl. oz.	86	22.0
(Hi-C)	6 fl. oz.	78	20.0
(Nehi)	6 fl. oz.	87	21.8
(Patio)	6 fl. oz.	96	24.0
(Schweppes)	6 fl. oz.	97	23.8
(Welch's) sparkling	6 fl. oz.	90	23.0
Half & half (Canada Dry)	6 fl. oz.		
	(6.5 oz.)	82	19.5
Hi-Spot (Canada Dry)	6 fl. oz.		
	(6.5 oz.)	75	18.7
Island lime (Canada Dry)	6 fl. oz.		
	(6.6 oz.)	97	24.8
Lemon (Hi-C)	6 fl. oz.	75	18.0
Lemonade (Shasta)	6 fl. oz.	71	19.0
Lemon lime (Shasta)	6 fl. oz.	69	19.0
Mello Yello	6 fl. oz.	86	22.0
Mr. PiBB	6 fl. oz.	71	19.0
Mt. Dew	6 fl. oz.	89	22.0
Orange:			
(Canada Dry) Sunripe	6 fl. oz.		
	(6.6 oz.)	97	24.7
(Fanta)	6 fl. oz.	88	23.0

(USDA): United States Department of Agriculture
(HEW/FAO):   Health, Education and Welfare/Food and Agriculture
            Organization
* Prepared as Package Directs

Food and Description	Measure or Quantity	Calories	Carbo-hydrates (grams)
(Hi-C)	6 fl. oz.	77	20.0
(Nehi)	6 fl. oz.	95	23.8
(Patio)	6 fl. oz.	96	24.0
(Schweppes) sparkling	6 fl. oz.	89	22.1
(Shasta)	6 fl. oz.	86	23.5
(Sunkist)	6 fl. oz.	96	7.6
(Welch's)	6 fl. oz.	90	23.5
Peach (Nehi)	6 fl. oz.	92	23.0
Pineapple (Canada Dry)	6 fl. oz.(6.5 oz.)	82	19.5
Punch (Hi-C)	6 fl. oz.	77	20.0
Purple Passion (Canada Dry)	6 fl. oz. (6.5 oz.)	90	22.5
Quinine or tonic water			
(Canada Dry)	6 fl. oz.	67	16.5
(Schweppes)	6 fl. oz.	66	16.5
(Shasta)	6 fl. oz.	59	16.0
Rondo (Schweppes)	6 fl. oz.	76	19.5
Root beer:			
Barrelhead (Canada Dry)	6 fl. oz.(6.5 oz.)	82	19.5
(Dad's)	6 fl. oz.	83	20.7
(Fanta)	6 fl. oz.	78	20.0
(Nehi)	6 fl. oz.	87	21.8
On Tap	6 fl. oz.	81	20.4
(Patio)	6 fl. oz.	83	21.0
(Ramblin')	6 fl. oz.	88	23.0
Rooti (Canada Dry)	6 fl. oz.	82	19.5
(Schweppes)	6 fl. oz.	79	19.3
(Shasta)	6 fl. oz.	75	20.5
Seltzer (Canada Dry)	6 fl. oz.	0	0.
7UP	6 fl. oz.	60	18.1
Sprite	6 fl. oz.	71	18.0
Strawberry:			
(Canada Dry)	6 fl. oz.	90	22.5
(Nehi)	6 fl. oz.	87	21.8
(Shasta)	6 fl. oz.	72	19.5
Tahitian Treat (Canada Dry)	6 fl. oz.	97	24.0
Teem	6 fl. oz.	74	18.6
Upper 10 (Royal Crown)	6 fl. oz.	76	19.0
Whiskey sour (Canada Dry)	6 fl. oz.	67	16.5
Wink (Canada Dry)	6 fl. oz. (6.5 oz.)	90	22.5
Dietetic:			
Bubble Up	6 fl. oz.	1	.2

Food and Description	Measure or Quantity	Calories	Carbo-hydrates (grams)
Cherry:			
(No-Cal) black	6 fl. oz.	1	Tr.
(Shasta) black	6 fl. oz.	Tr.	Tr.
Chocolate (No-Cal)	6 fl. oz.		
	(6.2 oz.)	1	Tr.
Coffee (No-Cal)	6 fl. oz.		
	(6.2 oz.)	1	Tr.
Cola:			
(Canada Dry)	6 fl. oz.		
	(6.2 oz.)	0	0.
Coca Cola, regular or caffeine free	6 fl. oz.	Tr.	.1
Diet Rite (Royal Crown)	6 fl. oz.	Tr.	.1
(No-Cal)	6 fl. oz.		
	(6.2 oz.)	0	0.
Pepsi, diet, light or caffeine free	6 fl. oz.	Tr.	Tr.
RC 100	6 fl. oz.	Tr.	.1
(Shasta)	6 fl. oz.	Tr.	Tr.
Cream:			
(No-Cal)	6 fl. oz.	0	0.
(Shasta)	6 fl. oz.	Tr.	Tr.
Dr. Pepper	6 fl. oz.		
	(6.4 oz.)	Tr.	.4
Fresca	6 fl. oz.	2	Tr.
Ginger Ale:			
(Canada Dry)	6 fl. oz.		
	(6.2 oz.)	1	0.
(No-Cal)	6 fl. oz.		
	(6.2 oz.)	1	0.
(Shasta)	6 fl. oz.	Tr.	Tr.
Grape (Shasta)	6 fl. oz.	Tr.	Tr.
Grapefruit (Shasta)	6 fl. oz.	Tr.	.2
Lemon-lime:			
(No-Cal)	6 fl. oz.	1	Tr.
(Shasta)	6 fl. oz.	Tr.	Tr.
Mr. PiBB	6 fl. oz.	Tr.	Tr.

(USDA): United States Department of Agriculture
(HEW/FAO):   Health, Education and Welfare/Food and Agriculture
                        Organization
* Prepared as Package Directs

Food and Description	Measure or Quantity	Calories	Carbo-hydrates (grams)
Orange:			
(Canada Dry)	6 fl. oz. (6.2 oz.)	1	Tr.
(No-Cal)	6 fl. oz.	1	0.
(Shasta)	6 fl. oz.	Tr.	Tr.
Quinine or tonic			
(Canada Dry: No-Cal)	6 fl. oz.	3	Tr.
RC 100 (Royal Crown) caffeine free	6 fl. oz.	Tr.	1.
Root beer:			
Barrelhead (Canada Dry)	6 fl. oz. (6.2 oz.)	1	0.
(Dad's)	6 fl. oz.	Tr.	.2
(No-Cal)	6 fl. oz.	1	0.
(Ramblin')	6 fl. oz.	Tr.	.2
(Shasta)	6 fl. oz.	Tr.	Tr.
7UP	6 fl. oz.	2	0.
Sprite	6 fl. oz.	1	Tr.
Strawberry (Shasta)	6 fl. oz.	Tr.	Tr.
Tab, regular or caffeine free	6 fl. oz.	Tr.	.2
SOLE, frozen:			
Raw, meat only (USDA)	4 oz.	90	0.
Frozen:			
(Mrs. Paul's) fillets, breaded & fried	6-oz. serving	280	19.0
(Van de Kamp's):			
Regular, batter dipped, french fried	2-oz. piece	140	12.0
Today's Catch	4 oz.	80	0.
(Weight Watchers) in lemon sauce	9⅛-oz. meal	200	17.0
SOUFFLE:			
Cheese:			
Home recipe (USDA)	1 cup (collapsed)	207	5.9
Frozen (Stouffer's)	6-oz. serving	355	14.0
Corn, frozen (Stouffer's)	4-oz. serving	155	19.0
SOUP:			
Canned, regular pack:			
*Asparagus (Campbell), condensed, cream of	8-oz. serving	90	11.0

Food and Description	Measure or Quantity	Calories	Carbo-hydrates (grams)
Bean:			
(Campbell):			
Chunky, with ham, old fashioned:			
Small	11-oz. can	290	37.0
Large	19¼-oz. can	500	64.0
*Condensed, with bacon	8-oz. serving	150	21.0
Semi-condensed, Soup For One,			
with ham	11-oz. serving	220	31.0
(Grandma Brown's)	8-oz . serving	182	29.1
Bean, black:			
*(Campbell) condensed	8-oz. serving	110	17.0
(Crosse & Blackwell) with			
sherry	6½-oz. serving	80	18.0
Beef:			
(Campbell):			
Chunky:			
Regular:			
Small	10¾-oz. can	190	23.0
Large	19-oz. can	340	40.0
With noodles	10¾-oz. can	300	23.0
*Condensed:			
Regular	8-oz. serving	80	10.0
Broth:			
Plain	8-oz. serving	16	1.0
& barley	8-oz. serving	60	10.0
& noodles	8-oz. serving	60	9.0
Consomme	8-oz. serving	25	2.0
Mushroom	8-oz. serving	70	6.0
Noodle	8-oz. serving	70	7.0
Teriyaki	8-oz. serving	70	9.0
(College Inn) broth	1 cup (8.3 oz.)	18	1.0
(Swanson)	7½-oz. can	20	1.0
Celery:			
*(Campbell) condensed,			
cream of	8-oz. serving	100	8.0

(USDA): United States Department of Agriculture
(HEW/FAO): Health, Education and Welfare/Food and Agriculture
        Organization
* Prepared as Package Directs

Food and Description	Measure or Quantity	Calories	Carbo-hydrates (grams)
*(Rokeach):			
Prepared with milk	10-oz. serving	190	19.0
Prepared with water	10-oz. serving	90	12.0
*Cheddar cheese (Campbell)	8-oz. serving	130	10.0
Chicken:			
(Campbell):			
Chunky:			
Regular:			
Small	10¾-oz. can	200	20.0
Large	19-oz. can	360	36.0
Old fashioned	10¾-oz. can	170	21.0
& rice	19-oz. can	280	30.0
Vegetable	19-oz. can	340	38.0
*Condensed:			
Alphabet	8-oz. serving	80	10.0
Broth:			
Plain	8-oz. serving	35	3.0
& rice	8-oz. serving	50	8.0
& vegetables	8-oz. serving	25	4.0
Cream of	8-oz. serving	110	9.0
& dumplings	8-oz. serving	90	9.0
Gumbo	8-oz. serving	60	8.0
Mushroom, creamy	8-oz. serving	110	9.0
Noodle	8-oz. serving	70	8.0
NoodleOs	8-oz. serving	70	9.0
& rice	8-oz. serving	60	7.0
& stars	8-oz. serving	50	7.0
Vegetable	8-oz. serving	70	8.0
*Semi-condensed,			
Soup For One:			
& noodles, golden	11-oz. serving	130	14.0
Vegetable, full			
flavored	11-oz. serving	120	13.0
(College Inn) broth	1 cup (8.3 oz.)	35	0.
(Swanson) broth	7¼-oz. can	35	3.0
Chili beef (Campbell):			
Chunky:			
Small	11-oz. can	300	37.0
Large	19½-oz. can	520	66.0
*Condensed	8-oz. serving	130	17.0
Chowder:			
Beef'n vegetable (Hormel)			
Short Orders	7½-oz. can	120	15.0

Food and Description	Measure or Quantity	Calories	Carbo-hydrates (grams)
Chicken'n corn (Hormel)			
Short Orders	7½-oz. can	130	15.0
Clam:			
Manhattan style:			
(Campbell):			
Chunky:			
Small	10¾-oz. can	160	24.0
Large	19-oz. can	300	44.0
*Condensed	8-oz. serving	70	11.0
(Crosse & Blackwell)	6½-oz. serving	50	9.0
New England Style:			
*(Campbell):			
Condensed:			
Made with milk	8-oz. serving	150	17.0
Made with water	8-oz. serving	80	11.0
Semi-condensed,			
Soup For One:			
Made with milk	11-oz. serving	200	23.0
Made with water	11-oz. serving	130	18.0
(Crosse & Blackwell)	6½-oz. serving	90	14.0
Ham'n potato (Hormel)			
Short Orders	7½-oz. can	130	14.0
Consomme madrilene			
(Crosse & Blackwell)	6½-oz. serving	25	4.0
Crab (Crosse & Blackwell)	6½-oz. serving	50	8.0
Gazpacho:			
*(Campbell) condensed	8-oz. serving	50	9.0
(Crosse & Blackwell)	6½-oz. serving	30	1.0
Ham'n butter bean			
(Campbell) *Chunky*	10¾-oz. can	280	33.0
Lentil (Crosse & Blackwell)			
with ham	6½-oz. serving	80	13.0
*Meatball alphabet			
(Campbell) condensed	8-oz. serving	100	12.0
Mexicali bean (Campbell)			
Chunky	19½-oz. can	420	70.0

(USDA): United States Department of Agriculture
(HEW/FAO):   Health, Education and Welfare/Food and Agriculture
                        Organization
* Prepared as Package Directs

Food and Description	Measure or Quantity	Calories	Carbo-hydrates (grams)
Minestrone:			
(Campbell):			
Chunky	19-oz. can	300	42.0
*Condensed	8-oz. serving	80	11.0
(Crosse & Blackwell)	6½-oz. serving	90	18.0
Mushroom:			
*(Campbell):			
Condensed:			
Cream of	8-oz. serving	100	9.0
Golden	8-oz. serving	80	10.0
Semi-condensed,			
Soup For One, cream			
of, savory	11-oz. serving	180	15.0
(Crosse & Blackwell) cream			
of, bisque,	6½-oz. serving	90	8.0
*(Rokeach) cream of			
Prepared with milk	10-oz. serving	240	20.0
Prepared with water	10-oz. serving	150	13.0
*Mushroom barley			
(Campbell)	8-oz. serving	80	12.0
*Noodle (Campbell):			
Curly, & chicken	8-oz. serving	70	9.0
& ground beef	8-oz. serving	90	10.0
*Onion (Campbell):			
Regular	8-oz. serving	70	9.0
Cream of:			
Made with water	8-oz. serving	100	12.0
Made with water & milk	8-oz. serving	160	15.0
*Oyster stew (Campbell):			
Made with milk	8-oz. serving	140	10.0
Made with water	8-oz. serving	70	5.0
*Pea, green (Campbell)	8-oz. serving	150	25.0
Pea, split:			
(Campbell):			
Chunky, with ham:			
Small	10¾-oz. can	230	33.0
Large	19-oz. can	400	58.0
*Condensed, with ham &			
bacon	8-oz. serving	170	24.0
(Grandma Brown's)	8-oz. serving	184	28.2
*Pepper pot (Campbell)	8-oz. serving	90	9.0
*Potato (Campbell) cream of:			
Made with water	8-oz. serving	70	11.0
Made with water & milk	8-oz. serving	130	14.0

Food and Description	Measure or Quantity	Calories	Carbo- hydrates (grams)
*Scotch broth (Campbell) condensed	8-oz. serving	80	9.0
Shav (Gold's)	8-oz. serving	11	2.1
Shrimp:			
*(Campbell) condensed, cream of:			
Made with milk	8-oz. serving	160	22.0
Made with water	8-oz. serving	90	8.0
(Crosse & Blackwell)	6½-oz. serving	90	7.0
Sirloin burger (Campbell) *Chunky:*			
Small	10¾-oz. can	220	23.0
Large	19-oz. can	400	40.0
Steak & potato (Campbell) *Chunky:*			
Small	10¾-oz. can	190	23.0
Large	19-oz. can	340	42.0
Tomato:			
(Campbell):			
Condensed:			
Regular:			
Made with milk	8-oz. serving	160	22.0
Made with water	8-oz. serving	90	17.0
Bisque	8-oz. serving	120	23.0
Garden	8-oz. serving	80	18.0
& rice, old fashioned	8-oz. serving	110	22.0
Semi-condensed, *Soup for One*, Royale	11-oz. serving	180	35.0
*(Rokeach):			
Plain:			
Made with milk	10-oz. serving	190	27.0
Made with water	10-oz. serving	90	20.0
& rice	10-oz. serving	160	25.0
Turkey (Campbell):			
Chunky	18¾-oz. can	360	36.0
*Condensed:			
Noodle	8-oz. serving	60	8.0
Vegetable	8-oz. serving	70	8.0

(USDA): United States Department of Agriculture
(HEW/FAO):   Health, Education and Welfare/Food and Agriculture
 Organization
* Prepared as Package Directs

Food and Description	Measure or Quantity	Calories	Carbo-hydrates (grams)
Vegetable:			
(Campbell):			
Chunky:			
Regular:			
Small	10¾-oz. can	140	23.0
Large	19-oz. can	260	42.0
Beef, old fashioned:			
Small	10¾-oz. can	180	20.0
Large	19-oz. can	360	18.0
Mediterranean	19-oz. can	340	48.0
*Condensed:			
Regular	8-oz. serving	80	12.0
Beef	8-oz. serving	70	8.0
Old fashioned	8-oz. serving	60	10.0
Vegetarian	8-oz. serving	70	12.0
*Semi-condensed, *Soup For One:*			
Barley, with beef	11-oz. serving	150	20.0
Old world	11-oz. serving	130	18.0
*(Rokeach) vegetarian	10-oz. serving	90	15.0
Vichyssoise (Crosse & Blackwell) cream of	6½-oz. serving	70	5.0
*Won ton (Campbell)	8-oz. serving	40	5.0
Canned, dietetic pack:			
Beef (Campbell) *Chunky,* & mushroom, low sodium	10¾-oz. can	200	23.0
Chicken:			
(Campbell) low sodium:			
Chunky, regular	7½-oz. can	150	14.0
Vegetable	10¾-oz. can	240	21.0
*(Dia-Mel) & noodle	8-oz. serving	50	11.0
Corn (Campbell) low sodium	10¾-oz. can	190	31.0
Mushroom:			
(Campbell) cream of, low sodium	7¼-oz. can	130	10.0
(Dia-Mel) cream of	8-oz. serving	85	9.0
Pea, green (Campbell) low sodium	7½-oz. can	160	23.0
Pea, split (Campbell) low sodium	10¾-oz. can	220	35.0
Tomato:			
(Campbell) low sodium:			
Regular	7¼-oz. can	140	24.0
With tomato pieces	10½-oz. can	200	32.0

Food and Description	Measure or Quantity	Calories	Carbo-hydrates (grams)
(Dia-Mel)	8-oz. serving	50	11.0
Turkey (Campbell) low sodium	7¼-oz. can	70	8.0
Vegetable:			
(Campbell) low sodium:			
Regular	7¼-oz. can	90	15.0
Beef	7¼-oz. can	90	9.0
Chunky	10¾-oz. can	180	22.0
(Dia-Mel) & beef	8-oz. serving	70	12.0
Frozen:			
*Barley & mushroom (Mother's Own)	8-oz. serving	50	8.0
Chowder, clam, New England style (Stouffer's)	8-oz. serving	200	19.0
Pea, split:			
*(Mother's Own)	8-oz. serving	130	20.0
(Stouffer's) with ham	8¼-oz. serving	190	27.0
Spinach (Stouffer's) cream of	8-oz. serving	230	17.0
*Vegetable (Mother's Own)	8-oz. serving	40	Tr.
*Won ton (La Choy)	½ of 15-oz. pkg.	50	6.0
Mix, regular:			
Beef:			
Carmel Kosher	6 fl. oz.	12	1.8
*(Lipton) *Cup-A-Soup:*			
Regular, & noodle	6 fl. oz.	50	8.0
Lots-A-Noodles	7 fl. oz.	120	21.0
*(Weight Watchers) broth	6 fl. oz.	10	1.0
*Chicken:			
Carmel Kosher	6 fl. oz.	12	1.8
(Lipton):			
Regular & rice	8 fl. oz.	12	1.8
Cup-A-Broth	6 fl. oz.	25	4.0
Cup-A-Soup:			
Regular	6 fl. oz.	80	9.0
& noodles with meat	6 fl. oz.	45	6.0
& rice	6 fl. oz.	45	7.0
& vegetable	6 fl. oz.	40	7.0

(USDA): United States Department of Agriculture
(HEW/FAO): Health, Education and Welfare/Food and Agriculture Organization
* Prepared as Package Directs

Food and Description	Measure or Quantity	Calories	Carbo-hydrates (grams)
Country style:			
Hearty	6 fl. oz.	70	11.0
Supreme	6 fl. oz.	100	11.0
Lots-A-Noodles	7 fl. oz.	130	23.0
*Noodle (Lipton):			
With chicken broth	8 fl. oz.	60	8.0
With chicken meat	8 fl. oz.	50	1.0
Giggle Noodle	8 fl. oz.	80	12.0
Ring-O-Noodle	8 fl. oz.	60	9.0
Ripple Noodle	8 fl. oz.	80	13.0
*Mushroom:			
Carmel Kosher	6 fl. oz.	12	2.4
(Lipton):			
Regular:			
Beef	8 fl. oz.	40	7.0
Onion	8 fl. oz.	40	6.0
Cup-A-Soup, cream of	6 fl. oz.	80	10.0
*Onion:			
Carmel Kosher	6 fl. oz.	12	2.4
(Lipton):			
Regular:			
Plain	8 fl. oz.	35	6.0
Beefy	8 fl. oz.	30	4.0
Cup-A-Soup	6 fl. oz.	30	5.0
*Pea, green (Lipton)			
Cup-A-Soup	6 fl. oz.	120	16.0
*Pea, Virginia (Lipton)			
Cup-A-Soup, country style	6 fl. oz.	140	18.0
*Tomato (Lipton)			
Cup-A-Soup	6 fl. oz.	80	17.0
*Vegetable:			
(Lipton):			
Regular:			
Beef	8 fl. oz.	50	8.0
Spring	6 fl. oz.	40	7.0
Cup-A-Soup:			
Regular:			
Beef	6 fl. oz.	50	8.0
Spring	6 fl. oz.	40	7.0
Country Style, harvest	6 fl. oz.	100	20.0
Lots-A-Noodles, garden	7 fl. oz.	130	23.0
(Southland) frozen	⅕ of 16-oz. pkg.	60	12.0

Food and Description	Measure or Quantity	Calories	Carbo-hydrates (grams)
*Mix, dietetic (Estee):			
Chicken, cream of	6½-fl. oz. serving	50	8.0
Mushroom, cream of	6½-fl. oz. serving	50	9.0
Tomtato:			
Cream of	6½-fl. oz. serving	60	10.0
Vegetable	6½-fl. oz. serving	60	13.0
SOUP GREENS (Durkee)	2½-oz. jar	216	43.0
SOURSOP, raw (USDA):			
Whole	1 lb. (weighed with skin & seeds)	200	50.3
Flesh only	4 oz.	74	18.5
SOUSE (USDA)	1 oz.	51	.3
SOUTHERN COMFORT:			
80 proof	1 fl. oz.	79	3.4
86 proof	1 fl. oz.	84	3.5
100 proof	1 fl. oz.	97	3.5
SOYBEAN:			
(USDA):			
Young seeds:			
Raw	1 lb. (weighed in pod)	322	31.7
Boiled, drained	4 oz.	134	11.5
Canned:			
Solids & liq.	4 oz.	85	7.1
Drained solids	4 oz.	117	8.4
Mature seeds:			
Raw	1 lb.	1828	152.0
Raw	1 cup (7.4 oz.)	846	70.4
Cooked	4 oz.	147	12.2

(USDA): United States Department of Agriculture
(HEW/FAO):   Health, Education and Welfare/Food and Agriculture
                        Organization
* Prepared as Package Directs

Food and Description	Measure or Quantity	Calories	Carbo-hydrates (grams)
Oil roasted:			
(Soy Ahoy) regular, or garlic	1 oz.	152	4.8
(Soytown)	1 oz.	152	4.8
SOYBEAN CURD OR TOFU (USDA):			
Regular	4 oz.	82	2.7
Cake	4.2-oz. cake	86	2.9
SOYBEAN FLOUR (See **FLOUR**)			
SOYBEAN GRITS, high fat (USDA)	1 cup (4.9 oz.)	524	46.0
SOYBEAN MILK (USDA):			
Fluid	4 oz.	37	1.5
Powder	1 oz.	122	7.9
SOYBEAN PROTEIN (USDA)	1 oz.	91	4.3
SOYBEAN PROTEINATE (USDA)	1 oz.	88	2.2
SOYBEAN SPROUT (See **BEAN SPROUT**)			
SOY SAUCE (See **SAUCE**, Soy)			
SPAGHETTI. (Plain spaghetti products are essentially the same in calorie value and carbohydrate content on the same weight basis. The longer the cooking, the more water is absorbed and this affects the nutritive value):			
Cooked USDA):			
8–10 minutes, "Al Dente"	1 cup (5.1 oz.)	216	43.9
14–20 minutes, tender	1 cup (4.9 oz.)	155	32.2

Food and Description	Measure or Quantity	Calories	Carbo-hydrates (grams)
Canned, regular pack:			
(Franco-American):			
With meatballs in tomato sauce, *SpaghettiOs*	7⅜-oz. can	210	25.0
With meatballs, in tomato sauce	7⅜-oz. can	220	22.0
In meat sauce	7½-oz. can	220	26.0
With sliced franks in tomato sauce, *SpaghettiOs*	7⅜-oz. can	220	26.0
In tomato & cheese sauce, *SpaghettiOs*	7⅜-oz. can	170	33.0
In tomato sauce with cheese	7⅜-oz. can	180	36.0
(Hormel) *Short Orders*, & meatballs in tomato sauce	7½-oz. can	210	26.0
(Libby's) & meatballs in tomato sauce	7½-oz. serving	189	27.5
Canned, dietetic:			
(Dia-Mel) & meatballs	8-oz. serving	220	24.0
(Featherweight) & meatballs	7½-oz. serving	200	28.0
Frozen:			
(Banquet) & meat sauce	8-oz. pkg.	270	35.0
(Green Giant) & meatballs, twin pouch	10-oz. entree	396	53.9
(Morton):			
Casserole, & meat	8-oz. casserole	220	31.0
Dinner, & meatball	11-oz. dinner	360	61.0
(Stouffer's):			
Regular, & meat sauce	14-oz. pkg.	445	62.0
Lean Cuisine	11½-oz. pkg.	280	38.0
(Swanson) *TV Brand:*			
Dinner	12½-oz. dinner	370	46.0
Entree, in tomato sauce with breaded veal	9-oz. entree	310	32.0

(USDA): United States Department of Agriculture
(HEW/FAO): Health, Education and Welfare/Food and Agriculture
        Organization
* Prepared as Package Directs

Food and Description	Measure or Quantity	Calories	Carbo-hydrates (grams)
SPAGHETTI SAUCE, CANNED:			
Regular pack:			
Garden Style (Ragu)	4-oz. serving	80	14.0
Home style (Ragu):			
Plain or mushroom	4-oz. serving	70	12.0
Meat flavored	4-oz. serving	80	12.0
Marinara:			
(Prince)	4-oz. serving	80	12.4
(Ragu)	4-oz. serving	120	12.0
Meat or meat flavored:			
(Prego)	4-oz. serving	160	22.0
(Prince)	½ cup (4.9 oz.)	101	11.0
(Ragu):			
Regular	4-oz. serving	80	11.0
Extra Thick & Zesty	4-oz. serving	100	14.0
Meatless or plain:			
(Hain) Italian style	4-oz. serving	72	14.2
(Prego)	4-oz. serving	160	22.0
(Prince)	½ cup (4.6 oz.)	90	11.4
(Ragu):			
Regular	4-oz. serving	80	11.0
Extra Thick & Zesty	4-oz. serving	100	15.0
Mushroom:			
(Hain)	4-oz. serving	80	14.3
(Prego)	4-oz. serving	140	22.0
(Prince)	4-oz. serving	77	11.3
(Ragu):			
Regular	4-oz. serving	90	9.0
Extra Thick & Zesty	4-oz. serving	110	13.0
Dietetic pack (Featherweight)	⅔ cup	30	10.0
SPAGHETTI SAUCE MIX:			
*(Durkee):			
Regular	½ cup	45	10.4
With mushrooms	1⅓ cups	104	24.0
*(French's):			
Italian style	⅝ cup	100	15.0
With mushrooms	⅝ cup	100	13.0
Thick, homemade style	⅞ cup	170	24.0
(McCormick)	1½-oz. pkg.	128	25.1
*(Spatini)	½ cup	84	8.4

Food and Description	Measure or Quantity	Calories	Carbo-hydrates (grams)
SPAM, luncheon meat (Hormel):			
Regular, smoke flavored or with cheese chunks	1-oz. serving	85	0.
Deviled	1 T.	35	0.
SPANISH MACKEREL, raw (USDA):			
Whole	1 lb. (weighed whole)	490	0.
Meat only	4 oz.	201	0.
SPECIAL K, cereal (Kellogg's)	1 cup (1 oz.)	110	21.0
SPINACH:			
Raw (USDA):			
Untrimmed	1 lb. (weighed with large stems & roots)	85	14.0
Trimmed or packaged	1 lb.	118	19.5
Trimmed, whole leaves	1 cup (1.2 oz.)	9	1.4
Trimmed, chopped	1 cup (1.8 oz.)	14	2.2
Boiled (USDA) whole leaves, drained	1 cup (5.5 oz.)	36	5.6
Canned, regular pack: (USDA):			
Solids & liq.	½ cup (4.1 oz.)	21	3.5
Drained solids	½ cup	27	4.0
(Del Monte) solids & liq.	½ cup (4.1 oz.)	25	4.0
(Libby's) solids & liq.	½ cup (4.2 oz.)	27	3.6
(Sunshine) whole leaf, solids & liq.	½ cup (4.1 oz.)	24	2.9
Canned, dietetic or low calorie (USDA) low sodium:			
Solids & liq.	4 oz.	24	3.9
Drained solids	4 oz.	29	4.5
(Blue Boy) solids & liq.	4-oz. serving	22	2.4
(Del Monte) No Salt Added, Solids & liq.	½ cup	25	4.0

(USDA): United States Department of Agriculture
(HEW/FAO):   Health, Education and Welfare/Food and Agriculture
Organization
* Prepared as Package Directs

Food and Description	Measure or Quantity	Calories	Carbo-hydrates (grams)
(Featherweight) low sodium	½ cup	35	4.0
Frozen:			
(Birds Eye):			
Chopped or leaf	⅓ of pkg. (3.3 oz.)	28	3.4
Creamed	⅓ of pkg. (3 oz.)	60	4.9
& water chestnuts with selected seasonings	⅓ of 10-oz. pkg.	32	5.0
(Green Giant):			
Creamed	½ cup	70	8.0
Cut or leaf, in butter sauce	½ cup	50	6.0
Harvest Fresh	½ cup	30	4.0
(McKenzie) chopped or cut	⅓ of pkg.	20	3.0
(Stouffer's):			
Creamed	½ of 9-oz. pkg.	190	9.0
Souffle	4-oz. serving	135	12.0
SPLEEN, raw (USDA):			
Beef & calf	4 oz.	118	0.
Hog	4 oz.	121	0.
Lamb	4 oz.	130	0.
SQUAB, pigeon, raw (USDA):			
Dressed	1 lb. (weighed with feet, inedible viscera & bones)	569	0.
Meat & skin	4 oz.	333	0.
Meat only	4 oz.	161	0.
Light meat only, without skin	4 oz.	142	0.
Giblets	1 oz.	44	.3
SQUASH SEEDS, dry (USDA):			
In hull	4 oz.	464	12.6
Hulled	1 oz.	157	4.3
SQUASH, SUMMER:			
Fresh (USDA):			
Crookneck & straightneck, yellow:			
Whole	1 lb. (weighed untrimmed)	89	19.1

Food and Description	Measure or Quantity	Calories	Carbo-hydrates (grams)
Boiled, drained:			
Diced	½ cup (3.6 oz.)	15	3.2
Slices	½ cup (3.1 oz.)	13	2.7
Scallop, white & pale green:			
Whole	1 lb. (weighed untrimmed)	93	22.7
Boiled, drained, mashed	½ cup (4.2 oz.)	19	4.5
Zucchini & cocazelle, green:			
Whole	1 lb. (weighed untrimmed)	73	15.5
Boiled, drained slices	½ cup (2.7 oz.)	9	1.9
Canned (Del Monte) zucchini, in tomato sauce	½ cup (4 oz.)	30	8.0
Frozen:			
(Birds Eye):			
Regular	⅓ of 10-oz. pkg.	22	3.9
Zucchini	⅓ of 10-oz. pkg.	19	3.3
(McKenzie):			
Crookneck	⅓ of pkg. (3.3 oz.)	18	4.0
Zucchini	3.3 oz.	16	3.0
(Mrs. Paul's) sticks, batter dipped, french fried	⅓ of 9-oz. pkg.	180	23.1
(Southland):			
Crookneck:			
Plain	⅕ of 16-oz. pkg.	20	4.0
With onions	⅕ of 16-oz. pkg.	20	5.0
Zucchini:			
With onions	⅕ of 16-oz. pkg.	15	3.0
Sliced	⅕ of 16-oz. pkg.	15	3.3

SQUASH, WINTER:
Fresh (USDA):
  Acorn:

Whole	1 lb. (weighed with skin & seeds)	152	38.6

(USDA): United States Department of Agriculture
(HEW/FAO):   Health, Education and Welfare/Food and Agriculture
              Organization
* Prepared as Package Directs

Food and Description	Measure or Quantity	Calories	Carbo-hydrates (grams)
Baked, flesh only, mashed	½ cup (3.6 oz.)	56	14.3
Boiled, mashed	½ cup (4.1 oz.)	39	9.7
Butternut:			
Whole	1 lb. (weighed with skin & seeds)	171	44.4
Baked, flesh only	4 oz.	77	19.8
Boiled, flesh only	4 oz.	46	11.8
Hubbard:			
Whole	1 lb. (weighed with skin & seeds)	117	28.1
Baked, flesh only	4 oz.	57	13.3
Boiled, flesh only, diced	½ cup (4.2 oz.)	35	8.1
Boiled, flesh only, mashed	½ cup (4.3 oz.)	37	8.4
Frozen:			
(USDA) heated	½ cup (4.2 oz.)	46	11.0
(Birds Eye)	⅓ of pkg. (3.3 oz.)	43	9.2
(Southland) butternut	⅓ of 20-oz. pkg.	60	16.0
SQUID, raw (USDA) meat only	4 oz.	95	1.7
STARCH (See **CORNSTARCH**)			
*START, instant breakfast drink	½ cup	51	12.7
STEAK & GREEN PEPPERS, frozen:			
(Green Giant) twin pouch, with rice & vegetables	9-oz. entree	250	32.0
(Swanson) in Oriental style sauce	8½-oz. entree	180	12.0
STOCK BASE (French's):			
Beef	1 tsp. (4 grams)	8	2.0
Chicken	1 tsp. (3 grams)	8	3.0
STOMACH, PORK, scalded (USDA)	4 oz.	172	0.
STRAINED FOOD (See **BABY FOOD**)			

Food and Description	Measure or Quantity	Calories	Carbo-hydrates (grams)
STRAWBERRY:			
Fresh (USDA):			
Whole	1 lb. (weighed with caps & stems)	161	36.6
Whole, capped	1 cup (5.1 oz.)	53	2.1
Canned (USDA) unsweetened or low calorie, water pack, solids & liq.	4 oz.	25	6.4
Frozen (Birds Eye):			
Halves:			
Regular	⅓ of 16-oz. pkg.	164	34.9
Quick thaw in lite syrup	½ of 10-oz. pkg.	68	15.8
Whole:			
Regular	¼ of 16-oz. pkg.	89	21.4
In lite syrup	¼ of 16-oz. pkg.	61	14.4
Quick thaw	1.2 of 10-oz. pkg.	125	30.1
STRAWBERRY DRINK (Hi-C):			
Canned	6 fl. oz.	89	22.0
*Mix	6 fl. oz.	68	17.0
STRAWBERRY JELLY:			
Sweetened (Smucker's)	1 T. (.7 oz.)	53	13.5
Dietetic:			
(Diet Delight)	1 T. (.6 oz.)	12	3.0
(Estee)	1 T.	18	4.8
(Featherweight)	1 T.	16	4.0
STRAWBERRY KRISPIES,			
cereal (Kellogg's)	¾ cup (1 oz.)	110	25.0
STRAWBERRY NECTAR,			
canned (Libby's)	6 fl. oz.	60	14.0

(USDA): United States Department of Agriculture
(HEW/FAO): Health, Education and Welfare/Food and Agriculture Organization
* Prepared as Package Directs

Food and Description	Measure or Quantity	Calories	Carbo-hydrates (grams)
STRAWBERRY PRESERVE OR JAM:			
Sweetened:			
(Smucker's)	1 T. (.7 oz.)	53	13.5
(Welch's)	1 T.	52	13.5
Dietetic or low calorie:			
(Dia-Mel)	1 T. (.6 oz.)	6	0.
(Featherweight): calorie reduced	1 T.	16	4.0
(Louis Sherry) wild	1 T. (.6 oz.)	6	0.
(S-W) *Nutradiet*, red label	1 T.	12	3.0
STRAWBERRY SHORTCAKE, cereal (General Mills)	1 cup (1 oz.)	110	25.0
STUFFING MIX:			
*Beef, *Stove Top*	½ cup	181	21.5
Chicken:			
(Pepperidge Farm)	1 oz.	120	22.0
Stove Top	½ cup	178	20.2
Cornbread:			
(Pepperidge Farm)	1 oz.	110	22.0
Stove Top	½ cup	174	21.6
Cube or herb seasoned (Pepperidge Farm)	1 oz.	110	22.0
*New England Style, *Stove Top*	½ cup	180	20.8
*Pork, *Stove Top*	½ cup	176	20.3
*With rice, *Stove Top*	½ cup	183	23.2
*San Francisco Style, *Stove Top*	½ cup	175	19.9
Seasoned (Pepperidge Farm) pan style	1 oz.	110	23.0
&Turkey, *Stove Top*	½ cup	177	20.7
White bread (Mrs. Cubbison's)	1 oz.	101	20.5
STURGEON (USDA)			
Raw:			
Section	1 lb. (weighed with skin & bones)	362	0.
Meat only	4 oz.	107	0.

Food and Description	Measure or Quantity	Calories	Carbo-hydrates (grams)
Smoked	4 oz.	169	0.
Steamed	4 oz.	181	0.
SUCCOTASH:			
Canned, solids & liq.:			
(Libby's):			
Cream style	½ cup (4.6 oz.)	111	22.8
Whole kernel	¼ of 16-oz. can	82	16.0
(Stokely-Van Camp)	½ cup (4.5 oz.)	85	17.5
Frozen (Birds Eye)	⅓ of 10-oz. pkg.	104	20.7
SUCKER, CARP (USDA) raw:			
Whole	1 lb. (weighed whole)	196	0.
Meat only	4 oz.	126	0.
SUCKER, including **WHITE MULLET** (USDA) raw:			
Whole	1 lb. (weighed whole)	203	0.
Meat only	4 oz.	118	0.
SUET, raw (USDA)	1 oz.	242	0.
SUGAR, beet or cane (there are no differences in calories and carbohydrates among brands) (USDA):			
Brown:			
Regular	1 lb.	1692	437.3
Brownulated	1 cup (5.4 oz.)	567	146.5
Firm-packed	1 cup (7.5 oz.)	791	204.4
Firm-packed	1 T. (.5 oz.)	48	12.5
Confectioner's:			
Unsifted	1 cup (4.3 oz.)	474	122.4
Unsifted	1 T. (8 grams)	30	7.7
Sifted	1 cup (3.4 oz.)	366	94.5

(USDA): United States Department of Agriculture
(HEW/FAO):   Health, Education and Welfare/Food and Agriculture
                      Organization
* Prepared as Package Directs

Food and Description	Measure or Quantity	Calories	Carbo-hydrates (grams)
Sifted	1 T. (6 grams)	23	5.9
Stirred	1 cup (4.2 oz.)	462	119.4
Stirred	1 T. (8 grams)	29	7.5
Granulated	1 lb.	1746	451.3
Granulated	1 cup (6.9 oz.)	751	194.0
Granulated	1 T. (.4 oz.)	46	11.9
Granulated	1 lump (1⅛″ × ¾″ × ⅜″, 6 grams)	23	6.0
Maple	1 lb.	1579	408.0
Maple	1¾″ × 1¼″ × ½″ piece (1.2 oz.)	104	27.0
SUGAR APPLE, raw (USDA):			
Whole	1 lb. (weighed with skin & seeds)	192	48.4
Flesh only	4 oz.	107	26.9
SUGAR CORN POPS, cereal (Kellogg's)	1 cup (1 oz.)	110	26.0
SUGAR CRISP, cereal (Post)	⅞ cup (1 oz.)	112	25.6
SUGAR PUFFS, cereal (Malt-O-Meal)	⅞ cup (1 oz.)	110	26.0
SUGAR SMACKS cereal (Kellogg's)	¾ cup (1 oz.)	110	25.0
SUGAR SUBSTITUTE:			
(Estee)	1 tsp. (4 grams)	12	3.0
(Featherweight) liquid or tablet	3 drops or 1 tablet	0	0.
Sprinkle Sweet (Pillsbury)	1 tsp.	2	.5
Sweet'n It (Dia-Mel) liquid	5 drops	0	0.
*Sweet *10* (Pillsbury)	⅛ tsp.	0	0.
*SUKIYAKI DINNER, canned (La Choy) bi-pack	¾ cup	70	9.0
SUNFLOWER SEED:			
(USDA):			
In hulls	4 oz. (weighed in hull)	343	12.2
Hulled	1 oz.	159	5.6

Food and Description	Measure or Quantity	Calories	Carbo- hydrates (grams)
(Fisher):			
In hull, roasted, salted	1 oz.	86	3.0
Hulled, roasted:			
Dry, salted	1 oz.	164	5.6
Oil, salted	1 oz.	167	5.6
(Flavor House) dry roasted	1 oz.	179	4.0
(Frito-Lay's)	1 oz.	181	4.7
(Planter's):			
Dry roasted	1 oz.	160	5.0
Unsalted	1 oz.	170	5.0
SUNFLOWER SEED FLOUR, (See **FLOUR**)			
SUZY Q (Hostess):			
Banana	2¼-oz. piece	242	38.4
Chocolate	2¼-oz. piece	237	36.4
SWAMP CABBAGE (USDA):			
Raw, whole	1 lb. (weighed untrimmed)	107	19.8
Boiled, trimmed, drained	4 oz.	24	4.4
SWEETBREADS (USDA):			
Beef:			
Raw	1 lb.	939	0.
Braised	4 oz.	363	0.
Calf:			
Raw	1 lb.	426	0.
Braised	4 oz.	363	0.
Hog (See **PANCREAS**)			
Lamb:			
Raw	1 lb.	426	0.
Braised	4 oz.	198	0.
SWEET POTATO:			
Baked (USDA) peeled after baking	5″ × 2″ potato (3.9 oz.)	155	35.8

(USDA): United States Department of Agriculture
(HEW/FAO):   Health, Education and Welfare/Food and Agriculture
Organization
* Prepared as Package Directs

Food and Description	Measure or Quantity	Calories	Carbo-hydrates (grams)
Candied, home recipe (USDA)	3½″ × 2¼″ piece (6.2 oz.)	294	59.8
Canned (USDA):			
In syrup	4-oz. serving	129	31.2
Vacuum or solid pack	½ cup (3.8 oz.)	118	27.1
Frozen:			
(Mrs. Paul's) candied:			
Regular	4-oz. serving	180	44.0
N' apples	4-oz. serving	150	36.0
(Stouffer's) & apples	5-oz. serving	160	31.0
SWEET POTATO PIE (USDA)			
home recipe	⅙ of 9″ pie (5.4 oz.)	324	36.0
***SWEET & SOUR ORIENTAL,**			
canned (La Choy):			
Chicken	½ of 15-oz. can	240	50.0
Pork	½ of 15-oz. can	260	48.0
SWEET & SOUR PORK,			
frozen:			
(La Choy)	12-oz. entree	360	64.0
(Van de Kamp's) & rice	11-oz. serving	460	61.0
SWISS STEAK, frozen:			
(Green Giant)	1 meal	350	37.0
(Swanson) *TV Brand*	10-oz. dinner	350	36.0
SWORDFISH (USDA):			
Raw, meat only	1 lb.	535	0.
Broiled, with butter or margarine	3″ × 3″ × ½″ steak (4.4 oz.)	218	0.
Canned, solids & liq.	4 oz.	116	0.
SYRUP (See also **TOPPING**):			
Regular:			
Apricot (Smucker's)	1 T. (.6 oz.)	50	13.0
Blackberry (Smucker's)	1 T. (.6 oz.)	50	13.0
Chocolate or chocolate-flavored:			
Bosco	1 T. (.7 oz.)	55	13.3
(Hershey's)	1 T. (.7 oz.)	52	11.7

Food and Description	Measure or Quantity	Calories	Carbo- hydrates (grams)
Cane (USDA)	1 T. (.7 oz.)	55	14.0
Corn, *Karo*, dark or light	1 T. (.7 oz.)	58	14.5
Maple:			
(USDA)	1 T. (.7 oz.)	50	13.0
Karo, imitation	1 T.	57	14.2
Pancake or waffle:			
(Aunt Jemima)	1 T. (.7 oz.)	53	13.1
Golden Griddle	1 T. (.7 oz.)	54	13.3
Karo	1 T. (.7 oz.)	58	14.4
Log Cabin	1 T. (.7 oz.)	56	14.0
Mrs. Butterworth's	1 T. (.7 oz.)	55	13.0
Strawberry (Smucker's)	1 T.	50	13.0
Dietetic or low calorie:			
Blueberry:			
(Dia-Mel)	1 T. (.5 oz.)	1	0.
(Featherweight)	1 T.	14	3.0
Chocolate or chocolate- flavored:			
(Dia-Mel) *Choco-Syp*	1 T.	6	1.0
(Diet Delight)	1 T. (.6 oz.)	8	2.0
(No-Cal)	1 T.	6	0.
Coffee (No-Cal)	1 T.	6	1.2
Cola (No-Cal)	1 T.	0	Tr.
Maple (S&W) *Nutradiet*, imitation	1 T.	12	3.0
Pancake or waffle:			
(Aunt Jemima)	1 T. (.6 oz.)	29	7.3
(Dia-Mel)	1 T. (.5 oz.)	1	Tr.
(Diet Delight)	1 T. (.6 oz.)	6	4.0
(Featherweight)	1 T.	12	3.0
(S&W) *Nutradiet*, red label	1 T.	12	3.0
(Tillie Lewis) *Tasti Diet*	1 T. (.5 oz.)	4	1.0

(USDA): United States Department of Agriculture
(HEW/FAO):   Health, Education and Welfare/Food and Agriculture
                    Organization
* Prepared as Package Directs

Food and Description	Measure or Quantity	Calories	Carbo-hydrates (grams)

T

TACO:
  *(Ortega) — 1 taco — 150 — 15.0
  *Mix:

Food and Description	Measure or Quantity	Calories	Carbo-hydrates (grams)
TACO:			
*(Ortega)	1 taco	150	15.0
*Mix:			
*(Durkee)	½ cup	321	3.7
(French's)	1¼-oz. pkg.	120	24.0
(McCormick)	1½-oz. pkg.	123	23.7
Shell:			
Old El Paso	1 shell (.4 oz.)	52	6.0
(Ortega)	1 shell	50	7.7
TAMALE:			
Canned:			
(Hormel) beef:			
Regular	1 tamale	70	4.0
Hot & Spicy	1 tamale	70	4.5
Short Orders	7½-oz. can	270	17.0
Old El Paso,			
with chili gravy	1 tamale	116	11.5
Frozen (Hormel) beef	1 tamale (3.1 oz.)	130	13.0
TAMARIND, fresh (USDA):			
Whole	1 lb. (weighed with peel, membrane & seeds)	104	24.6
Juice	½ cup (4.4 oz.)	51	12.0
TANG:			
Grape, regular	6 fl. oz.	93	23.2
Orange:			
Regular	6 fl. oz.	87	21.8
Dietetic	6 fl. oz.	2	.5
TANGELO, fresh (USDA):			
Whole	1 lb. (weighed with peel,		

Food and Description	Measure or Quantity	Calories	Carbo-hydrates (grams)
	membrane & seeds)	104	24.6
Juice	½ cup (4.4 oz.)	51	12.0
TANGERINE or MANDARIN ORANGE:			
Fresh (USDA):			
Whole	1 lb. (weighed with peel, membrane & seeds)	154	38.9
Whole	4.1-oz. tangerine (2⅜" dia.)	39	10.0
Sections (without membranes)	1 cup (6.8 oz.)	89	22.4
Canned, regular pack (Del Monte) solids & liq.	¼ of 22-oz. can	100	25.0
Canned, dietetic or low calories, solids & liq.:			
(Diet Delight) juice pack	½ cup (4.3 oz.)	50	13.0
(Featherweight) water pack	½ cup	35	8.0
(S&W) *Nutradiet*	½ cup	28	7.0
TANGERINE DRINK, canned (Hi-C)	6 fl. oz.	90	23.0
***TANGERINE JUICE,** frozen (Minute Maid)	6 fl. oz.	85	20.8
TAPIOCA, dry, *Minute,* quick cooking	1 T. (.3 oz.)	32	7.9
TAQUITO, frozen (Van de Kamp's) beef	8-oz. serving	490	47.0
TARO, raw (USDA):			
Tubers, whole	1 lb. (weighed with skin)	373	90.3

(USDA): United States Department of Agriculture
(HEW/FAO):   Health, Education and Welfare/Food and Agriculture
                        Organization
* Prepared as Package Directs

Food and Description	Measure or Quantity	Calories	Carbo-hydrates (grams)
Tubers, skin removed	4 oz.	111	26.9
Leaves & stems	1 lb.	181	33.6
TARRAGON (French's)	1 tsp. (1.4 grams)	5	.7
TASTEEOS, cereal (Ralston Purina)	1¼ cups (1 oz.)	110	22.0
TAUTUG or BLACKFISH, raw (USDA):			
Whole	1 lb. (weighed whole)	149	0.
Meat only	4 oz.	101	0.
***TEA:**			
Bag:			
(Lipton):			
Plain or flavored	1 cup	2	Tr.
Herbal:			
Almond pleasure, dessert mint, gentle orange or cinnamon apple	1 cup	2	0.
Quietly chamomile or toasty spice	1 cup	4	Tr.
(Sahadi):			
Herbal	6 fl. oz.	2	0.
Spearmint	6 fl. oz.	4	Tr.
Instant (Lipton) 100% tea	8 fl.oz.	0	0.
TEA, ICED:			
Canned:			
Regular:			
(Lipton)	6 fl. oz.	67	16.5
(Shasta)	6 fl. oz.	61	16.5
Dietetic (Lipton) lemon flavored	6 fl. oz.	2	0.
*Mix:			
Regular:			
Country Time, sugar & lemon flavored	8 fl. oz.	121	30.2
(Lipton)	8 fl. oz.	60	16.0

Food and Description	Measure or Quantity	Calories	Carbohydrates (grams)
(Nestea) lemon & sugar flavored	8 fl. oz.	90	25.6
Dietetic:			
Crystal Light	8 fl. oz.	2	.2
(Lipton) lemon flavored	8 fl. oz.	2	0.
(Nestea) light	6 fl. oz.	4	1.0
TEAM, cereal (Nabisco)	1 cup (1 oz.)	110	24.0
TEQUILA SUNRISE COCKTAIL (Mr. Boston) 12½% alcohol	3 fl. oz.	120	14.4
TERIYAKI, frozen (Stouffer's) beef with rice & vegetables	10-oz. serving	365	26.0
*TEXTURED VEGETABLE PROTEIN, *Morningstar Farms:*			
Breakfast link	1 link	73	1.3
Breakfast patties	1 patty (1.3 oz.)	100	3.5
Breakfast strips	1 strip (.3 oz.)	37	.7
*Grillers	1 patty (2.3 oz.)	190	6.0
THURINGER:			
(Eckrich):			
Sliced	1-oz. slice	90	1.0
Smoky Tange	1-oz. serving	80	1.0
(Hormel):			
Packaged, sliced	1 slice	70	0.
Whole:			
Regular or tangy, chub	1 oz.	90	0.
Beefy	1-oz. serving	100	0.
Old Smokehouse	1-oz. serving	90	1.0
(Louis Rich) turkey	1-oz. slice	50	Tr.
(Oscar Mayer):			
Regular	.8-oz. slice	75	.2
Beef	.8-oz. slice	72	.7

(USDA): United States Department of Agriculture
(HEW/FAO): Health, Education and Welfare/Food and Agriculture
              Organization
* Prepared as Package Directs

Food and Description	Measure or Quantity	Calories	Carbo- hydrates (grams)
THYME (French's)	1 tsp.	5	1.0
TIGER TAILS (Hostess)	2¼-oz. piece	227	38.9
TOASTER CAKE OR PASTRY:			
Pop-Tarts (Kellogg's):			
Regular:			
Blueberry or cherry	1.8-oz. pastry	210	36.0
Brown sugar cinnamon	1¾-oz. pastry	210	33.0
Strawberry	1.8-oz. pastry	200	37.0
Frosted:			
Blueberry or strawberry	1 pastry	200	38.0
Brown sugar cinnamon	1 pastry	210	34.0
Cherry chocolate fudge	1 pastry	200	36.0
Chocolate-vanilla creme	1 pastry	210	37.0
Concord grape, dutch apple or raspberry	1 pastry	210	36.0
Toastees (Howard Johnson):			
Blueberry	1 piece	121	48.0
Corn	1 piece	112	51.3
Oatmeal	1 piece	95	53.2
Orange	1 piece	127	54.8
Raisin bran	1 piece	104	55.4
Toaster Strudel (Pillsbury):			
Blueberry	1 piece	190	28.0
Cinnamon	1 piece	190	26.0
Raspberry or strawberry	1 piece	190	27.0
Toast-R-Cake (Thomas'):			
Blueberry	1 piece	116	17.7
Bran	1 piece	113	18.5
Corn	1 piece	118	17.4
TOASTIES, cereal (Post)	1¼ cups (1 oz.)	107	24.4
TOASTY O's, cereal (Malt-O-Meal)	1¼ cup (1 oz.)	110	20.0
TOFU (See **SOYBEAN CURD**)			
TOMATO:			
Fresh (USDA):			
Green:			
Whole, untrimmed	1 lb. (weighed with core & stem end)	99	21.1

Food and Description	Measure or Quantity	Calories	Carbo-hydrates (grams)
Trimmed, unpeeled	4 oz.	27	5.8
Ripe:			
Whole:			
Eaten with skin	1 lb.	100	21.3
Peeled	1 lb. (weighed with skin, stem ends & hard core)	88	18.8
Peeled	1 med. (2" × 2½", 5.3 oz.)	33	7.0
Peeled	1 small (1¾" × 2½", 3.9 oz.)	24	5.2
Sliced, peeled	½ cup (3.2 oz.)	20	4.2
Boiled (USDA)	½ cup (4.3 oz.)	31	6.7
Canned, regular pack, solids & liq.:			
(Contadina):			
Sliced, baby	½ cup (4.2 oz.)	50	10.0
Pear shape	½ cup (4.2 oz.)	25	6.0
Stewed	½ cup (4.3 oz.)	35	9.0
Whole, peeled	½ cup (4.2 oz.)	25	5.0
(Del Monte):			
Stewed	4 oz.	35	8.0
Wedges	½ cup (4 oz.)	30	8.0
Whole, peeled	½ cup (4 oz.)	25	5.0
(Stokely-Van Camp) stewed	½ cup (4.2 oz.)	35	7.5
Canned, dietetic pack, solids & liq.:			
(Del Monte) No Salt Added	½ cup (4 oz.)	35	8.0
(Diet Delight) whole, peeled	½ cup (4.3 oz.)	25	5.0
(Featherweight)	½ cup	20	4.0
(S&W) Nutradiet, green label:			
Stewed	½ cup	30	8.0
Whole	½ cup	25	5.0

(USDA): United States Department of Agriculture
(HEW/FAO): Health, Education and Welfare/Food and Agriculture Organization
* Prepared as Package Directs

Food and Description	Measure or Quantity	Calories	Carbo-hydrates (grams)
TOMATO JUICE, CANNED:			
Regular pack:			
(Campbell)	6 fl. oz.	35	8.0
(Del Monte)	6 fl. oz.		
	(6.4 oz.)	36	7.4
(Libby's)	6 fl. oz.	35	8.0
Musselman's	6 fl. oz.	30	7.0
(Ocean Spray)	6 fl. oz.	35	7.0
Dietetic pack:			
(Diet Delight)	6 fl. oz.	35	7.0
(Featherweight)	6 fl. oz.	35	8.0
(S&W) *Nutradiet*, green label	6 fl. oz.	35	8.0
TOMATO JUICE COCKTAIL, canned:			
(Ocean Spray) *Firehouse Jubilee*	6 fl. oz.	44	9.1
Snap-E-Tom	6 fl. oz.		
	(6.5 oz.)	40	7.0
TOMATO PASTE, canned:			
Regular pack:			
(Contadina):			
Regular	6 oz.	150	35.0
Italian:			
Plain	6 oz.	210	36.0
With mushroom	6 oz.	180	36.0
(Del Monte)	6-oz. can	150	35.0
Dietetic (Featherweight) low sodium	6-oz. can	150	35.0
TOMATO & PEPPER, HOT CHILI:			
Old El Paso, Jalapeno	1-oz. serving	6	1.1
(Ortega) Jalapeno	1 oz.	7	1.1
TOMATO, PICKLED			
(Claussen) green	1 piece (1 oz.)	6	1.1
TOMATO PUREE, canned:			
Regular (Contadina)	½ cup (4.2 oz.)	50	11.0
Dietetic (Featherweight) low sodium	1 cup	90	20.0

Food and Description	Measure or Quantity	Calories	Carbo-hydrates (grams)
TOMATO SAUCE, canned:			
(Contadina):			
Regular	½ cup (4.4 oz.)	45	9.0
Italian style	½ cup (4.4 oz.)	40	8.0
(Del Monte):			
Regular or No Salt Added	½ cup (4 oz.)	35	4.0
With onions	½ cup (4 oz.)	50	11.5
(Hunt's) with cheese	4-oz. serving	70	10.0
TOMCOD, ATLANTIC, raw (USDA):			
Whole	1 lb. (weighed whole)	136	0.
Meat only	4 oz.	87	0.
TOM COLLINS (Mr. Boston)			
12½% alcohol	3 fl. oz.	105	
TONGUE (USDA):			
Beef, medium fat:			
Raw, untrimmed	1 lb.	714	1.4
Braised	4 oz.	277	.5
Calf:			
Raw, untrimmed	1 lb.	454	3.1
Braised	4 oz.	181	1.1
Hog:			
Raw, untrimmed	1 lb.	741	1.7
Braised	4 oz.	287	.6
Lamb:			
Raw, untrimmed	1 lb.	659	1.7
Braised	4 oz.	288	.6
Sheep:			
Raw, untrimmed	1 lb.	877	7.9
Braised	4 oz.	366	2.7
TONGUE, CANNED:			
(USDA):			
Pickled	1 oz.	76	Tr.

(USDA): United States Department of Agriculture
(HEW/FAO): Health, Education and Welfare/Food and Agriculture
                Organization
* Prepared as Package Directs

Food and Description	Measure or Quantity	Calories	Carbo- hydrates (grams)
Potted or deviled	1 oz.	82	.2
(Hormel) cured	1 oz.	63	0.
TOPPING:			
Regular:			
Butterscotch (Smucker's)	1 T. (.7 oz.)	70	16.5
Caramel (Smucker's)	1 T.	70	16.5
Chocolate fudge (Hershey's)	1 T.	49	7.3
Pecans in syrup (Smucker's)	1 T.	65	14.0
Pineapple (Smucker's)	1 T. (.7 oz.)	65	16.0
Dietetic, chocolate (Diet Delight)	1 T. (.6 oz.)	16	3.6
TOPPING, WHIPPED:			
Regular:			
Cool Whip (Birds Eye):			
Dairy	1 T.	16	1.2
Non-dairy	1 T.	13	1.0
Dover Farms, dairy	1 T. (.2 oz.)	17	1.2
Lucky Whip, aerosol	1 T.	12	.5
Whip Topping (Rich's)	¼ oz.	20	1.2
Dietetic (Featherweight)	1 T.	3	.5
*Mix:			
Regular, *Dream Whip*	1 T. (.2 oz.)	9	.9
Dietetic:			
(D-Zerta)	1 T.	4	.2
(Estee)	1 T. (.1 oz.)	4	Tr.
TOP RAMEN, beef (Nissin Foods)	3-oz. serving	390	50.5
TORTILLA:			
(Amigos)	6" × ⅛" tortilla	111	19.7
Old El Paso, corn	1 oz.	76	15.3
TOSTADA, frozen (Van de Kamp's)	8½-oz. serving	530	37.0
TOSTADA SHELL:			
Old El Paso	1 shell (.4 oz.)	50	6.4
(Ortega)	1 shell (.4 oz.)	50	6.0

Food and Description	Measure or Quantity	Calories	Carbo-hydrates (grams)
TOTAL, cereal (General Mills):			
Regular	1 cup (1 oz.)	110	23.0
Corn	1 cup (1 oz.)	110	24.0
TOWEL GOURD, raw (USDA):			
Unpared	1 lb. (weighed with skin)	69	15.8
Pared	4 oz.	20	4.6
TRIPE:			
Beef (USDA):			
Commercial	4 oz.	113	0.
Pickled	4 oz.	70	0.
Canned (Libby's)	¼ of 24-oz. can	290	1.1
TRIPLE SEC LIQUEUR (Mr. Boston)	1 fl. oz.	79	8.5
TRIX, cereal (General Mills)	1 cup (1 oz.)	110	25.0
TROUT (USDA):			
Brook, fresh:			
Whole	1 lb. (weighed whole)	224	0.
Meat only	4 oz.	115	0.
Lake (See **LAKE TROUT**)			
Rainbow:			
Fresh, meat with skin	4 oz.	221	0.
Canned	4 oz.	237	0.
TUNA:			
Raw (USDA) meat only:			
Bluefin	4 oz.	164	0.
Yellowfin	4 oz.	151	0.

(USDA): United States Department of Agriculture
(HEW/FAO):   Health, Education and Welfare/Food and Agriculture
                    Organization
* Prepared as Package Directs

Food and Description	Measure or Quantity	Calories	Carbo-hydrates (grams)
Canned in oil:			
(Bumble Bee):			
Chunk, light, drained	6½-oz. can	309	0.
Solids, white, drained	7-oz. can	333	0.
(Carnation) solids & liq.	6½-oz. can	427	0.
(Star Kist) solid, white,			
solids & liq.	7-oz. serving	503	0.
Canned in water:			
(Breast O'Chicken)	6½-oz. can	211	0.
(Bumble Bee):			
Chunk, light, solids & liq.	6½-oz. can	234	0.
Solid, white, solids & liq.	7-oz. can	252	0.
(Featherweight) light, chunk	6½-oz. can	210	0.
(Star Kist) light	7-oz. can	220	0.
TUNA HELPER			
(General Mills):			
Country dumplings	⅕ of pkg.	230	31.0
Creamy noodle	⅕ of pkg.	280	31.0
Noodles/cheese	⅕ of pkg.	200	18.0
TUNA PIE, frozen:			
(Banquet)	8-oz. pie	510	48.0
(Morton)	8-oz. pie	370	36.0
TUNA SALAD:			
Home recipe,			
(USDA) made with tuna,			
celery, mayonnaise, pickle,			
onion and egg salad	4-oz. serving	193	4.0
Canned (Carnation)	¼ of 7½-oz. can	100	3.3
TURBOT, GREENLAND			
(USDA) raw:			
Whole	1 lb. (weighed whole)	344	0.
Meat only	4 oz.	166	0.
TURKEY:			
Raw (USDA):			
Ready-to-cook	1 lb. (weighed with bones)	722	0.
Dark meat	4 oz.	145	0.
Light meat	4 oz.	132	0.
Skin only	4 oz.	459	0.

Food and Description	Measure or Quantity	Calories	Carbo-hydrates (grams)
Barbecued (Louis Rich) breast, half	1 oz.	40	0.
Roasted (USDA):			
Flesh, skin & giblets	From 13½-lb. raw, ready-to-cook turkey	9678	0.
Flesh & skin	From 13½-lb. raw, ready-to-cook turkey	7872	0.
Flesh & skin	4 oz.	253	0.
Meat only:			
Chopped	1 cup (5 oz.)	268	0.
Diced	4 oz.	200	0.
Light	4 oz.	200	0.
Light	1 slice (4″ × 2″ × ¼″, 3 oz.)	75	0.
Dark	1 slice (2½″ × 1⅝″ × ¼″, .7 oz.)	43	0.
Skin only	1 oz.	128	0.
Giblets, simmered (USDA)	2 oz.	132	.9
Canned:			
(Hormel) chunk	6¾-oz. serving	230	0.
(Swanson) chunk	2½-oz. serving	120	0.
(Hormel) breast			
Regular	1 slice	30	0.
Smoked	1 slice	25	0.
(Louis Rich):			
Turkey bologna	1-oz. slice	60	1.0
Turkey breast:			
Oven roasted	1-oz. slice	30	0.
Smoked	.7-oz. slice	25	0.
Turkey cotto salami	1-oz. slice	50	Tr.
Turkey ham:			
Chopped	1-oz. slice	45	Tr.
Cured	1-oz. slice	35	Tr.
Turkey pastrami	1-oz. slice	35	Tr.
(Oscar Mayer) breast	¾-oz. slice	21	0.

(USDA): United States Department of Agriculture
(HEW/FAO): Health, Education and Welfare/Food and Agriculture Organization
* Prepared as Package Directs

Food and Description	Measure or Quantity	Calories	Carbo-hydrates (grams)
Smoked (Louis Rich):			
Breast	1 oz.	35	0.
Drumsticks	1 oz. (without bone)	40	Tr.
Wing drumettes	1 oz. (without bone)	45	Tr.
TURKEY DINNER OR ENTREE, FROZEN:			
(Banquet):			
American Favorites	11-oz. dinner	320	41.0
Extra Helping	9-oz. dinner	723	98.0
(Green Giant) twin pouch with white & wild rice stuffing	9-oz. entree	460	34.0
(Morton):			
Regular:			
Dinner	11-oz. dinner	340	35.0
Entree	5-oz. entree	120	5.0
Country Table, sliced	15-oz. dinner	520	80.0
King size	19-oz. dinner	580	65.0
(Stouffer's) casserole, with gravy and dressing	9¾-oz. serving	370	29.0
(Swanson):			
Regular, with gravy & dressing	9¼-oz. entree	310	25.0
Hungry Man:			
Dinner	18¾-oz. dinner	600	70.0
Entree	13¼-oz. entree	370	37.0
3-course	16-oz. dinner	430	56.0
TV Brand:			
Dinner	11½-oz. dinner	340	40.0
Entree	8¾-oz. entree	220	23.0
(Weight Watchers) sliced, 3-compartment, with gravy and stuffing	15¼-oz. meal	380	32.0
TURKEY GIZZARD (USDA):			
Raw	4 oz.	178	1.2
Simmered	4 oz.	222	1.2
TURKEY PIE, frozen:			
(Banquet):			
Regular	8-oz. pie	526	32.0
Supreme	8-oz. pie	430	41.0

Food and Description	Measure or Quantity	Calories	Carbo-hydrates (grams)
(Morton)	8-oz. pie	340	31.0
(Stouffer's)	10-oz. pie	460	35.0
(Swanson):			
Regular	8-oz. pie	430	39.0
Hungry Man	16-oz. pie	730	61.0
TURKEY, POTTED (USDA)	1 oz.	70	0.
TURKEY SALAD, canned			
(Carnation)	¼ of 7½-oz. can	110	3.1
TURKEY TETRAZINI, frozen:			
(Stouffer's)	6-oz. serving	240	17.0
(Weight Watchers) boil-in-bag	10-oz. pkg.	310	28.0
TURMERIC (French's)	1 tsp.	7	1.3
TURNIP (USDA):			
Fresh:			
Without tops	1 lb. (weighed with skins)	117	25.7
Pared, diced	½ cup (2.4 oz.)	20	4.4
Pared, slices	½ cup (2.3 oz.)	19	4.2
Boiled, drained:			
Diced	½ cup (2.8 oz.)	18	3.8
Mashed	½ cup (4 oz.)	26	5.6
TURNIP GREENS, leaves & stems:			
Fresh (USDA):	1 lb. (weighed untrimmed)	107	19.0
Boiled (USDA):			
In small amount water, short time, drained	½ cup (2.5 oz.)	14	2.6
In large amount water, long time, drained	½ cup (2.5 oz.)	14	2.4
Canned:			
(USDA) solids & liq.	½ cup (4.1 oz.)	21	3.7

(USDA): United States Department of Agriculture
(HEW/FAO):   Health, Education and Welfare/Food and Agriculture
                    Organization
* Prepared as Package Directs

Food and Description	Measure or Quantity	Calories	Carbo-hydrates (grams)
(Stokely-Van Camp) chopped	½ cup (4.1 oz.)	23	3.5
(Sunshine) solids & liq.:			
Chopped	½ cup (4.1 oz.)	19	2.5
& diced turnips	½ cup (4.1 oz.)	21	3.2
Frozen:			
(Birds Eye):			
Chopped	⅓ of 10-oz. pkg.	20	3.0
Chopped, with sliced turnips	⅓ of 10-oz. pkg.	20	3.0
(McKenzie or Seabrook Farms):			
Chopped	⅓ of 10-oz. pkg.	25	3.4
Diced	1-oz. serving	4	.8
(Southland):			
Chopped	⅕ of 16-oz. pkg.	20	4.0
With diced turnips	⅕ of 16-oz. pkg.	20	5.0
TURNOVER:			
Frozen (Pepperidge Farm):			
Apple	1 turnover	310	35.0
Blueberry	1 turnover	320	32.0
Cherry	1 turnover	310	32.0
Peach	1 turnover	320	34.0
Raspberry	1 turnover	320	37.0
Refrigerated (Pillsbury):			
Apple	1 turnover	170	23.0
Blueberry	1 turnover	170	22.0
Cherry	1 turnover	170	24.0
TURTLE, GREEN (USDA):			
Raw:			
In shell	1 lb. (weighed in shell)	97	0.
Meat only	4 oz.	101	0.
Canned	4 oz.	120	0.
TWINKIE (Hostess):			
Regular	1½-oz. piece	155	26.0
Devil's food	1½-oz. piece	150	24.7

Food and Description	Measure or Quantity	Calories	Carbo-hydrates (grams)

V

VALPOLICELLA WINE
  (Antinori) red | 3 fl. oz. | 84 | 6.3

VANDERMINT, liqueur | 1 fl. oz. | 90 | 10.2

VANILLA EXTRACT (Virginia
Dare) pure, 35% alcohol | 1 tsp. | 10 | DNA

VEAL, medium fat (USDA):
  Chuck:

Raw	1 lb. (weighed with bone)	628	0.
Braised, lean & fat	4 oz.	266	0.
Flank:			
Raw	1 lb. (weighed with bone)	1410	0.
Stewed, lean & fat	4 oz.	442	0.
Foreshank:			
Raw	1 lb. (weighed with bone)	368	0.
Stewed, lean & fat	4 oz.	245	0.
Loin:			
Raw	1 lb. (weighed with bone)	681	0.
Broiled, medium done, chop, lean & fat	4 oz.	265	0.
Plate:			
Raw	1 lb. (weighed with bone)	828	0.
Stewed, lean & fat	4 oz.	344	0.

(USDA): United States Department of Agriculture
(HEW/FAO):   Health, Education and Welfare/Food and Agriculture
                        Organization
* Prepared as Package Directs

Food and Description	Measure or Quantity	Calories	Carbo- hydrates (grams)
Rib:			
Raw, lean & fat	1 lb. (weighed with bone)	723	0.
Roasted, medium done, lean & fat	4 oz.	305	0.
Round & rump:			
Raw	1 lb. (weighed with bone)	573	0.
Broiled, steak or cutlet, lean & fat	4 oz. (weighed with bone)	245	0.
VEAL DINNER, frozen:			
(Banquet) parmigiana:			
Casserole	2-lb. pkg.	1385	125.0
Cookin' Bag	5-oz. pkg.	293	23.0
Dinner:			
Extra Helping	20-oz. dinner	1092	116.0
International Favorites	11-oz. dinner	413	43.0
(Morton) parmigiana:			
Regular:			
Dinner	11-oz. dinner	250	27.0
Entree	5-oz. pkg.	130	14.0
Family Meal	2-lb. pkg.	1200	100.0
King Size	20-oz. dinner	600	83.0
(Swanson) parmigiana:			
Hungry Man	20½-oz. dinner	700	61.0
TV Brand	12¼-oz. dinner	450	46.0
(Weight Watchers) patty, parmigiana, 2-compartment meal	9-oz. meal	250	12.0
VEAL STEAK, FROZEN			
(Hormel):			
Regular	4-oz. serving	130	2.0
Breaded	4-oz. serving	240	13.0
VEGETABLE BOUILLON			
(Herb-Ox):			
Cube	1 cube	6	.6
Packet	1 packet	12	2.2

VEGETABLE FAT (See **FAT**)

Food and Description	Measure or Quantity	Calories	Carbo-hydrates (grams)
VEGETABLE FLAKES			
(French's)	1 T.	12	3.0
VEGETABLE JUICE COCKTAIL:			
Regular, *V-8:*			
Regular	6 fl. oz.	35	8.0
Spicy hot	6 fl. oz.	40	8.0
Dietetic:			
(Featherweight) low sodium	6 fl. oz.	35	8.0
(S&W) *Nutradiet*, low			
sodium, green label	6 fl. oz.	35	8.0
V-8, low sodium	6 fl. oz.	40	9.0
VEGETABLES, MIXED:			
Canned, regular pack:			
(Del Monte) solids & liq.	½ cup (4 oz.)	40	7.0
(La Choy) drained:			
Chinese	⅓ of 14-oz. can	12	2.0
Chop Suey	½ cup (4.7 oz.)	10	2.0
(Libby's) solids & liq.	½ cup (4.2 oz.)	40	9.8
Canned, dietetic pack			
(Featherweight) low sodium	½ cup (4 oz.)	40	8.0
Frozen:			
(Birds Eye):			
Regular:			
Broccoli, cauliflower & carrots in butter sauce	⅓ of 10-oz. pkg.	51	5.7
Broccoli, cauliflower & carrots in cheese sauce	⅓ of 10-oz. pkg.	72	7.9
Broccoli, cauliflower & red pepper	⅓ of 10-oz. pkg.	31	4.7
Carrots, peas & onions, deluxe	⅓ of 10-oz. pkg.	52	10.0
Medley, in butter sauce	⅓ of 10-oz. pkg.	62	9.7
Mixed	⅓ of 10-oz. pkg.	68	13.3
Mixed, with onion sauce	⅓ of 8-oz. pkg.	103	11.7

(USDA): United States Department of Agriculture
(HEW/FAO):   Health, Education and Welfare/Food and Agriculture
            Organization
* Prepared as Package Directs

Food and Description	Measure or Quantity	Calories	Carbo- hydrates (grams)
Pea & potatos in cream sauce	⅓ of 8-oz. pkg.	164	15.6
Farm Fresh:			
Broccoli, carrots & water chestnuts	⅕ of 16-oz. pkg.	36	6.5
Broccoli, cauliflower & carrot strips	⅕ of 16-oz. pkg.	30	5.3
Broccoli, corn & red pepper	⅕ of 16-oz. pkg.	58	10.9
Broccoli, green bean, onion & red pepper	⅕ of 16-oz. pkg.	31	5.4
Brussels sprouts, cauliflower & carrots	⅕ of 16-oz. pkg.	38	6.5
Cauliflower, green beans & carrots	⅕ of 16-oz. pkg.	42	8.1
Green beans, corn, carrot & pearl onion	⅕ of 16-oz. pkg.	49	10.1
Green beans, cauliflower & carrots	⅕ of 16-oz. pkg.	32	6.1
Pea, carrot & pearl onion	⅕ of 16-oz. pkg.	59	10.7
International:			
Bavarian style beans Epaetzle	⅓ of 10-oz. pkg.	112	11.5
Chinese style	⅓ of 10-oz. pkg.	85	8.4
Far Eastern style	⅓ of 10-oz. pkg.	84	8.4
Italian style	⅓ of 10-oz. pkg.	114	11.4
Japanese style	⅓ of 10-oz. pkg.	102	10.4
Mexican style	⅓ of 10-oz. pkg.	133	16.1
New England style	⅓ of 10-oz. pkg.	129	14.2
San Francisco style	⅓ of 10-oz. pkg.	99	10.9
Stir Fry:			
Chinese style	⅓ of 10-oz. pkg.	36	6.9
(Green Giant): Japanese style	⅓ of 10-oz. pkg.	32	5.9
Regular:			
Broccoli, carrot fanfare	½ cup	25	5.0
Broccoli, cauliflower & carrots in cheese sauce	½ cup	60	8.0
Broccoli, cauliflower supreme	½ cup	20	4.0
Cauliflower, green bean festival	½ cup	16	3.0

Food and Description	Measure or Quantity	Calories	Carbo-hydrates (grams)
Corn, broccoli bounty	½ cup	60	11.0
Mixed, butter sauce	½ cup	80	12.0
Mixed, polybag	½ cup	50	10.0
Pea, pea pod & water chestnut in butter sauce	½ cup	80	10.0
Pea & cauliflower medly	½ cup	40	7.0
Harvest Fresh	½ cup	60	13.0
Harvest Get Togethers:			
Broccoli-cauliflower medley	½ cup	60	10.0
Broccoli fanfare	½ cup	80	14.2
Cauliflower-carrot bonanza	½ cup	60	7.0
Chinese style	½ cup	60	7.0
Japanese style	½ cup	45	8.0
(Le Sueur) peas, onions & carrots in butter sauce	½ cup	90	11.0
(La Choy) Chinese	⅓ of 10-oz. pkg.	25	5.0
(McKenzie)	3.3-oz. serving	65	13.0
(Southland):			
California blend	⅕ of 16-oz. pkg.	35	7.0
Gumbo	⅕ of 16-oz. pkg.	45	10.0
Oriental	⅕ of 16-oz. pkg.	30	6.0
Stew	4 oz.	60	14.0
VEGETABLES IN PASTRY, frozen (Pepperidge Farm):			
Asparagus with mornay sauce or broccoli with cheese	½ of 7½-oz. pkg.	250	18.0
Broccoli with cheese	½ of 7½-oz. pkg.	250	19.0
Cauliflower & cheese sauce	½ of 7½-oz. pkg.	220	20.0
Mushroom dijon	½ of 7½-oz. pkg.	230	19.0

(USDA): United States Department of Agriculture
(HEW/FAO):   Health, Education and Welfare/Food and Agriculture
                    Organization
* Prepared as Package Directs

Food and Description	Measure or Quantity	Calories	Carbo-hydrates (grams)
Spinach almondine	½ of 7½-oz. pkg.	260	19.0
Zucchini provencal	½ of 7½-oz. pkg.	210	21.0
VEGETABLE STEW, canned			
Dinty Moore (Hormel)	⅓ of 24-oz. can	170	20.0
"VEGETARIAN FOODS":			
Canned or dry:			
Chicken, fried (Loma Linda) with gravy	1½-oz. piece	96	3.4
Chili (Worthington)	½ cup (4.9 oz.)	177	13.2
Choplet (Worthington)	1 choplet (1.6 oz.)	50	1.7
Dinner cuts (Loma Linda) drained:			
Regular	1 piece (1.5 oz.)	54	1.6
No Salt Added	1 piece (1.5 oz.)	44	2.6
Franks, big (Loma Linda)	1.9-oz. frank	100	4.1
Franks, sizzle (Loma Linda)	2.2-oz. frank	167	4.6
FriChik (Worthington)	1 piece (1.6 oz.)	75	2.5
Granburger (Worthington)	1 oz.	96	5.8
Linkettes (Loma Linda)	1.3-oz. link	74	2.2
Little links (Loma Linda) drained	.8-oz. link	45	1.5
Non-Meatballs (Worthington)	1 meatball (.6 oz.)	32	1.9
Numete (Worthington)	½″ slice (2.4 oz.)	145	7.1
Nuteena (Loma Linda)	½″ slice (2.4 oz.)	165	7.6
Peanuts & soya (USDA)	4 oz.	269	15.2
Prime Stakes	1 slice	171	7.8
Proteena (Loma Linda)	½″ slice	144	6.5
Protose (Worthington)	½″ slice	176	8.1
Redi-burger (Loma Linda)	½″ slice (2.4 oz.)	132	8.8
Sandwich spread (Loma Linda)	1 T.	24	1.7
Savorex (Loma Linda)	1 T.	32	2.0
Skallops (Worthington) drained	½ cup (3 oz.)	89	3.0
Soyalac (Loma Linda):			
Concentrate, liquid	1 cup (9 oz.)	177	17.0
Ready to use	1 cup (8.5 oz.)	166	15.9

Food and Description	Measure or Quantity	Calories	Carbo-hydrates (grams)
Soyameat (Worthington):			
Beef, sliced	1 slice (1 oz.)	44	2.6
Chicken, diced	1 oz.	40	1.4
Soyamel, any kind (Worthington)	1 oz.	120	12.2
Stew pack (Loma Linda) drained	1 piece (.2 oz.)	7	.6
Super Links (Worthington)	1 link(1.9 oz.)	110	3.7
Swiss steak with gravy (Loma Linda)	1 steak (2¾ oz.)	138	8.9
Tender bits (Loma Linda) drained	1 piece	23	1.1
Tender rounds (Loma Linda)	1-oz. piece	39	2.4
Vege-burger (Loma Linda):			
Regular	½ cup	116	4.3
No Salt Added	½ cup	119	7.0
Vegelona (Loma Linda)	½" slice (2.4 oz.)	102	7.0
Vega-links (Worthington)	1 link (1.1 oz.)	55	2.8
Vita-Burger (Loma Linda)	1 T. (¼ oz.)	23	2.1
Wheat protein (USDA)	4 oz.	170	10.8
Worthington 209	1 slice (1.1 oz.)	58	2.2
Frozen:			
Beef pie (Worthington)	8-oz. pie	278	41.8
Bologna (Loma Linda)	1 oz.	77	2.8
Bolono (Worthington)	¾-oz. slice	23	1.0
Chicken (Loma Linda)	1-oz. slice	57	1.5
Chicken, fried (Loma Linda)	2-oz. serving	188	3.6
Chicken pie (Worthington)	8-oz. pie	346	37.5
Chic-Ketts (Worthington)	1 oz.	53	2.2
Corned beef, sliced (Worthington)	1 slice (.5 oz.)	32	1.9
Fillets (Worthington)	1½-oz. piece	90	4.6
FriPats (Worthington)	1 patty	204	5.2
Meatballs (Loma Linda)	1 meatball (¾ oz.)	46	2.2
Meatless salami (Worthington)	¾-oz. slice	44	1.2

(USDA): United States Department of Agriculture
(HEW/FAO):   Health, Education and Welfare/Food and Agriculture Organization
* Prepared as Package Directs

Food and Description	Measure or Quantity	Calories	Carbo-hydrates (grams)
Prosage (Worthington):			
Links	1 link	60	1.5
Patty	1.3-oz. piece	96	2.8
Roll	⅜" slice (1.2 oz.)	86	2.0
Roast beef (Loma Linda)	1 oz.	65	1.3
Salami (Loma Linda)	1-oz. slice	65	1.7
Sausage, breakfast (Loma Linda)	⅓" slice (1 oz.)	72	1.4
Smoked beef, slices (Worthington)	1 slice	14	1.1
Stakelets (Worthington)	3-oz. piece	164	9.4
Tuno (Worthington)	2-oz. serving	81	3.4
Turkey (Loma Linda)	1 oz.	61	1.6
Wahm roll (Worthington)	1 slice (.8 oz.)	36	1.9
VENISON (USDA) raw, lean, meat only	4 oz.	143	0.
VERMOUTH:			
Dry & extra dry (Lejon; Noilly Pratt)	1 fl. oz.	33	1.0
Sweet (Lejon; Taylor)	1 fl. oz.	45	3.8
VICHY WATER (Schweppes)	Any quantity	0	0.
VINEGAR:			
Cider:			
(USDA)	1 T. (.5 oz.)	2	.9
(USDA)	½ cup (4.2 oz.)	17	7.1
Distilled:			
(USDA)	1 T. (.5 oz.)	2	.8
(USDA)	½ cup (4.2 oz.)	14	6.0
Red, red with garlic or white wine (Regina)	1 T. (.5 oz.)	Tr.	Tr.
VINESPINACH or BASELLA (USDA) raw	4 oz.	22	3.9
VODKA, unflavored (See **DISTILLED LIQUOR**)			

Food and Description	Measure or Quantity	Calories	Carbo-hydrates (grams)

W

WAFFELOS, cereal
(Ralston Purina) · · · · · 1 cup (1 oz.) · · · 110 · · · 25.0

WAFFLE:
Home recipe (USDA) · · · 7″ waffle
· · · · · · · · · · · · · · · · (2.6 oz.) · · · 209 · · · 28.1
Frozen:
(Aunt Jemima) jumbo · · 1 waffle · · · 86 · · · 14.5
(Eggo):
Regular · · · · · · · · 1 waffle · · · 120 · · · 16.0
Apple cinnamon · · · 1 waffle · · · 150 · · · 20.0
Blueberry · · · · · · 1 waffle · · · 130 · · · 16.0
Buttermilk · · · · · · 1 waffle · · · 110 · · · 15.0
Home style · · · · · 1 waffle · · · 120 · · · 18.0
Roman Meal:
Regular · · · · · · · · 1 waffle · · · 140 · · · 16.5
Golden Delight · · · 1 waffle · · · 131 · · · 15.1

WAFFLE MIX (See also
**PANCAKE & WAFFLE
MIX**) (USDA):
Complete mix:
Dry · · · · · · · · · · · 1 oz. · · · 130 · · · 18.5
*Prepared with water · · 2.6-oz. waffle · · · 229 · · · 30.2
Incomplete mix:
Dry · · · · · · · · · · · 1 oz. · · · 101 · · · 21.5
*Prepared with egg & milk · 2.6-oz. waffle · · · 206 · · · 27.2
*Prepared with egg & milk · 7.1-oz. waffle
· · · · · · · · · · · · · · · · (9″ × 9″ × ⅝″,
· · · · · · · · · · · · · · · · 1⅛ cups) · · · 550 · · · 72.4

WAFFLE SYRUP (See **SYRUP**)

(USDA): United States Department of Agriculture
(HEW/FAO):   Health, Education and Welfare/Food and Agriculture
· · · · · · · · · · · Organization
* Prepared as Package Directs

Food and Description	Measure or Quantity	Calories	Carbo-hydrates (grams)
WALNUT:			
(USDA):			
Black, in shell, whole	1 lb. (weighed in shell)	627	14.8
Black, shelled, whole	4 oz. (weighed whole)	712	16.8
Black, chopped	½ cup (2.1 oz.)	377	8.9
English or Persian, shelled, whole	1 lb. (weighed in shell)	1327	32.2
English or Persian, shelled, whole	4 oz.	738	17.9
English or Persian, halves	½ cup (1.8 oz.)	356	6.5
(California) halves & pieces	½ cup (1.8 oz.)	356	6.5
(Fisher):			
Black	½ cup (2.1 oz.)	374	8.8
English	½ cup (2.1 oz.)	389	9.5
WATER CHESTNUT, CHINESE:			
Raw (USDA):			
Whole	1 lb. (weighed unpeeled)	272	66.5
Peeled	4 oz.	90	21.5
Canned (La Choy) sliced, drained	¼ of 8-oz. can	16	3.9
WATERCRESS, raw (USDA):			
Untrimmed	½ lb. (weighed untrimmed)	40	6.2
Trimmed	½ cup (.6 oz.)	3	.5
WATERMELON, fresh (USDA):			
Whole	1 lb. (weighed with rind)	54	13.4
Wedge	4″ × 8″ wedge (2 lb. measured with rind)	111	27.3
Diced	½ cup	21	5.1

Food and Description	Measure or Quantity	Calories	Carbohydrates (grams)
WAX GOURD, raw (USDA):			
Whole	1 lb. (weighed with skin & cavity contents)	41	9.4
Flesh only	4 oz.	15	3.4
WEAKFISH (USDA):			
Raw, whole	1 lb. (weighed whole)	263	0.
Broiled, meat only	4 oz.	236	0.
WELSH RAREBIT:			
Home recipe	1 cup (8.2 oz.)	415	14.6
Frozen (Stouffer's)	5-oz. serving	355	17.0
WESTERN DINNER, frozen:			
(Banquet) American Favorites	11-oz. dinner	513	43.0
(Morton)	11.8-oz. dinner	400	32.0
(Swanson):			
Hungry Man	17¾-oz. dinner	820	73.0
TV Brand	11¾-oz. dinner	430	45.0
WHEATENA, cereal	¼ cup	112	22.5
WHEAT FLAKES CEREAL			
(Featherweight) low sodium	1¼ cups (1 oz.)	100	23.0
WHEAT GERM:			
(USDA)	1 oz.	103	13.2
(Elam's) raw	1 T. (.3 oz.)	28	3.2
WHEAT GERM CEREAL			
(Kretschmer):			
Regular	¼ cup (1 oz.)	99	8.8
Brown sugar & honey	¼ cup (1 oz.)	114	17.0
WHEAT HEARTS, cereal			
(General Mills)	1 oz. dry	110	21.0

(USDA): United States Department of Agriculture
(HEW/FAO):   Health, Education and Welfare/Food and Agriculture
             Organization
* Prepared as Package Directs

Food and Description	Measure or Quantity	Calories	Carbo-hydrates (grams)
WHEATIES, cereal (General Mills)	1 cup (1 oz.)	110	23.0
WHEAT & OATMEAL CEREAL, hot (Elam's)	1 oz.	105	18.8
WHEAT, ROLLED (USDA):			
Uncooked	1 cup (3.1 oz.)	296	66.3
Cooked	1 cup (7.7 oz.)	163	36.7
WHEAT, SHREDDED, cereal (See **SHREDDED WHEAT**)			
WHEAT, WHOLE GRAIN (USDA) hard red spring	1 oz.	94	19.6
WHEAT, WHOLE-MEAL, cereal (USDA):			
Dry	1 oz.	96	20.5
Cooked	4 oz.	51	10.7
WHEY (USDA):			
Dry	1 oz.	99	20.8
Fluid	1 cup (8.6 oz.)	63	12.4
WHISKEY (See **DISTILLED LIQUOR**)			
WHISKEY SOUR COCKTAIL (Mr. Boston) 12½% alcohol	3 fl. oz.	120	14.4
WHITE CASTLE:			
Bun	.8-oz. bun	65	12.4
Cheeseburger (meat & cheese only)	1.54-oz. serving	120	5.2
Fish sandwich (fish only, without tartar sauce & bun)	1.5-oz. serving	127	7.8
French fires	2.6-oz. serving	225	15.1
Hamburger (meat only, no bun)	1.2-oz. serving	95	5.2
WHITEFISH, LAKE (USDA):			
Raw, meat only	4 oz.	176	0.

Food and Description	Measure or Quantity	Calories	Carbo-hydrates (grams)
Baked, stuffed, home recipe, with bacon, butter, onion, celery & breadcrumbs	4 oz.	244	6.6
Smoked	4 oz.	176	0.
WIENER WRAP (Pillsbury)			
plain or cheese	1 piece	60	10.0
WILD BERRY DRINK, canned			
(Hi-C)	6 fl. oz.	88	22.0
WINCHELL'S DONUT HOUSE:			
Buttermilk:			
Bar	2.1-oz. piece	243	54.4
Old fashioned	2-oz. piece	249	56.0
Cake, devil's food, iced	2-oz. piece	241	54.0
Cinnamon crumb	2-oz. piece	240	60.1
Iced, chocolate	2-oz. piece	227	55.0
Raised, glaze	1¾-oz. piece	212	48.5
WINE, COOKING (Regina):			
Burgundy or sauterne	¼ cup	2	Tr.
Sherry	¼ cup	20	5.0

Food and Description	Measure or Quantity	Calories	Carbo- hydrates (grams)

Y

YAM (USDA):
  Raw:

Whole	1 lb. (weighed with skin)	394	90.5
Flesh only	4 oz.	115	26.3

  Canned & frozen (See
    SWEET POTATO)

YAM BEAN, raw (USDA):

Unpared tuber	1 lb. (weighed unpared)	225	52.2
Pared tuber	4 oz.	62	14.5

YEAST:
  Baker's:
    Compressed:

(USDA)	1 oz.	24	3.1
(Fleischmann's)	¾-oz. cake	19	1.9

    Dry:

(USDA)	1 oz.	80	11.0
(USDA)	7-gram pkg.	20	2.7
(Fleischmann's)	¼ oz. (pkg. or jar)	24	2.9

YOGURT:
  Regular:
    Plain:

(Bison)	8-oz. container	160	16.8
(Colombo):			
Regular	8-oz. container	150	13.0
Natural Lite	8-oz. container	110	17.0
(Dannon)	8-oz. container	150	17.0
(Friendship)	8-oz. container	170	15.0
Yoplait	6-oz. container	130	14.0
Plain with honey, *Yoplait,*			
Custard Style	6-oz. container	160	23.0

Food and Description	Measure or Quantity	Calories	Carbo-hydrates (grams)
Apple:			
(Bison) dutch	8-oz. container	262	45.9
(Colombo) spiced	8-oz. container	240	39.0
(Dannon) dutch	8-oz. container	260	49.0
Mélangé	6-oz. container	180	31.0
(New Country) crisp	8-oz. container	210	40.0
(Sweet'N Low) dutch	8-oz. container	150	33.0
Yoplait	6-oz. container	190	32.0
Apple-cinnamon, *Yoplait,*			
Breakfast Yogurt	6-oz. container	240	40.0
Apricot (Bison)	8-oz. container	262	45.9
Banana (Dannon)	8-oz. container	260	49.0
Banana-strawberry			
(Colombo)	8-oz. container	235	38.0
Berry:			
(New Country) mixed	8-oz. container	210	40.0
Yoplait, Breakfast Yogurt	6-oz. container	230	39.0
Blueberry:			
(Bison):			
Regular	8-oz. container	262	45.9
Light	6-oz. container	162	28.1
(Colombo)	8-oz. container	250	38.0
(Dannon)	8-oz. container	260	49.0
(Friendship)	8-oz. container	230	44.0
Mélangé	6-oz. container	180	31.0
(New Country) supreme	8-oz. container	210	40.0
(Riché)	6-oz. container	180	33.0
(Sweet'n Low)	8-oz. container	150	33.0
Yoplait:			
Regular	6-oz. container	190	32.0
Custard Style	6-oz. container	180	30.0
Boysenberry:			
(Bison)	8-oz. container	262	45.9
(Dannon)	8-oz. container	260	49.0
(Sweet'n Low)	8-oz. container	150	33.0
Yoplait	6-oz. container	190	32.0

(USDA): United States Department of Agriculture
(HEW/FAO):   Health, Education and Welfare/Food and Agriculture
             Organization
* Prepared as Package Directs

Food and Description	Measure or Quantity	Calories	Carbo-hydrates (grams)
Cherry:			
(Bison):			
Regular	8-oz. container	262	45.9
Light	6-oz. container	162	28.1
(Colombo) black	8-oz. container	230	34.0
(Dannon)	8-oz. container	260	49.0
(Friendship)	8-oz. container	230	44.0
Mélangé	6-oz. container	180	31.0
(New Country) supreme	8-oz. container	210	40.0
(Riché)	6-oz. container	180	33.0
(Sweet'n Low)	8-oz. container	150	33.0
Yoplait	6-oz. container	190	32.0
Cherry-vanilla (Colombo)	8-oz. container	250	40.0
Citrus, *Yoplait, Breakfast Yogurt*	6-oz. container	250	43.0
Coffee:			
(Colombo)	8-oz. container	200	29.0
(Dannon)	8-oz. container	200	32.0
(Friendship)	8-oz. container	210	35.0
Yoplait, Custard Style	6-oz. container	180	30.0
Date walnut raisin (Bison)	8-oz. container	262	45.9
Fruit crunch (New Country)	8-oz. container	210	40.0
Granola strawberry (Colombo)	8-oz. container	240	40.0
Guava (Colombo)	8-oz. container	240	40.0
Hawaiian salad (New Country)	8-oz. container	210	40.0
Honey vanilla (Colombo)	8-oz. container	220	30.0
Lemon:			
(Dannon)	8-oz. container	200	32.0
(New Country) supreme	8-oz. container	210	40.0
(Sweet'n Low)	8-oz. container	150	33.0
Yoplait:			
Regular	6-oz. container	190	32.0
Custard Style	6-oz. container	180	30.0
Orange, *Yoplait*	6-oz. container	190	32.0
Orange supreme (New Country)	8 oz. container	210	40.0
Orchard, *Yoplait, Breakfast Yogurt*	6-oz. container	240	40.0
Peach:			
(Bison)	8-oz. container	262	45.9
(Dannon)	8-oz. container	260	49.0

Food and Description	Measure or Quantity	Calories	Carbo- hydrates (grams)
(Friendship)	8-oz. container	230	44.0
(Meadow Gold)			
sundae style	8-oz. container	260	48.0
(New Country) 'n cream	8-oz. container	210	40.0
(Riché)	6-oz. container	180	33.0
(Sweet'N Low)	8-oz. container	150	33.0
Yoplait	6-oz. container	190	32.0
Peach melba (Colombo)	8-oz. container	230	37.0
Pina colada:			
(Colombo)	8-oz. container	240	40.0
(Dannon)	8-oz. container	260	49.0
(Friendship)	8-oz. container	230	44.0
Pineapple:			
(Bison) light	6-oz. container	162	28.1
Mélangé	6-oz. container	180	31.0
Yoplait	6-oz. container	190	32.0
Raspberry:			
(Bison):			
Regular	8-oz. container	262	45.9
Light	6-oz. container	162	28.1
(Colombo)	8-oz. container	250	39.0
(Dannon) red	8-oz. container	260	49.0
(Friendshop)	8-oz. container	230	44.0
Mélangé	6-oz. container	180	31.0
(New Country)	8-oz. container	210	40.0
(Riché)	6-oz. container	180	33.0
(Sweet'n Low)	8-oz. container	150	33.0
Yoplait:			
Regular	6-oz. container	190	32.0
Custard Style	6-oz. container	180	30.0
Strawberry:			
(Bison):			
Regular	8-oz. container	262	45.9
Light	6-oz. container	162	28.1
(Colombo)	8-oz. container	230	36.0
(Dannon)	8-oz. container	260	49.0
(Friendship)	8-oz. container	230	44.0

Food and Description	Measure or Quantity	Calories	Carbohydrates (grams)
(Meadow Gold) sundae style	8-oz. container	270	49.0
Mélangé	6-oz. container	180	31.0
(New Country)	8-oz. container	210	40.0
(Riché)	6-oz. container	180	33.0
(Sweet'n Low)	8-oz. container	150	33.0
Yoplait:			
Regular	6-oz. container	190	32.0
Custard Style	6-oz. container	180	30.0
Strawberry-banana:			
(Riché)	6-oz. container	180	33.0
(Sweet'n Low)	8-oz. container	190	33.0
Strawberry colada (Colombo)	8-oz. container	230	36.0
Tropical, *Yoplait, Breakfast Yogurt*	6-oz. container	250	43.0
Tropical fruit (Sweet'N Low)	8-oz. container	150	33.0
Vanilla:			
(Dannon)	8-oz. container	200	32.0
(Friendship)	8-oz. container	210	35.0
(New Country) french	8-oz. container	210	40.0
Yoplait, Custard Style	6-oz. container	180	30.0
Frozen, hard:			
Banana (Dannon)			
Danny-in-a-Cup	8-oz. cup	210	42.0
Boysenberry (Dannon)			
Danny-On-A-Stick, carob coated	2½-fl.-oz. bar	140	15.0
Boysenberry swirl (Bison)	¼ of 16-oz. container	116	24.0
Cherry vanilla (Bison)	¼ of 16-oz. container	116	24.0
Chocolate:			
(Bison)	¼ of 16-oz. container	116	24.0
(Colombo) bar, chocolate coated	1 bar	145	17.0
(Dannon):			
Danny-in-a-Cup	8-fl.-oz. cup	190	32.0
Danny-On-A-Stick:			
Uncoated	2½-fl.-oz. bar	60	10.0
Chocolate coated	2½-fl.-oz. bar	130	12.0
Chocolate chip (Bison)	¼ of 16-oz. container	116	24.0

Food and Description	Measure or Quantity	Calories	Carbo-hydrates (grams)
Chocolate chocolate chip (Colombo)	4-oz. serving	150	28.0
Mocha (Colombo) bar	1 bar	80	14.0
Pina colada:			
(Colombo)	4-oz. serving	110	20.0
(Dannon):			
Danny-in-a-Cup	8-oz. cup	230	44.0
Danny-On-A-Stick, uncoated	2½-fl.-oz. bar	65	14.0
Raspberry, red (Dannon):			
Danny-in-a-cup	8-oz. container	210	42.0
Danny-On-A-Stick, chocolate coated	2½-fl.-oz. bar	130	15.0
Raspberry swirl (Bison)	¼ of 16-oz. container	116	24.0
Strawberry:			
(Bison)	¼ of 16-oz. container	116	24.0
(Colombo):			
Regular	4-oz. serving	110	20.0
Bar	1 bar	80	14.0
(Dannon):			
Danny-in-a-Cup	8-fl.-oz. container	210	42.0
Danny-On-A-Stick, chocolate coated	2½-fl.-oz. bar	130	15.0
Vanilla:			
(Bison)	¼ of 16-oz. container	116	24.0
(Colombo):			
Regular	4-oz. serving	110	20.0
Bar, chocolate coated	1 bar	145	17.0
(Dannon):			
Danny-in-a-Cup	8 fl. oz.	180	33.0
Danny-On-A-Stick	2½-fl.-oz. bar	60	11.0
Frozen, soft:			
(Colombo) all flavors	6-fl.-oz. serving	130	24.0
(Dannon) *Danny-Yo*	3½-fl.-oz. serving	115	21.0

(USDA): United States Department of Agriculture
(HEW/FAO):   Health, Education and Welfare/Food and Agriculture
             Organization
* Prepared as Package Directs

Food and Description	Measure or Quantity	Calories	Carbo-hydrates (grams)

Z

ZINFANDEL WINE (Inglenook)
Vintage, 12% alcohol | 3 fl. oz. | 49 | .3

ZITI, FROZEN (Weight Watchers) one-compartment meal | 11¼-oz. pkg. | 284 | 30.0

ZWEIBACK:
(USDA) | 1 oz. | 120 | 21.1
(Gerber) | 7-gram piece | 30 | 5.1
(Nabisco) | 1 piece | 30 | 5.0

CANADIAN SUPPLEMENT

Food and Description	Measure or Quantity	Calories	Carbo-hydrates (grams)

A

AWAKE (General Foods)
orange | 4 fl. oz. | 52 | 13.3

B

BACON BITS, *Bac-O-Bits*
(General Mills) | 1 oz. | 119 | 8.0

BEAN, BAKED, canned
(Campbell) in tomato sauce | 8-oz. serving | 251 | 44.0

BEAN, GREEN, frozen
(McCain):
French style | ⅓ of 10-oz. pkg. | 29 | 5.6
Whole | 3.3-oz. serving | 34 | .6

BEAN, LIMA, frozen (McCain) | 3.3-oz. serving | 107 | 18.6

BEAN, YELLOW OR WAX,
frozen (McCain) | ⅓ of 10.6-oz. pkg. | 34 | 6.8

(USDA): United States Department of Agriculture
(HEW/FAO):   Health, Education and Welfare/Food and Agriculture
                    Organization
* Prepared as Package Directs

Food and Description	Measure or Quantity	Calories	Carbo-hydrates (grams)
BEEF DINNER OR ENTREE, frozen (Swanson):			
Regular, sliced	8½-oz. entree	248	16.4
Hungry Man, sliced	17-oz. dinner (482 gms.)	631	67.5
TV Brand:			
Chopped sirloin	10-oz. dinner (283 gms.)	445	39.9
Sliced	11½-oz. dinner	433	34.0
BEEF PIE, frozen (Swanson):			
Regular	8-oz. pie (227 grams)	443	37.0
Hungry Man	16-oz. pie (454 grams)	631	51.3
BEEF STEW:			
Canned, regular pack (Bounty)	8-oz. serving	180	15.9
Frozen (EfficienC)	8-oz. entree (227 grams)	202	15.8
BROCCOLI, frozen (McCain):			
Chopped	⅓ of 10.6-oz. pkg.	36	5.2
Spears	⅓ of 10.6-oz. pkg.	40	5.7
BRUSSELS SPROUT, frozen (McCain)	⅓ of 10.6-oz. pkg.	68	11.2
BUTTER, dietetic, *Meadowlight*	1 T. (14 grams)	51	.2
BUTTERSCOTCH CHIPS (Baker's)	6.2-oz. pkg.	915	103.0

C

CAKE, frozen:			
Banana (McCain)	⅛ of 19-oz. cake	218	35.5

Food and Description	Measure or Quantity	Calories	Carbo- hydrates (grams)
Banana-nut loaf (Pepperidge Farm)	⅙ of 11½-oz. cake	199	28.3
Carrot-nut loaf (Pepperidge Farm)	⅙ of 11½-oz. cake	227	24.4
Chocolate:			
(McCain):			
Regular	⅛ of 19-oz. cake	199	28.9
Fiesta	⅛ of 19-oz. cake	249	29.9
(Pepperidge Farm)	⅙ of 13-oz. cake	213	30.2
Coconut (Pepperidge Farm)	⅙ of 13-oz. cake	230	31.3
Devil's food (Pepperidge Farm)	⅙ of 13-oz. cake	223	32.0
Maple spice (Pepperidge Farm)	⅙ of 13-oz. cake	213	32.2
Marble (McCain)	⅛ of 19-oz. cake	219	34.2
Neapolitan Fiesta (McCain)	⅛ of 19-oz. cake	252	29.7
Pound (Pepperidge Farm)	⅙ of 10.4-oz. cake	198	24.0
Shortcake (McCain):			
Raspberry	⅛ of 25-oz. cake	269	44.4
Strawberry	⅛ of 25-oz. cake	207	37.6
Vanilla:			
(McCain)	⅛ of 18-oz. cake	211	31.7
(Pepperidge Farm) layer	⅙ of 13-oz. cake	222	32.0
CAKE ICING, regular (General Mills):			
Chocolate	¹/₁₂ of container	162	25.0
Vanilla	½ of container	166	28.0
*CAKE ICING MIX, regular (General Mills):			
Chocolate, fudge	¹/₁₂ of pkg.	134	28.6
White:			
Fluffy	¹/₁₂ of pkg.	58	14.9
Traditional	¹/₁₂ of pkg.	140	29.8

(USDA): United States Department of Agriculture
(HEW/FAO):   Health, Education and Welfare/Food and Agriculture
                     Organization
* Prepared as Package Directs

Food and Description	Measure or Quantity	Calories	Carbo-hydrates (grams)
*CAKE MIX, regular (General Mills):			
Angel food:			
Regular	1/16 of cake	111	26.2
Confetti	1/16 of cake	114	26.8
Raspberry	1/16 of cake	115	27.0
Cherry chip, layer	1/12 of cake	198	37.6
Chocolate, layer:			
German	1/12 of cake	200	35.9
Milk	1/12 of cake	199	35.0
Sour cream, fudge	1/12 of cake	195	35.4
Devil's food, layer	1/12 of cake	199	35.8
Lemon, layer	1/12 of cake	202	36.1
Orange, layer	1/12 of cake	201	36.8
Pound, golden	1/12 of cake	210	28.0
White, layer:			
Regular	1/12 of cake	190	34.5
Sour cream	1/12 of cake	191	34.1
CANDY, regular (Rowntree Mackintosh):			
Aero:			
Regular	1.4-oz. bar	206	23.5
Peppermint	1.1-oz. bar	168	18.1
Chocolate bar with whole almonds	1.1-oz. bar	171	16.2
Coffee Crisp	1.7-oz. bar	246	28.1
Crispettes, coffee or orange	15-gram piece	79	9.6
Kit Kat	1.5-oz. bar (42 grams)	222	26.6
Maple Buds	1.1-oz. bar (31 grams)	162	18.9
Mint, chocolate covered, After Eight	.3-oz. piece (8.4 grams)	37	6.2
Mirage	1.4-oz. bar (39 grams)	208	23.5
Smarties	1.5-oz. bar (44 grams)	207	32.1
Toffee	2-oz. serving	255	40.1
CARROT, frozen (McCain):			
Diced, sticks or whole	3½-oz. serving	34	7.1
Sliced	3½-oz. serving	48	9.6

Food and Description	Measure or Quantity	Calories	Carbo-hydrates (grams)
CAULIFLOWER, frozen			
(McCain)	3½-oz. serving	77	13.2
CEREAL (General Mills):			
Boo*Berry	1 cup (1 oz.)	111	24.0
Cherrios:			
Regular	1¼ cups (1 oz.)	109	20.2
Honey nut	¾ cup (1 oz.)	110	23.0
Cocoa Puffs	1 cup (1 oz.)	107	24.2
Corn flakes, *Country*	1¼ cups (1 oz.)	109	24.0
Count Chocula	1 cup (1 oz.)	105	24.1
Frankenberry	1 cup (1 oz.)	110	24.5
Golden Grahams	1 cup (1 oz.)	110	23.6
Lucky Charms	1 cup (1 oz.)	112	24.4
Total	1¼ cups (1 oz.)	100	23.0
Trix	1 cup (1 oz.)	107	24.4
Wheaties	1¼ cups (1 oz.)	100	23.0
CHICKEN A LA KING, frozen:			
(EfficienC)	7-oz. entree (198 grams)	257	9.3
(Swanson)	9¾-oz. entree	284	9.9
CHICKEN DINNER OR ENTREE, frozen (Swanson):			
Regular	7-oz. entree	410	27.0
Hungry Man:			
Boneless	19-oz. dinner	685	60.4
Fried	15-oz. dinner	1058	96.9
TV Brand	11½-oz. entree	575	44.7
CHICKEN PIE, frozen (Swanson):			
Regular	8-oz. pie (227 grams)	503	52.9
Hungry Man	16-oz. pie (454 grams)	731	57.7

(USDA): United States Department of Agriculture
(HEW/FAO):   Health, Education and Welfare/Food and Agriculture
            Organization
* Prepared as Package Directs

Food and Description	Measure or Quantity	Calories	Carbo-hydrates (grams)
CHICKEN STEW:			
Canned (Bounty)	8-oz. serving	186	15.5
Frozen (EfficienC)	8-oz. entree	238	12.9
CHILI OR CHILI CON CARNE, canned, with beans (Bounty)	8-oz. serving	270	21.8
CHOCOLATE, BAKING (Baker's):			
Unsweetened	1-oz. square	143	8.8
Milk, chips	6.2-oz. pkg.	857	115.0
Semi-sweet:			
Regular	1-oz. square	136	16.8
Chips	6.2-oz. pkg.	798	120.0
Sweet	1-oz. square	138	18.8
CLAMATO JUICE DRINK, canned (Mott's)	6 fl. oz.	75	18.0
COCOA:			
Dry, unsweetened (Fry's)	1 T. (5 grams)	23	2.8
*Mix, regular (Cadbury's) instant	6 fl. oz.	116	23.0
COCONUT, packaged (Baker's):			
Angel Flake	½ of 7-oz. pkg.	438	44.4
Premium Shred	½ of 7-oz. pkg.	453	46.0
COFFEE, instant, *General Foods International Coffee:*			
Amaretto	6 fl. oz.	46	DNA
Irish Mocha Mint	6 fl. oz.	46	6.4
Orange Cappucino	6 fl. oz.	55	9.5
Suisse Mocha	6 fl. oz.	49	6.8
Vienna Royale	6 fl. oz.	57	10.0
COOKIE OR BISCUIT, regular:			
Animal (Christie's) *Barnum*	1 piece (2.7 grams)	13	2.1
Arrowroot (Christie's)	1 piece (6.6 grams)	29	5.3

Food and Description	Measure or Quantity	Calories	Carbo-hydrates (grams)
Chew Chews (Christie's)	1 piece (.7 oz.)	93	15.7
Chocolate:			
(Cadbury's):			
Fingers	1 oz.	148	20.0
Wafer	1 oz.	162	18.2
(Christie's) wafer	1 piece (4.5 grams)	20	3.5
Chocolate chip (Christie's)			
Chips Ahoy!	1 piece (.5 oz.)	76	10.3
Coffee Break (Christie's)	1 piece (11.2 grams)	53	7.7
Date Lunch (Christie's)	1 piece (.6 oz.)	60	13.2
Fig Newtons (Christie's)	1 piece (.6 oz.)	60	13.4
Fudgee-O (Christie's)	1 piece (13 grams)	6	9.0
Hey-Days (Christie's)	1 piece (.7 oz.)	81	10.8
Hoo-Rays (Christie's)	1 piece (.6 oz.)	.78	11.3
Jelly shortcake (Christie's)	1 piece (.4 oz.)	44	6.7
Lemon puff (Christie's)	1 piece (6.5 grams)	35	4.0
Maple leaf creams (Christie's)	1 piece (.4 oz.)	53	7.3
Midget snaps (Christie's)	1 piece (5.3 grams)	21	4.5
Miniatures (Christie's)	1 piece (.3 oz)	40	6.4
Mint (Christies'):			
Cream	1 piece (.4 oz.)	58	7.6
Sandwich	1 piece (.6 oz.)	92	12.4
Neapolitan wafer (Christie's)	1 piece (4 grams)	21	2.8
Oatmeal (Christie's)	1 piece (.4 oz.)	53	8.0
Oreo (Christie's)	1 piece (.4 oz.)	57	8.3
Pantry (Christie's)	1 piece	55	9.9
Pirate (Christie's)	1 piece (10.6 grams)	53	7.2
Sandwich (Cadbury's):			
Chocolate	1 oz.	153	18.5
Coffee	1 oz.	155	18.9
Orange	1 oz.	154	19.4

(USDA): United States Department of Agriculture
(HEW/FAO): Health, Education and Welfare/Food and Agriculture Organization
* Prepared as Package Directs

Food and Description	Measure or Quantity	Calories	Carbo-hydrates (grams)
Social Tea (Christie's)	1 piece (4.5 grams)	20	3.6
Soft (Christie's):			
Apple or raspberry	1 piece (.7 oz.)	89	13.8
Date	1 piece (.7 oz.)	89	14.2
Granola	1 piece (.7 oz.)	86	13.4
Sugar (Christie's) raisin	1 piece (.5 oz.)	.65	9.3
Sultana (Christie's)	1 piece (.4 oz.)	43	9.7
Tea Treats (Christie's)	1 piece (.2 oz.)	25	3.8
Vanilla Wafer (Christie's)	1 piece (3.7 grams)	17	2.6
CORN, frozen (McCain) whole kernel	¼ of 12.4-oz. pkg.	74	14.7
CRACKER, PUFFS & CHIPS:			
Bacon Dipper (Christie's)	1 piece (2.1 grams)	10	1.3
Bits & Bites (Christie's):			
Regular	1 piece (.4 grams)	2	.3
Cheese flavor	1 piece (.3 grams)	1	.2
Bugles (General Mills)	1 piece (.9 grams)	5	.5
Canadian Harvest (Christie's)	1 piece (.1 oz.)	14	1.8
Cheese or cheese flavored:			
Cheddees (Christie's)	1 piece (.5 grams)	3	.2
Cheese Bits (Christie's)	1 piece (.8 grams)	3.6	.5
Cheese Willikers (General Mills)	1 piece (1.1 grams)	6	.6
& green onion (Christie's)	1 piece (.1 oz.)	14	1.8
Nips (Christie's)	1 piece (1.1 grams)	5	.6
Premium Plus (Christie's)	1 pieced (3.2 grams)	13	2.1
Swiss cheese (Christie's)	1 piece (2 grams)	10	1.2

Food and Description	Measure or Quantity	Calories	Carbo-hydrates (grams)
Tid Bits (Christie's)	1 piece (.3 grams)	1	.2
Corn chip (Christie's)	1 piece (.9 grams)	6	.6
Crisp-I-Taters (General Mills)	1 piece (.6 grams)	3	.3
Escort (Christie's)	1 piece (4.4 grams)	23	2.6
Flings (Christie's)	1 piece (.8 grams)	5	.3
Graham (Christie's):			
Country Maid	1 piece (5.5 grams)	25	3.9
Honey Maid	1 piece	27	4.8
Montclair	1 piece (.3 oz.)	39	6.8
Hovis Cracker (Christie's)	1 piece (5.7 grams)	28	3.4
Meal Mates (Christie's)	1 piece (5.3 grams)	23	3.7
Milk Lunch (Christie's)	1 piece (7.2 grams)	31	5.2
Mini chips (Christie's)	1 piece (.4 grams)	2	.3
Onion crisp (Christie's) with sesame	1 piece (3.8 grams)	17	2.5
Onion, french, thins (Christie's)	1 piece (2.1 grams)	10	1.4
Pizza Cracker (Christie's)	1 piece (.1 oz.)	7	1.1
Ritz (Christie's):			
Regular	1 piece (.1 oz.)	17	2.2
Cheese	1 piece (.1 oz.)	14	1.9
Rusk, Holland (Christie's)	1 piece (9.2 grams)	36	7.0
Rye, buffet (Christie's)	1 piece (3.4 grams)	16	2.4

(USDA): United States Department of Agriculture
(HEW/FAO):   Health, Education and Welfare/Food and Agriculture
             Organization
* Prepared as Package Directs

Food and Description	Measure or Quantity	Calories	Carbo-hydrates (grams)
Saltine, *Premium* (Christie's):			
Old fashioned	1 piece (6.6 grams)	30	4.4
Plus, with or without salt	1 piece (.1 oz.)	13	2.1
Sociables (Christie's)	1 piece (2.6 grams)	13	1.6
Sour cream & chive (Christie's)	1 piece	12	1.6
Tortilla chip (Christie's) nacho or taco flavor	1 piece (2.2 grams)	11	1.4
Triangle thins (Christie's)	1 piece (1.7 grams)	8	1.0
Triscuit Wafers (Christie's)	1 piece (4.7 grams)	21	3.3
Triticale Crackers (Christie's)	1 piece (.1 oz.)	15	1.8
Vegetable thins (Christie's)	1 piece (1.7 grams)	8	1.1
Wheat thins (Christies):			
Regular	1 piece (2.1 grams)	10	1.4
Ground	1 piece (5.8 grams)	24	4.5
Wheatsworth (Christie's)	1 piece (3.4 grams)	16	2.0
Whistles (General Mills)	1 piece (.8 grams)	4	.7
CRANAPPLE JUICE DRINK (Ocean Spray)	8 fl. oz.	180	44.0
CRANBERRY JUICE COCKTAIL, canned (Ocean Spray)	8 fl. oz.	160	40.0
CRANBERRY SAUCE, canned (Ocean Spray) jellied or whole	2 fl. oz. serving	90	22.0

Food and Description	Measure or Quantity	Calories	Carbo- hydrates (grams)

D

DOUGHNUT, frozen (McCain)			
chocolate iced	¼ of 9-oz. pkg.	266	24.1

F

FIDDLEHEAD GREENS,			
frozen (McCain)	⅓ of 10½-oz. pkg.	26	3.3
FLOUR:			
Bisquick (General Mills)	¼ cup	126	19.9
Five Roses:			
All-purpose or u .bleached	¼ cup	104	21.0
Whole wheat	¼ cup	105	21.3
(Swansdown) cake	½ cup (2 oz.)	204	44.4

G

***GELATIN DESSERT MIX:**			
Regular (Jell-O)	½ cup	81	19.4
Dietetic (D-Zerta):			
Lemon	½ cup	8	0.
Orange or strawberry	½ cup	9	.1
Raspberry	½ cup	9	0.
GRAPE DRINK, canned,			
Welch's	8 fl. oz. (8.4 oz.)	112	30.0

(USDA): United States Department of Agriculture
(HEW/FAO):   Health, Education and Welfare/Food and Agriculture
            Organization
* Prepared as Package Directs

Food and Description	Measure or Quantity	Calories	Carbohydrates (grams)
GRAPEFRUIT JUICE, canned (Ocean Spray)	8 fl. oz.	95	21.0
GRAPE JUICE, canned, *Welch's,* purple or white	8 fl. oz.	160	40.0
GRAVY, canned (Franco-American):			
Beef	2-oz. serving	44	3.6
Chicken	2-oz. serving	50	3.1
Mushroom	2-oz. serving	28	2.8
Onion	2-oz. serving	40	2.7

H

Food and Description	Measure or Quantity	Calories	Carbohydrates (grams)
***HAMBURGER HELPER** (General Mills):			
Beef flavored dinner	1 cup	328	26.2
Cheeseburger	1 cup	334	35.2
Chili tomato dinner	1 cup	334	35.2
Hash	1 cup	300	26.8
Lasagna	1 cup	332	35.2
Noodle Romanoff	1 cup	241	26.4
Potato Stroganoff	1 cup	323	28.5
Short cut spaghetti	1 cup	330	24.7
Tomato Roma	1 cup	334	35.2
HAM DINNER OR ENTREE, frozen (Swanson) *TV Brand*	10½-oz. dinner	365	42.0

I

Food and Description	Measure or Quantity	Calories	Carbohydrates (grams)
ICE CREAM CONE (Christie's):			
Regular	1 piece (4.5 grams)	19	3.7
Sugar	1 piece (12.5 grams)	49	10.3

Food and Description	Measure or Quantity	Calories	Carbo-hydrates (grams)
ICE CREAM CUP (Christie's)	1 cup (5.8 grams)	23	4.7
ICE MAGIC (General Foods) chocolate or chocolate mint	.6-oz. serving	111	6.0

J

JELL-O PUDDING POPS (General Foods):			
Chocolate	2.1-oz. pop	88	16.7
All other flavors	2.1-oz. pop	87	15.9

K

***KOOL-AID** (General Foods):			
Regular, sugar added after bought	8 fl. oz.	106	28.0
Pre-sweetened, with sugar:			
All except lemonade, orange and sunshine punch	8 fl. oz.	86	22.3
Lemonade	8 fl. oz.	85	22.1
Orange	8 fl. oz.	85	22.2
Sunshine punch	8 fl. oz.	85	22.3
Dietetic, sugar free:			
Cherry, grape or strawberry	8 fl. oz.	2	.2
Orange	8 fl. oz.	3	.3
Tropical Punch	8 fl. oz.	2	.3

(USDA): United States Department of Agriculture
(HEW/FAO):   Health, Education and Welfare/Food and Agriculture
                        Organization
* Prepared as Package Directs

Food and Description	Measure or Quantity	Calories	Carbo-hydrates (grams)

L

Food and Description	Measure or Quantity	Calories	Carbo-hydrates (grams)
LASAGNA, frozen:			
(EfficienC)	9.2-oz. entree	325	30.5
(Swanson)	12-oz. entree	445	39.4
LEMONADE, canned, *Country Time*	10 fl. oz.	248	29.5

M

Food and Description	Measure or Quantity	Calories	Carbo-hydrates (grams)
MACARONI:			
Dry (Catelli)	3 oz.	306	63.8
Canned (Franco-American) and beef	8-oz. serving	225	25.0
Frozen (Swanson) and beef	8-oz. casserole	211	24.4
MACARONI & CHEESE:			
Canned (Franco-American)	8 oz.	220	25.0
Frozen:			
(EfficienC)	8-oz. entree	308	64.5
(Swanson)	8-oz. casserole	328	29.2
Mix (Catelli)	3 oz.	425	77.4
MEATBALL, frozen (Swanson) and gravy	9-oz. entree	378	17.6
***MUFFIN MIX** (General Mills):			
Apple cinnamon	1 muffin	159	26.4
Blueberry	1 muffin	118	19.3
Butter pecan	1 muffin	159	21.3
Corn	1 muffin	156	24.8
Honey bran	1 muffin	154	26.2

Food and Description	Measure or Quantity	Calories	Carbo-hydrates (grams)

N

NOODLE, dry (Catelli):
Egg	3 oz.	316	61.3
Lasagna, spinach	3 oz.	304	63.2

O

ONION, frozen (McCain) rings, battered or breaded	3 oz.	167	24.1

P

PANCAKE, frozen (EfficienC)	1.7-oz. pancake	112	17.8
PATTY SHELL, frozen (Pepperidge Farm) regular	1.7-oz. shell (47.2 grams)	215	13.4
PEA, green, frozen (McCain)	¼ of 12.4-oz. pkg.	72	11.9
PEA & CARROT, frozen (McCain)	⅓ of 10½-oz. pkg.	65	11.6
PIE, frozen (McCain):			
Banana cream	⅙ of 14-oz. pie	149	20.3

(USDA): United States Department of Agriculture
(HEW/FAO):   Health, Education and Welfare/Food and Agriculture
              Organization
* Prepared as Package Directs

Food and Description	Measure or Quantity	Calories	Carbo-hydrates (grams)
Chocolate cream	⅙ of 14-oz. pie	197	22.5
Coconut cream	⅙ of 14-oz. pie	201	19.9
Lemon cream	⅙ of 14-oz. pie	210	29.0
Mincemeat	⅛ of 24-oz. pie	237	35.0
Pecan	⅛ of 20-oz. pie	307	36.4
Pumpkin	⅛ of 22-oz. pie	168	19.1
Raisin	3½-oz. serving	277	42.7
*PIE CRUST MIX:			
(Christie's) graham	1 shell (14.1 oz.)	2097	243.2
(General Mills)	⅙ of double-crust shell	302	24.1
*PIE MIX (General Mills)			
Boston cream	⅛ of pie	265	47.9
PIZZA, frozen (McCain):			
Deluxe:			
Regular	5″ pie (15 oz.)	268	29.0
Tendercrisp	5″ pie (17 oz.)	269	29.0
Pepperoni, regular or tendercrisp	5″ pie	293	29.0
PORK DINNER or ENTREE, frozen (Swanson) *TV Brand,* loin of	11-oz. dinner	505	44.5
POTATO, frozen (McCain):			
Country style	2-oz. serving	83	12.4
Diced, all-purpose	2-oz. serving	42	9.
French fries	2-oz. serving	83	12.4
Hasbhrowns, western style	2-oz. serving	129	16.5
Puffs	⅓ of 8.8-oz. pkg.	157	20.9
Superfries	2-oz. serving	41	11.8
PRETZEL (Christie's) *Mr. Salty:*			
Sticks	1 piece (3.9 grams)	15	3.1
Twists	1 piece (6.9 grams)	26	5.4
PRUNE NECTAR, canned, *Welch's*	8 fl. oz. (8.6 oz.)	200	45.0

Food and Description	Measure or Quantity	Calories	Carbo-hydrates (grams)
PUDDING OR PIE FILLING:			
Canned, regular pack (Laura Secord):			
Chocolate:			
Regular	5-oz. serving	199	32.4
Fudge	5-oz. serving	199	32.7
Vanilla	5-oz. serving	192	29.4
*Mix:			
Regular:			
Banana cream (Jell-O):			
Regular	½ cup	150	27.7
Instant	½ cup	163	30.9
Butter pecan (Jell-O):			
Regular	½ cup	147	27.2
Instant	½ cup	159	28.7
Butterscotch (Jello-O):			
Regular	½ cup	168	32.8
Instant	½ cup	169	32.8
Caramel (Jell-O):			
Regular	½ cup	168	32.8
Instant	½ cup	169	32.7
Chocolate (Jell-O):			
Plain:			
Regular	½ cup	163	31.0
Instant	½ cup	165	31.5
Cream, regular	½ cup	158	28.4
Fudge, instant	½ cup	162	30.6
Coconut cream (Jell-O) regular	½ cup	159	25.0
Custard (Bird's)	½ cup	98	17.0
Lemon (Jell-O) instant	½ cup	163	31.3
Pistachio (Jell-O) instant	½ cup	166	30.3
Tapioca:			
(Jell-O) instant	½ cup	149	27.7
Minit (General Foods)	½ cup	140	21.9
Vanilla (Jell-O):			
Regular	½ cup	150	27.7
Instant	½ cup	149	27.6

(USDA): United States Department of Agriculture
(HEW/FAO): Health, Education and Welfare/Food and Agriculture
Organization
* Prepared as Package Directs

Food and Description	Measure or Quantity	Calories	Carbohydrates (grams)
Dietetic (D-Zerta):			
Butterscotch	½ cup	68	11.8
Chocolate	½ cup	77	13.3
Vanilla	½ cup	69	11.9

Q

QUENCH (General Foods): | | | |
Canned			
Regular:			
Fruit punch	9.5 fl. oz.	115	30.2
Grape	9.5 fl. oz.	139	37.0
Lemonade	9.5 fl. oz.	111	29.5
Orange	9.5 fl. oz.	121	33.0
Dietetic:			
Fruit punch or grape	8½ fl. oz.	5	.5
Lemonade	8½ fl. oz.	8	.9
Orange	8½ fl. oz.	7	.7
*Mix, regular:			
Fruit punch	8½ fl. oz.	116	30.4
Grape or lemonade	8½ fl. oz.	115	30.4
Lemon-lime	8½ fl. oz.	115	30.5
Orange	8½ fl. oz.	115	30.2

R

ROLL OR BUN, frozen (McCain): | | | |
| Danish, iced | 2-oz. serving | 241 | 25.3 |
| Honey | 2-oz. serving | 121 | 28.0 |

S

SALISBURY STEAK, frozen: (EfficienC) | 5¾-oz. entree | 274 | 5.4 |

Food and Description	Measure or Quantity	Calories	Carbo-hydrates (grams)
(Swanson):			
Regular	5½-oz. entree	330	26.6
Hungry Man	17-oz. dinner	805	65.1
TV Brand	11½-oz. dinner	427	37.8
*SOUP, canned, regular pack:			
Asparagus (Campbell)			
condensed, cream of	7-oz. serving	71	9.3
Bean (Campbell) condensed,			
with bacon	7-oz. serving	133	17.0
Beef (Campbell) condensed:			
Broth	7-oz. serving	22	1.9
Mushroom	7-oz. serving	51	4.5
Noodle	7-oz. serving	58	7.2
With vegetables & barley	7-oz. serving	86	9.1
Celery (Campbell) condensed,			
cream of	7-oz. serving	66	6.4
Cheddar cheese (Campbell)			
condensed	7-oz. serving	124	8.4
Chicken (Campbell) condensed:			
Alphabet	7-oz. serving	64	8.1
Broth	7-oz. serving	27	.7
Cream of:			
Made with milk	7-oz. serving	144	11.1
Made with water	7-oz. serving	76	3.6
Creamy, & mushroom	7-oz. serving	77	7.3
Gumbo	7-oz. serving	48	7.3
Noodle	7-oz. serving	54	7.1
NoodleOs	7-oz. serving	59	7.8
With rice	7-oz. serving	42	4.9
& stars	7-oz. serving	49	6.1
Vegetable	7-oz. serving	60	7.6
Chowder, clam (Campbell)			
condensed:			
Manhattan style	7-oz. serving	64	9.1
New England style	7-oz. serving	71	9.4
Consomme (Campbell)			
condensed	7-oz. serving	29	2.3

(USDA): United States Department of Agriculture
(HEW/FAO):   Health, Education and Welfare/Food and Agriculture
                        Organization
* Prepared as Package Directs

Food and Description	Measure or Quantity	Calories	Carbo-hydrates (grams)
Meatball alphabet (Campbell) condensed	7-oz. serving	53	8.8
Minestrone (Campbell) condensed	7-oz. serving	71	9.1
Mushroom (Campbell) condensed:			
Cream of	7-oz. serving	114	7.5
Golden	7-oz. serving	70	6.8
Noodle (Campbell) condensed, & ground beef	7-oz. serving	80	8.1
Onion (Campbell) condensed:			
Regular	7-oz. serving	36	2.9
Cream of, made with water	7-oz. serving	74	8.6
Ox Tail (Campbell) condensed	7-oz. serving	83	8.7
Oyster stew (Campbell) condensed	7-oz. serving	31	2.7
Pea, French Canadian style (Campbell) condensed	7-oz. serving	139	20.1
Pea, green:			
(Campbell) condensed	7-oz. serving	115	18.4
(Habitant)	1 cup (259 grams)	176	24.2
Potato (Campbell) condensed, cream of, made with water	7-oz. serving	58	9.1
Scotch broth (Campbell) condensed	7-oz. serving	74	8.6
Shrimp (Campbell) condensed	7-oz. serving	74	6.2
Tomato (Campbell) condensed:			
Regular	7-oz. serving	69	12.2
Bisque of	7-oz. serving	101	18.3
& rice, old fashioned	7-oz. serving	87	14.6
Turkey (Campbell) condensed:			
Noodle	7-oz. serving	63	6.5
Vegetable	7-oz. serving	64	7.0
Vegetable:			
(Campbell) condensed:			
Regular	7-oz. serving	67	11.0
Beef	7-oz. serving	62	6.3
Country style	7-oz. serving	50	6.7
Cream of, made with water	7-oz. serving	91	8.4
Hearty	7-oz. serving	81	15.6

Food and Description	Measure or Quantity	Calories	Carbo-hydrates (grams)
Old fashioned	7-oz. serving	61	7.8
Vegetarian	7-oz. serving	62	10.3
(Habitant)	1 cup (9 oz.)	74	13.2
SPINACH, frozen (McCain)	⅓ of 12-oz. pkg.	37	4.3
SPAGHETTI, canned (Franco-American)			
& ground beef	8-oz. serving	218	32.7
In tomato sauce	8-oz. serving	159	31.4
SpaghettiOs	8-oz. serving	173	32.9
SQUASH, frozen (McCain)	¼ of 14-oz. pkg.	25	4.7
STRUDEL, frozen (Pepperidge Farm):			
Apple	⅙ of strudel (2.3 oz.)	78	10.0
Blueberry	⅙ of strudel (2.3 oz.)	93	11.0
SWISS STEAK DINNER OR ENTREE, frozen (Swanson) *TV* Brand	11¼-oz. dinner	374	38.2

T

***TANG** (General Foods):			
Apple	4.2 fl. oz.	69	18.2
Grapefruit	4.2 fl. oz.	52	14.6
Orange	4.2 fl. oz.	56	15.0
Orange & grapefruit	4.2 fl. oz.	55	14.6
Pineapple & grapefruit	4.2 fl. oz.	66	17.4

(USDA): United States Department of Agriculture
(HEW/FAO): Health, Education and Welfare/Food and Agriculture Organization
* Prepared as Package Directs

Food and Description	Measure or Quantity	Calories	Carbo- hydrates (grams)
TOMATO SAUCE, canned, regular pack (Catelli):			
Plain	½ cup (80 grams)	44	5.9
With meat	½ cup (80.5 grams)	71	4.5
TOPPING, WHIPPED, frozen, *Cool Whip* (Genearl Foods)	1 T. (.1 oz.)	13	1.0
TURKEY DINNER OR ENTREE, frozen:			
(EfficienC) sliced (Swanson):	5.2-oz. entree	157	4.4
Regular	8¾-oz. entree	304	28.7
Regular, sliced	9¼-oz. entree	265	22.5
Hungry Man	19-oz. dinner	647	67.9
TV Brand	11½-oz. dinner	397	43.3
TURKEY PIE, frozen (Swanson):			
Regular	8-oz. pie	442	40.1
Hungry Man	16-oz. pie	608	53.1
TURNOVER, frozen:			
Apple:			
(McCain)	2-oz. serving	122	18.9
(Pepperidge Farm)	2.7-oz. piece	258	23.9
Blueberry (Pepperidge Farm)	2.7-oz. piece	263	26.0
Blueberry/raspberry (McCain)	2-oz. serving	123	19.4
Raspberry (Pepperidge Farm)	2.7-oz. piece	274	28.9
Strawberry (Pepperidge Farm)	2.7-oz. piece	267	27.2

V

VEGETABLES, MIXED, frozen (McCain):			
Regular	⅓ of 10.6-oz. pkg.	67	12.6
Florentine style	⅕ of 17.6-oz. pkg.	41	7.2
Parisienne style	3-oz. serving	37	6.6

Food and Description	Measure or Quantity	Calories	Carbo-hydrates (grams)
V-8 JUICE:			
Regular	6 fl. oz.	36	6.5
Spicy hot	6 fl. oz.	38	DNA

W

***WHIP'N CHILL** (Jell-O):*			
Chocolate	½ cup	131	18.6
Lemon	½ cup	129	18.1
Strawberry	½ cup	129	17.7
Vanilla	½ cup	129	18.0

Y

YOGURT, regular (Laura Secord):			
Blueberry	4.5-oz. serving	120	19.5
Peach	4.5-oz. serving	119	19.1
Raspberry	4.5-oz. serving	120	19.4
Strawberry	4.5-oz. serving	122	18.3

(USDA): United States Department of Agriculture
(HEW/FAO):   Health, Education and Welfare/Food and Agriculture
                    Organization
* Prepared as Package Directs